D1042307

HEAL THYSELF

HEAL THYSELF

*Nicholas Culpeper
and the Seventeenth-Century Struggle
to Bring Medicine to the People*

BENJAMIN WOOLLEY

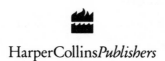

HarperCollins*Publishers*

FIRST EDITION

Published in Great Britain in 2004 under the title *The Herbalist* by HarperCollins Publishers.

Printed on acid-free paper

Library of Congress Cataloging-in-Publication Data is available upon request.

ISBN 0-06-009066-9

04 05 06 07 08   RPTUK/RRD   10 9 8 7 6 5 4 3 2 1

In memory of Joy Woolley,
1921–2003

CONTENTS

PREFACE

In the landscape of history, Nicholas Culpeper has not always been welcome. If monarchs, ministers, political notables and scientific luminaries are stately oaks or cultivated blooms, Culpeper is the Cleavers (or Goosegrass, or Barweed, or Hedgeheriff, or Hayruff, or Mutton Chops, or Robin-Run-in-the-Grass, to use any of its multitude of names), a common grass that is 'so troublesome an Inhabitant in Gardens', creeping into the herbaceous borders and snagging clothes. As a result, he has been weeded out of the historical record, and barely a trace of him is left. The only documentation relating to him that survives is a brief memoir, one letter, a couple of manuscript fragments, several tantalising mentions in official papers, and some pamphlets. His own voluminous writings brim with character, but are almost empty of biographical details. Official medical and botanical histories written while he lived and since have contributed nothing, and in some cases have taken a great deal away. For this reason, Nicholas's presence in history, and in the account that follows, is necessarily fleeting.

However, hidden in the undergrowth is a startling story, entangled with so many others, with the struggles of the wood-turner Nehemiah Wallington to survive the plague, with the mischievous prophesies of the astrologer William Lilly, with the Olympian struggles and self-belief of King Charles I, and most of all with the anatomical explorations and loyal ministrations of the King's doctor William Harvey, the Isaac Newton of medical science and model of medical professionalism. Like the Cleavers and other discarded weeds championed in his *Herbal*, Nicholas certainly had 'some Vices [but] also many Virtues'. His vices were well known, itemised by friends as well as his many enemies: smoking, drinking, 'consumption of the purse'. But he was also audacious and adventurous. He championed the poor and sick at a time when they were more vulnerable than ever. He took on an establishment fighting for survival and ferociously intent on preserving its privileges.

The heirs of that same establishment are inevitably the custodians of much of the material upon which this book relies, in particular the Royal College of Physicians, which provided generous access to its archives. Acknowledgement must also go to the Society of Apothecaries, the British Library, the Bodleian Library at Oxford, the Cambridge University Library, the Records Offices of the counties of East and West Sussex, Kent, Surrey, and of London, primarily the Guildhall Library, the Corporation of London and the Metropolitan Archives. Individual thanks are due to Briony Thomas and the Revd Roger Dalling for local information on Nicholas's childhood, to Dr Jonathan Wright for reading the manuscript and Dr Adrian Mathie for checking some of the medical information.

The dates given are new style unless otherwise stated. Spelling and punctuation have been modernised where appropriate. Notes at the back provide details on sources, clarifications and definitions of some of the medical and astrological terminology, and brief discussions of the historical evidence. One final note: the capitalised 'City' refers to the square mile that is the formally recognised city of London, a distinct political as well as urban entity with its own government and privileges, lying within the bounds of the ancient city walls. 'London' or the 'city' refers to the wider metropolitan area, embracing the city of Westminster to the west, Southwark on the south bank of the Thames, and the sprawling suburbs to the north and east.

HEAL
THYSELF

TANSY

Tanacetum vulgare

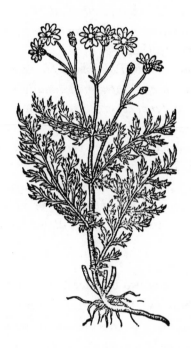

Dame Venus was minded to pleasure Women with Child by this Herb, for there grows not an Herb fitter for their uses than this is, it is just as though it were cut out for the purpose. The Herb bruised and applied to the Navel stays miscarriage, I know no Herb like it for that use. Boiled in ordinary Beer, and the Decoction drunk, doth the like, and if her Womb be not as she would have, this Decoction will make it as she would have it, or at least as she should have it.

*Let those Women that desire Children love this Herb,
'tis their best Companion, their Husband excepted.*

*The Herb fried with Eggs (as is accustomed in the Spring
time) which is called a Tansy, helpeth to digest, and carry
downward those bad Humours that trouble the Stomach:
The Seed is very profitably given to Children for the Worms,
and the Juice in Drink is as effectual. Being boiled in Oil
it is good for the sinews shrunk by Cramps, or pained with
cold, if thereto applied.*

*Also it consumes the Phlegmatic Humours, the cold and
moist constitution of Winter most usually infects the Body
of Man with, and that was the first reason of eating Tansies
in the Spring. At last the world being overrun with Popery,
a Monster called Superstition perks up his head ... and
now forsooth Tansies must be eaten only on Palm and
Easter Sundays, and their neighbour days; [the] Superstition of the time was found out, but the Virtue of the Herb
hidden, and now 'tis almost, if not altogether, left off.**

Tansy has a tall, leafy stem, two or three feet high, with ferny foliage and flowers like golden buttons.[1] Maud Grieve describes it as having 'a very curious and not altogether disagreeable odour, somewhat like camphor'. The name probably comes from the Greek *Athanaton*, meaning immortal, either because it flowers for so long, or because of its use in ancient times to preserve corpses. It was said to have been given to Ganymede ('the most beautiful of mortals', carried off by Zeus to Olympus to serve as cupbearer and catamite) to make him immortal.

The herb was long associated not only with immortality but birth, hence the link with Easter, when, according to Grieve, 'even archbishops and bishops played handball with men of their congregation, and a Tansy cake

---

* This and the following extracts introducing each chapter are taken from Culpeper's *The English Physitian*.

was the reward of the victors'. Richard Mabey, echoing Culpeper, writes that its original medicinal use at Easter time was to counteract the 'phlegm and worms' arising from the heavy consumption of seafood during Lent.

Though tansy has a strong, bitter taste, the cake was sweet. According to a traditional recipe, it was made by adding to seven beaten eggs a pint of cream, the juice of spinach and of a small quantity of tansy pounded in a mortar, a quarter of a pound of Naples biscuit (sponge fingers similar to macaroons, but made with ground pine nut kernels rather than almonds), sugar to taste, a glass of white wine, and nutmeg. The ingredients were combined, thickened in a saucepan over a gentle heat, poured into a lined cake tin, and baked.[2]

dark, gnarled yew stood next to the lych-gate, poisoning with a drizzle of noxious needles anything that grew beneath it. Rose bushes still in flower were scattered across the graveyard, planted, according to local tradition, by the betrothed on the graves of their dead lovers. A mound of fresh earth marked the spot where, a few days earlier, Maurice Sackville, the late rector of Ockley, had been interred. This was the scene beheld on 15 September 1615 by the Revd Nicholas Culpeper, Sackville's hastily-appointed successor. He had arrived just four days after Sackville's funeral from his old post as vicar of nearby Alciston. He was in his mid-thirties and, for a country parson, uncommonly well educated, boasting a degree from the University of Cambridge.[3]

Ockley was a modest but busy parish on the border of the counties of Surrey and Sussex, straddling Stane Street, the Roman road that still acted as the main thoroughfare from Chichester on the south coast to London. The church itself was a quarter of a mile from the village, perched on a hill, next to the remains of a castle and Ockley Manor, owned by Nicholas's cousin and patron Sir Edward Culpeper.[4]

Nicholas and Sir Edward were from branches of the same family that was joined three generations back, part of a voracious dynasty that grew like white bryony through the counties of Sussex, Kent, and Surrey. The origin of the Culpeper name is obscure. Some have speculated that it derived from the place where the first family members settled, perhaps Gollesberghe in Sandwich, Kent or Culspore in Hastings, Sussex. To most, however, it was more suggestive of politics than geography. 'Cole' was a prefix meaning a fraud, as in cole-prophet, a false prophet, or 'Colle tregetour', a magician or trickster mentioned by Geoffrey Chaucer in his poem *The House of Fame*.[5] Colepeper, one of innumerable spellings, would therefore mean a false pepperer, someone trading illicitly as a grocer outside the Fraternity of Pepperers, the guild incorporated in 1345 which later became the Grocers' Company. Or the 'pepper' could simply refer to the herb's association with offensiveness. Jack Straw, a supposed leader of the fourteenth-century Peasants' Revolt, was described by a contemporary writer as a 'culpeper', meaning mischief maker.[6]

Elements of the family had certainly lived up to this interpretation of the name. Wakehurst, the family's main seat in Sussex, had come to the Culpepers after the daughters of its original owners were abducted by brothers Richard (1435–1516) and Nicholas (1437–1510). A grandchild of their elder brother John, Sir Thomas Culpeper, was beheaded in 1541 for treason, accused of being the lover of Catherine Howard, Henry VIII's fifth wife, herself the daughter of Joyce Culpeper, Thomas's sixth cousin, once removed.

By the early seventeenth century, the leading Culpepers were eager for respectability. Edward Culpeper, the current occupant of Wakehurst and the great-great-grandchild of Richard, had risen to become a Sergeant-at-Law (a high-ranking barrister). But in those days, lawyers, like physicians and merchants, were not considered gentlemen. Titles and land were the real currency of social rank, and Edward was ruthless in his pursuit of both. In 1603, he bought himself one of the new knighthoods that James I sold on his succession to the English throne in order to finance an opulent court. Through legal action as well as acquisition, Edward also enlarged his estate at Wakehurst into one of the most extensive in Sussex, and built an impressive mansion in the middle of it to show off his new-found status. Among the many lucrative plots for which he litigated was one of 120 acres at Balcombe, on the south-west border of his Wakehurst estate. This had been the principal possession of the Revd Nicholas Culpeper's grandfather, leaving that branch of the family incurably reduced. Nicholas had inherited just £120 on his twenty-first birthday, enough to pay for his education at Cambridge University, where he received an MA in 1608. Thereafter he was dependent on the patronage of Sir Edward.

Now, as rector of Ockley, entitled to the living or 'benefice' generated by local church taxes, Nicholas could look forward to a comfortable, if undemanding, life. He had also become engaged to Mary, the twenty-year-old daughter of another rector, William Attersoll of Isfield, a village near Nicholas's old parish of Alciston and within the same deanery or church administrative district.[7] A month after Nicholas took up his position at Ockley, they were married at Isfield.

Nicholas's first few weeks in the parish were busy with funerals. Coffin after coffin was carried past the old yew into the church yard, six before Christmas, a high number for a village with a population of a hundred or so. One of them contained Katherine Sackville, wife of the late rector, suggesting that both had succumbed to a disease passing through the village. Nicholas must have been concerned about the infection lingering in the rectory he and his new wife had so recently occupied.[8]

Within the year, Nicholas too was dead, around the time of the first anniversary of his marriage to Mary, who was about to give birth to their first child. There is no record of what killed Nicholas, but there was a ready supply of possible causes. At around this time, the practice began of hiring old women – 'ancient Matrons' – to roam parishes as 'searchers of the dead', recording the number and causes of death for regularly published 'Bills of Mortality'. There was some controversy about this practice. According to John Graunt, who started analysing these figures in the 1660s, people questioned 'why the Accompt of Casualties is made', since death was a divine, not a demographic, matter; its time preordained; its cause the instrument by which God's will was performed. No intervention, physical or otherwise, could prevent it. 'This must not seem strange to you,' advised William Attersoll two years before his son-in-law's death, 'for the whole life of a Christian should be nothing but a meditation of death ... You must consider that nothing befalleth us by chance or fortune, all things are ruled and guided by the sovereign providence of almighty God.'[9]

Despite qualms about the searchers' work, they were diligent in their efforts and came up with an elaborate catalogue of causes: apoplexy, bleach, cancer, execution, fainting in the bath, gout, grief, itch, lethargy, lunacy, murder, palsy (paralysis), poison, sciatica, and 'suddenly'. But one class of cause prevailed over all these: infectious disease.

There was no concept of germs in the seventeenth century. Infection was a corruption of the air, a humidity or 'miasma' that exuded from the earth, a theory that lingers today in the belief in the benefits of 'fresh' or 'country' air. Some places were more prone to infection than others because they were near sources of this miasma, such as sewers and swamps. London, with its cramped streets, fetid streams, and cesspits, oozed contagion. But the countryside could be just as dangerous. Some settled rural populations – for example in remote parts of the West Country or on the chalk uplands of the Sussex Downs – had high levels of shared immunity to native bugs and lack of exposure to foreign ones. A village such as Hartland in Devon enjoyed infant mortality and life expectancy rates so low they would not be matched nationally until the 1920s. But other areas were as bad as any urban pesthole, notably large tracts of Sussex and Kent. 'Marish' and estuarine terrain, alluvial tracts, swampy low-lying basins, and sluggish rivers were suffused with 'marsh fever' or the 'ague' – malaria (from the Italian for 'bad air'). The disease was familiar, and its diagnosis precise, categorized according to the frequency of the feverish attacks that announced its onset: daily (quotidian), every other day (tertian), and every third day (quartan).[10] The convulsions produced by marsh fever, though distressing, were not usually fatal. However, they left sufferers more susceptible to enteric diseases – gut infections such as typhoid and dysentery. These were less clearly differentiated, but more deadly, frequently killing off one in ten of the population of a village in a single year.[11]

Just such a crisis seemed to overtake Ockley in 1615 and 1616. Autumn was the killing season for enteric infections, and nearly all of the twenty deaths in the parish during those years occurred between September and December. The summer of 1615 was particularly hot, and the stagnation of water supplies and sewers produced an epidemic of typhoid across the region.[12] Perhaps it was this that carried away Nicholas Culpeper. If so, the sickness would have taken three weeks to pass through its elaborate pageant of pain: innocuous aches at first, possibly accompanied by nosebleeds and diarrhoea; a fortnight or more of high fever and skin rashes, interrupted by brief remissions. This was the first phase. The second was a week of tortuous stomach pains and delirium.

If he was in this state, very little could be done for him. Mary would have been expected to mix up some palliative medicines, based on recipes she had learned from her mother, or from local women with more experience. Typical remedies known to soothe the symptoms of fever were flowers of camomile beaten into a pulp and mixed with cloves and vervain, to be applied, as one herbal unhelpfully reported, according to 'mother Bombies rule, to take just so many knots or sprigs, and no more, lest it fall out so that it do you no good'.[13]

A local 'wizard' or 'cunning woman' may have come to call. Bishop Latimer had noted in 1552 that 'A great many of us when we be in trouble or sickness . . . run hither to witches, or sorcerers . . . seeking aid and comfort in their hands'.[14] They were still a part of life in rural villages such as Ockham in the early 1600s, promising with remarkable assurance that they could heal a variety of ailments using a combination of magical rituals and semi-religious invocations or spells. Techniques included burning or burying animals alive, immersing sufferers in water flowing in a particular direction, dragging them through bushes, or touching them with a magical talisman or staff. Such methods were justified on the basis of no particular medical or magical theory, though many were inspired by the principle of sympathy – the idea that one thing (such as a disease) had an affinity with another that was similar or connected to it in some way. Thus, to cure a headache, a lock of hair might be taken from the victim and boiled in his or her urine.[15]

However, the Revd Nicholas Culpeper was very unlikely to have allowed such people near him. Their superstitious practices were closely associated with witchcraft, and a Christian minister would have considered them either fraudulent or diabolical. Mary's attitude may have been different. She was still a comparative stranger in the village, having been in the parish for little more than a year, and was heavily pregnant, expecting to give birth any day. In such a state of isolation and vulnerability, as Nicholas lay unconscious on his sickbed, she may have yielded to the temptation of letting a charismatic healer through the rectory door.

She may also have called for a doctor, though his chances of success were little better. The nearest large town, Horsham, was ten miles away, and the county town of Guildford a further five, so it would have taken some time and cost for him to come. Had one been summoned, his most likely treatment during the feverish stage of the illness would have been bleeding and purgation – in other words letting blood from the arm and prescribing toxic herbal emetics and laxatives to provoke violent vomiting and the evacuation of the bowels. Mary would have had to administer these medicines both orally and anally according to a strict timetable, and they would have intensified her weak husband's sufferings, forcing him to endure hours spending blood into a basin, retching over a bucket, and squatting on a chamber pot, until he was finally overcome.

The Revd Nicholas Culpeper was buried in his own graveyard on 5 October 1616. Less than a fortnight later, at 11 p.m. on 18 October 1616, in the dark of that dismal rectory, the venue for three deaths in thirteen months, his widow gave birth to their son. The boy, baptized six days later at Ockley church, was named Nicholas in honour of the father he would never know.

Sir Edward Culpeper's patronage apparently expired along with his relation, and Mary was forced to leave the rectory almost immediately. Some time that winter, mother and infant set off along Stane Street, headed for the village of Isfield in Sussex, forty miles away.

The handsome parish church of Isfield is at the confluence of the Rivers Uck and Ouse in Sussex. It sits alone in the middle of a water meadow that floods during wet seasons, bringing water lapping up to the church gate. The small village it serves is nearly a mile away to the south-east, on higher ground. According to local lore (now considered doubtful), it moved there following the Black Death in the fourteenth century, to escape the unhealthy miasma thought to rise from the marshy valley bottom.[16] This was the isolated domain of the man who was to be surrogate father to baby Nicholas, his grandfather William Attersoll.

The Revd William Attersoll was, like his recently deceased son-in-law, a Cambridge scholar, having taken his MA at Peterhouse in 1586. Now in his mid-forties, he had served as rector of Isfield since 1600 in a mood of resentment. The living was, by his estimation, 'poor'. So was the 'cottage' that acted as his rectory. A minister of his education deserved better.

The deficiencies of his situation were exacerbated by an ungrateful and ignorant congregation. He was surrounded by 'enemies to learning', he claimed, whose judgement was no more valid 'than the blind man of colours, or the deaf man of sounds'.[17]

The problem was his theology. Attersoll was a Puritan. The label is a difficult one, covering a multitude of opinions, not all consistent with one another. It was coined in the sixteenth century as a term of abuse (an Elizabethan equivalent of 'fundamentalist' or 'extremist') to refer to Protestant zealots.[18] Those marginalized as Puritan by some were happily accepted as mainstream Protestants by others. They are characterized as hair-shirted ascetics who wanted to ban Christmas and close theatres, yet some of the most theatrical figures of the Elizabethan age – courtiers such as Robert Devereux, Earl of Essex, and Sir Walter Raleigh – were associated with the term.

Attersoll's Puritanism was theologically absolute, and politically conservative. In 1606 he had published his first book, *The Badges of Christianity. Or, A treatise of the sacraments fully declared out of the word of God.* It was a critical examination of the role of various Christian rites based on a detailed examination of biblical principles. His idea was to purify religious ritual of a residue of Catholic tradition and restore it to the role ordained in the scriptures.

Like most rural communities, the villagers of Isfield were solidly anti-Catholic. However, it was nationalism, not religion, that fed their hatred of 'papists'. Isfield was just a few miles from the south coast, which had been in a state of alert for over half a century, in constant expectation of a Catholic invasion that might well have happened but for the famous defeat of the Spanish Armada in 1588. But on matters of religious practice, many wanted to keep the rituals that dated back to the Catholic era. Saints' days and sacraments were woven into the pattern of their lives. They enjoyed church ales (parish fund-raising events during which potent home brews were sold) and tansy cake. They were reassured by visitations of the sick and 'churching', a service for accepting the mother of a newborn back into the congregation after her confinement. Such ceremonies provided them with 'comfort and consolation', as Attersoll grudgingly acknowledged. But he believed comfort and consolation could never come from the cosy familiarity of empty pageants. It must come from reading the scriptures, intense self-examination, and devout prayer. He disapproved, for example, of the Catholic ritual of applying 'extreme unction', healing holy oil, even though it was still common practice and widely believed to cure illness. No 'material oil' could heal them, he protested, only the 'precious oil of the mercy of God'.[19] Illness was even to be welcomed. 'Sickness of the body is a physic of the soul,' Attersoll said.[20]

Life for the villagers was tough enough without having to put up with this, and around 1610 they attempted to oust their austere rector. 'The calling of a Minister, is a painful and laborious, a needful and troublesome calling,' Attersoll lamented.[21] Nevertheless, he was not prepared to go, and appealed for help to Sir Henry Fanshaw, another scholar and his mentor at Cambridge, who had since become an official in the Royal Court of Exchequer.

The manner of Fanshaw's intervention is unknown, but it was successful, and Attersoll would continue as rector of the parish for decades to come. Perhaps as a snub to his parishioners, and probably encouraged by the appearance of King James's Authorized Version of the Bible in 1611, he devoted more time than ever to biblical analysis, producing a number of hefty tomes over the next eight years: *The Historie of Balak the King and Balaam the False Prophet* (1610), an exposition on the Old Testament Book of Numbers that continued *The Pathway to Canaan* of 1609; *A Commentarie vpon the Epistle of Saint Pavle to Philemon* (1612); *The Neuu Couenant, or, A treatise of the sacraments* (1614); and a massive combined edition of his expositions on Numbers, the *Commentarie vpon the Fourth Booke of Moses*, in 1618. This was prolixity even by Puritan standards, in the case of the commentary on St Paul's letter to Philemon, five hundred plus pages arising from just one in the Bible.

He was working on the *Commentarie vpon the Fourth Booke of Moses* when his daughter Mary appeared at his doorstep, carrying his infant grandchild Nicholas. Attersoll was unlikely to have welcomed the interruption, particularly as he may have been expecting the Culpepers to provide for his widowed daughter. Sir Edward Culpeper had innumerable properties scattered across his Sussex estate, including many close to Attersoll's parish. Any one of these would have provided a comfortable home for Mary and her fatherless boy. Perhaps such offers had been made, and Mary had declined them in preference for her father. If that was so, the decision was one both he and she would come to regret.

Whatever the circumstances of Mary's arrival in Isfield, Attersoll had no option but to accommodate mother and child in the cramped rooms of his 'cottage' and assume responsibility as Nicholas's guardian. Being but a 'poor labourer in the Lord's vineyard', the extra cost of having to provide once more for a daughter and now a baby must have a put a strain on Attersoll's finances, and exacerbated the bile that had built up over his material circumstances.[22]

There is no mention of Attersoll's wife at the time Nicholas was in Isfield, suggesting that he was a widower and had been living alone. He had at least one son, also called William, but he was at Cambridge at the time of Mary's return to the household, preparing dutifully to follow his father into the Church. The university fees and maintenance costs would have added a further strain on the old man's fixed income.[23] This must have made the presence of a child in the midst of Attersoll's cloistered, scholastic world all the more disruptive.

He certainly did not like children. 'We see by common experience, that a little child coming into the world, is one of the miserablest and silliest creatures that can be devised, the very lively picture of the greatest infirmity that can be imagined, more weak in body, and less able to help himself, or shift for himself, then any of the beasts of the field.' Looking at an infant, all he could see was the image of men 'through sin & their revolt from God fallen down into the greatest misery, and lowest degree of all wretchedness'.[24]

Nevertheless, the care of children was a theme of great concern to him, because it related not only to the children of parents, but also to the children of God. Protestantism was a rebellion against the father-figure of the Pope (whose very title was derived from 'papa', the childish word for father). Some Protestants saw this as a liberation, allowing every Christian to find their own way to Christ, carrying the Bible and their sins with them, like Bunyan's burdened hero in *The Pilgrim's Progress*. But it worried Attersoll greatly. He saw 'godly' Protestants as being like the Israelites of the Old Testament, escaping the tyranny of the Pope just as the Jews had thrown off the tyranny of the Pharaoh. But the Jews had needed their Moses to guide them to the Promised Land.[25] This is what drew Attersoll to the study of Numbers, the fourth book of the Bible, and the penultimate section of the 'Pentateuch', the five books said to have been dictated directly to Moses by God. Numbers told the story of the Israelites in the Sinai desert, and Attersoll noted how, as they gathered there, they 'murmured' against Moses. Led by Korah, Datham, and Abi'ram, they became idolatrous, conspiring and threatening to destroy, as Attersoll put it, the 'order and discipline of the Church' – his intentionally anachronistic term for the religious organization around the Tabernacle, the portable structure used by the Israelites as their place of worship during the Exodus.[26] 'Thus . . . the wicked multitude usurped ecclesiastical authority,' Attersoll railed, 'and endeavoured to subvert the power of the Church-government, and to bring in a parity, that is, an horrible confusion.' The wicked multitude of his own parish had done the same thing, as had others across the country. All around there were rebellions and usurpations, and there was a social as well as religious need for figures of authority. 'Magistrates and rulers are needful to be set over the people of God,' he wrote. They are the 'father[s] of the country'. Similarly, though ministers of God like himself were no longer called padre, fatherhood was still their role: 'The Office of the Pastor and Minister of God, is an Office of power and authority under Christ.'[27]

And here before him was a little child who, like the Protestant children of God, was without a father. It was his responsibility to take on the role.

The model father was, of course, God. In some moods, this meant for Attersoll a New Testament God: embracing, protective, tolerant. Parents should offer their children 'good encouragement in well doing', he wrote, as little Nicholas played around his feet. 'We are bound to praise and commend them, to comfort them, and to cheer them up.' Of primary importance was education. Uncultivated childish minds 'bring forth cockle and darnel', weeds that grow in cornfields, 'in stead of good corn'. However, many parents 'do themselves through humane frailty and infirmity sometimes fail in the performance of this duty', he noted. They 'cocker', pamper, their children 'and are too choice and nice over them, they dare not offend them, or speak a word against them'. This 'overweening and suffering of them to have their will too much, God punisheth in their children' by making them rebellious. So, for the 'right ordering and good government' of the home, children must be taught, and their first lesson should be in godly discipline. Here, an Old Testament tone emerged. Youth must 'learn to bear the yoke of obedience', and it was the responsibility of parents to place it upon their shoulders: 'If we have been negligent in bringing [children] unto God, and let them run into all riot, and not restrained them, we have cause to lay it to our consciences, and to think with our selves, that we that gave them life, have also been instruments in their death.'[28]

Nicholas was in some respects a good student of Attersoll's lessons. As his work in later life would show, he read the classics and scriptures conscientiously, and became mathematically adept. Attersoll also had interesting and unexpected things to say on such matters as astrology and magic. He had an academic, if not practical, knowledge of the stars, noting that they mirrored the hierarchy of heaven and earth in that they 'are not all of one magnitude, but there is one glory of the Sun, another of the Moon, and another of the Stars for one star differeth from another star in glory'.[29]

Discipline was more of a problem. The sparse documentation that survives does not provide details, but young Nicholas did not accept the yoke of obedience willingly. 'The same affection that is between the Father and the Son, ought to be between the Minister & the people committed unto him,' Attersoll wrote optimistically in 1612.[30] Practical experience seemed to suggest a more negative equation. Just like the villagers of Isfield, Nicholas did not feel affection for his surrogate father, and would not do as he was told. Rumours persisted into his adulthood that Attersoll resorted to locking the boy up in his chamber, and leaving him in the dark.[31]

Lessons had to be learned, and Attersoll was uncompromising. The Bible was held over the boy, and its message battered into his head. God, like kings, expected unconditional obedience. Those set over us are put there by God, and it is his will that we submit to them, Attersoll believed. 'Evil parents are our parents, and evil Magistrates are Magistrates, and evil Ministers are Ministers', and, though he dare not write it, evil kings are kings – the position that underlay the belief of England's monarchs since Henry VIII in their divine right to rule and expectation of unquestioning obedience from their subjects. 'Servants are commanded to be subject to their masters, not only unto them that are good and gentle, but them that are froward [perverse], so ought children to yield obedience unto their fathers.'[32]

Underlying this tough message was Attersoll's belief in predestination. This was one of the central tenets of Protestant theology, and at the time Attersoll was writing accepted by both the established Church and Puritan radicals.[33] God, went the argument, must know in advance who will be saved – the 'elect', as theologians called them – and who will be damned. If he did not, then it meant he did not have perfect knowledge of the future, which suggested that his divine powers were limited. Attersoll found confirmation of this principle in the Book of Numbers. The book took its name from the census performed by Moses when the Israelites entered the wilderness of Sinai. 'We learn from hence,' argued Attersoll, 'that the Lord knoweth perfectly who [his people] are.' But his people, being but human and without perfect knowledge, do not know if they are among the elect. The signs were in their behaviour, which showed whether they tended towards godliness or wickedness. For example, rebellious acts, obstructions in the river of godly authority flowing from heaven, were symptoms of a wicked disposition.

In this fateful atmosphere, every act was subjected to providential scrutiny. The most trivial prank could mean the child was doomed, as deadly a sign as a cough indicating consumption. And whichever destiny was signified, salvation or damnation, nothing could be done about it. 'God keepeth a tally . . . & none are hidden from him, none escape his knowledge, or sight.'

No absolution could be provided, no repentance sought, no comfort or consolation given. Every time Nicholas broke the 'bands asunder' and cast off 'the cords of duty and discipline', and the admonishing finger directed him into the dark, it was not the bogeyman who awaited him there, but Satan.[34]

The daylight world of the scullery was Nicholas's escape from this predestinarian tyranny. This was where the women were, his adoring mother Mary, wives from the village, the maid. Here, salvation and damnation were replaced by blood and guts. Peeping over counter-tops, crouched in a corner, scurrying alongside blooming skirts, he could watch the preparation of meals and medicines, the skinning of a 'coney' (rabbit), its fur being dipped in beaten egg white and applied to heels that were 'kibed' or chapped by worn and ill-fitting shoes; cowslips being candied in layers of sugar; tangles of fibrous toadflax being laid in the water bowls to revive 'drooping' chickens.[35]

No fear of religious instruction here. Women were not expected to engage in such pursuits, at least not in Attersoll's household. He acknowledged that there were 'many examples of learned women', his own daughter perhaps among them; but the Bible 'requireth of them to be in subjection, not to challenge dominion' of male discourse. The 'frailness and weakness' of their sex made them 'easier to be seduced and deceived, and so fitter to be authors of much mischief'.[36] Their place was in the pantry, their role to preserve the frail body, while the male ministry of Attersoll administered to the soul.

Thus, in the company of women, Nicholas encountered the more practical arts of nurturing and healing. Food and physic, chores and hygiene, were inextricably entwined. Here Mary, her awareness sharpened by the tragedy in Ockley, would treat wounds and mix medicines, as well as feed the family and clean the house, using traditional recipes, ingredients and methods handed down the generations, or shared through the village.

The supplies needed to sustain this regime all came through the back door, and it was a young boy's job to go and fetch them. Outside lay one of the most beautiful and botanically rich areas of the country, a fertile valley on the southern fringes of the Ashdown Forest, the enchanted place into which future generations of children were enticed when A. A. Milne made it the setting for Winnie the Pooh's Hundred Acre Wood. This landscape became Nicholas's catechism, the meadows and woods his Sinai desert, the local names of medicinal flowers and shrubs his census of the elect. He attained an intimate botanical knowledge of Sussex, learning, for example, where to find such ingredients as 'fleur-de-luce' (elsewhere known as wild pansy, orris, love-in-idleness, and heartsease, the constituent of Puck's love potion in Shakespeare's *A Midsummer Night's Dream*) and 'langue-de-boeuf' (bugloss or borage), noting in later life how their 'Francified' names echoed the Norman invasion, which had taken place in 1066 at nearby Hastings.

He heard the women talk of the use of lady's mantle to revive sagging breasts, syrup of stinking arrach[37] to ward off 'strangulation of the mother' (period pains), honeysuckle ointment to soothe skin sunburned by summer days in the fields. They talked of 'kneeholm'

('holm' is the Old English for holly), 'dogwood', 'greenweed', and 'brakes', the local names for butcher's-broom, common alder, wold, and bracken. He discovered how every plant had its use, even one as predatory and toxic as brakes. Bracken was, and is, everywhere in Sussex. He would find it erupting in nearby woodland, wherever the undergrowth was disturbed by human activity, harassing stockmen who, during parched summers, would have to drive their animals away from grazing on its fronds, which are suffused with a form of cyanide. Yet the roots, bruised and boiled in mead or honeyed water, could be applied to boys' itching bottoms to get rid of threadworm. A shovel-load of the burning leaves carried through the house would drive away the gnats and other 'noisome' creatures that 'molest people lying in their beds' in such 'fenny' places as the Sussex lowlands.[38]

In the graveyard of his grandfather's church he would pick clary,[39] a wild sage, the leaves of which, battered and butter-fried, helped strengthen weak backs. Wandering further up the valley towards the neighbouring village of Barcombe, following the lazy course of the Ouse, negotiating the network of sluices and ditches draining off into the river, he would visit a clump of black alder trees standing next to the brooks and peel back the speckled outer bark to reveal the yellow phloem, or inner bark. Chewed, it turned spittle the colour of saffron; sucked too vigorously, or swallowed, it provoked violent vomiting; but boiled with handfuls of hops and fennel, the grated root of garden succory, or wild endive, and left for a few days, it turned into a bitter, black liquor which, taken every morning, drew down the excess of phlegm and bile that during winter accumulated in the body like the floodwater in the fields outside.

In these fields, he pored over the book of nature in the same fine detail as his grandfather combed the book of God inside. However, when Nicholas was ten, his days of wandering the countryside came to an abrupt end. Attersoll decided the boy needed a more formal education. He was packed off to a Sussex 'Free School' 'at the cost and charges of his mother' – probably the grammar school in Lewes, six miles away, or perhaps further afield, where he could no longer disturb his grandfather's work.

Attersoll had also decided upon a vocation for the boy. 'Every one must know & learn the duties of his own special calling,' he wrote, and, like Attersoll's more dutiful son William junior, Nicholas's was to be the Church. At school, he would learn Latin, a prerequisite for an education in divinity, and a preparation for university.[40]

Nicholas was sent to Cambridge in 1632, when he was sixteen years old. Little is known about his time there. He may have gone to his father's college, Queens', or to his grandfather's, Peterhouse.[41] In any case he would have followed the standard curriculum of the time, covering the seven 'liberal arts' – first the core subjects of grammar, logic, and rhetoric, followed by arithmetic, music, geometry, and astronomy. The way these subjects were taught rested on the authority of the text. Teachers would read out sections from set books, mostly by classical authors, all in Latin, elucidating where necessary. These were gospel. Students were not expected to question or challenge them, only to study and gloss them.

Nicholas's mother had given him £400 for his 'diet, schooling, and being at the university'. This was a lot of money, and it is not clear where she got it from – certainly not from the 'poor labourer' Attersoll, nor from her late husband's estate (Nicholas senior's short career more likely diminished than increased his £120 inheritance). Perhaps it was donated by a benefactor, a Culpeper relative such as Sir Edward's son William, who had recently inherited his father's title and estate and would later be described by Nicholas as a godfather figure. Or it may have come from a member of the local gentry to whom Attersoll dedicated his books, such as Sir John Shurley, owner of Isfield Manor.

Wherever it came from, £400 was enough for a comfortable life, leaving a sufficient surplus after board, lodging, and fees for a young student, later famous for his 'consumption of the purse', to develop an indulgence, such as smoking tobacco.

Nicholas's passion for smoking was legendary. Even friends accepted that he took 'too excessively' to tobacco. It was the rage in 1630s Cambridge, attracting 'smoky gallants, who have long time glutted themselves with the fond fopperies and fashions of our neighbour Countries' and were 'desirous of novelties'. Smoke-filled student chambers and taverns were an exhilarating change from the stuffy rooms of his grandfather's cottage, and so were the apothecary shops that acted as the main outlets for tobacco, with their snake-skins and turtleshells in the window, and smells of incense, herbs, and vinegars inside.

Tobacco had been in the country since Elizabethan times. Its introduction to England is attributed to Sir Walter Raleigh, but it was already known before Raleigh's voyages to America in the 1580s. In 1577, an English translation of an influential herbal by the Spanish physician Nicolas Monardes appeared under the poetic title *Ioyfull Nevves out of the Newe Founde Worlde*. An entry for 'the Tabaco, and of his great virtues' appeared prominently among a variety of exotic discoveries, such as 'Herbs of the Sun' (sunflowers), coca, and the 'Fig Tree from Hell'. Monardes dwelt mostly on tobacco's medicinal virtues (he claimed it was effective for treating headaches, chest complaints, and the worms), which he had exploited in his own practice in Seville. But he also included a detailed and scintillating report of a religious ritual performed by 'Indian priests' in America that had been observed by Spanish explorers. The priest would cast dried tobacco leaves upon a fire and 'receive the smoke of them at his mouth, and at his nose with a cane, and in taking of it [fall] down upon the ground, as a dead man'. 'In like sort,' Monardes added, 'the rest of the Indians for their pastime do take the smoke of the *Tabaco*, for to make them-selves drunk withal, and to see the visions, and things that do represent to them, wherein they do delight . . . And as the Devil is a deceiver, and hath the knowledge of the virtue of herbs, he did shew them the virtue of this herb, that by the means thereof, they might see their imaginations, and visions, that he hath represented

THE SECONDE PART *Fol.33.*

OF TH·IS BOOKE IȘ OF THE THIN·

ges that are brought from our Occidentall INDIAS, whiche ᴅoe ſerue foꝛ the bſe of 𝕸eᴅicine, where iȿ treateᴅ of the *Tabaco*, anᴅ of the *Saſſafras*, anᴅ of the *Carto Sanɗo*, anᴅ of manꝑ other ⍗earbeȿ anᴅ 𝔓lanteȿ, 𝕊æᴅeȿ anᴅ 𝕷ica= reȿ, that newlꝑ hath come from theſe parteȿ, of greate bertueȿ anᴅ maruetlouȿ effeɗes.

Made by the Doɗor M O N A R D V S, Phiſition of *Seuill.*

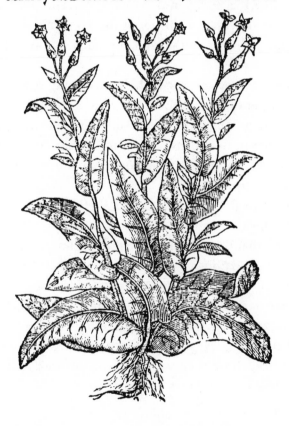

The tobacco plant featured in Nicolas Morandes's herbal.

to them, and by that means doth deceive them.' For this reason, Monardes placed the herb among a class of herbs 'which have the virtue in dreaming of things', hallucinogenics such as the root of 'solarto' (Belladonna or Deadly Nightshade), which, taken in wine, 'is very strange and furious ... and doth make him that taketh it dream of things variable'. Such properties encouraged English merchants with Spanish contacts to source samples of the herb for an eager market back home. The translator of *Ioyfull Nevves*, John Frampton, noted in the book's dedication to the poet and diplomat Edward Dyer how the 'medicines' Monardes mentioned 'are now by merchants and others brought out of the West Indies into Spain, and from Spain hither into England, by such as do daily traffic thither'.[42]

England, however, was at war with Spain during the latter years of the sixteenth century, and tobacco remained a rarity. That all changed in the 1620s, when bountiful supplies of a sweet, pungent variety, superior even by Spanish standards, began to be cultivated in England's newly-established colony of Virginia in North America, fuelling a surge in consumption.

The sudden spread of such a potent herb among the young alarmed the authorities. In the House of Commons, knights of the shires demanded that it be banned 'for the spoiling of the Subjects' Manners'. In his *Directions for Health*, first published in 1600 and one of the most popular medical books of the time, William Vaughan warned against the 'pleasing ease and sensible deliverance' experienced by young smokers, and, targeting his health-warning at the area that was likely to cause them greatest concern, urged them 'to take heed how they waste the oil of their vital lamps'. 'Repeat over these plain rhymes,' he instructed:

> Tobacco, that outlandish weed,
> It spends the brain, and spoils the seed:
> It dulls the sprite, it dims the fight,
> It robs a woman of her right.[43]

The sternest critic was King James himself. In 1604, he published his *Counterblaste to Tobacco*, in which he condemned the 'manifold abuses of this vile custom of tobacco taking'. 'With the report of a great discovery for a Conquest,' he wrote, recalling Sir Walter Raleigh's voyages to colonize Virginia, 'some two or three Savage men were brought in together with this Savage custom. But the pity is, the poor wild barbarous men died, but that vile barbarous custom is yet alive, yea in fresh vigour.'

The King was particularly affronted by the medicinal powers claimed for the plant. It had been advertised as a cure for the pox, for example, but for James 'it serves for that use but among the pocky Indian slaves'. He examined in detail its toxic effects, displaying an impressive grasp of prevailing medical theories. Following the intellectual fashion of the time, he also drew an important metaphorical conclusion about his own role in dealing with such issues: he was 'the proper Physician of his Politic-body' whose job was 'to purge it of all those diseases by Medicines meet for the same'.

But even the efforts of an absolute monarch could not stop the spread of this pernicious habit. 'Oh, the omnipotent power of tobacco!' he fumed, consigning it to the same class of intractabilities as religious extremism: 'If it could by the smoke thereof chase out devils . . . it would serve for a precious relic, both for the superstitious priests and the insolent Puritans, to call out devils withal.'[44]

His ravings had no effect on consumption. Imports of tobacco boomed: 2,300 pounds in 1615, 20,000 in 1619, 40,000 in 1620, 55,000 in 1621, two million pounds a year by 1640.[45] The more popular it became, the more James found that even he could not do without it. 'It is not unknown what dislike We have ever had of the use of Tobacco, as tending to a general and new corruption, both of men's bodies and manners,' the King announced in a proclamation of 1619; nevertheless, he considered 'it is . . . more tolerable, that the same should be imported amongst many other vanities and superfluities' because, without it, 'it doth manifestly tend to the diminution of our Customs'.[46] In other words, the health risks of smoking were less important than his need for money.

James's fiscal needs were certainly pressing. Since the reign of Elizabeth, finance had been a source of growing tension between the monarchy, Parliament, and members of the upper and 'middling' classes of society rich enough to pay taxes. Under England's often anomalous constitutional arrangements, the King, though an absolute monarch, had to summon a Parliament – representing the nobility and the bishops in the House of Lords, mostly the landowning, professional, and merchant classes in the Commons – if he wanted to raise taxes. James had several sources of private revenue, such as rents and fines, but their value had eroded during a period of escalating inflation.[47] Thus he was forced on several occasions to summon Parliament and haggle over his income, a process that tended to force some of the extravagances and corruptions of his court humiliatingly into the light. His response was to look for more private ways of raising money that did not require parliamentary consent. He borrowed heavily from the City of London, a ready source of money but provided, as events later showed, with strings. He started selling titles. He invented the lower rank of 'baronet', aimed at members of the gentry such as Sir Edward Culpeper, which offered the prestige of nobility without the prerogatives. He exploited feudal privileges such as 'wardships', a royal right to the income from estates inherited by under-age heirs. However, his most lucrative source of revenue was customs duties. These were notionally under the control of Parliament but, following a convention established in the reign of Edward IV, were granted to James for the duration of his reign. Taking advantage of the concession, he supplemented the income they generated with special duties or 'impositions' levied on particular goods. A test case brought in 1606 by a merchant who refused to pay the imposition on a hundredweight of currants affirmed that James was entitled to the money, on the grounds that the royal prerogative was 'absolute'. The custom duty due on tobacco was 2d. per pound weight in 1604.

James initially increased it more than fortyfold by adding an impost of 6s. 10d. a pound, a rate so punitive it proved unenforceable and had to be reduced. Exploiting another controversial privilege, he then granted a patent for control of the entire tobacco trade to a court favourite, who in return for the right to 'farm' the duties was expected to pay up to £15,000 a year into the royal exchequer. Later still, he allowed for the practice of 'garbling', imposing an obligation on merchants to have their goods checked and sealed by an official. It was claimed such a measure was needed to prevent the sale of bad or adulterated tobacco, but in practice it was used to increase revenue, as the officials began to charge a further 4d. per pound for passing each bale of tobacco. Such prescriptions set the tone not only of James's fiscal policy, but also that of his heir, Charles I – a purgative applied by these physicians of the 'Politic-body' that would result in the most dreadful convulsions.

As well as being embroiled in such political controversies, tobacco was associated with intellectual ones as well. Critics disapprovingly noted that the herb carried the endorsement of philosophers such as Giambattista della Porta. Della Porta's *Natural Magick* (first published in Latin in 1558 as *Magiae naturalis*) was one of a series of notorious sixteenth-century works that contained combustible mixes of herbalism, medicine, religion, magic, alchemy, and astrology. Such works had inspired a flowering of interest in magic in England, and particularly at Cambridge University, encouraged by Queen Elizabeth's magus Dr John Dee (who had noted the properties of tobacco in his copy of Monardes' herbal) and reflected in works such as Spenser's *Faerie Queene* and Shakespeare's *The Tempest*. In later years, tobacco also became associated with religious fanaticism. A sect called the Ranters thought that, since predestination meant that your fate in the next life was fixed, you may as well make the most of this one, and so smoking (along with drinking, feasting, and whoring) became elevated to a sacrament. Even the more sober Baptists were partial to a smoke during their services.[48]

Thus, a pipe of tobacco in the early seventeenth century took the smoker on a heady botanical, political, and philosophical, as well as recreational, trip. This made it all the more appealing to a young Cambridge undergraduate with a curious mind and a full pocket. It was also the reason why the university authorities tried to ban smoking. They failed, or even had the reverse effect, and Nicholas was one among many who enjoyed flouting the prohibition.

Anticipating future generations of students, Nicholas may even have grown his own. He was certainly well acquainted in later life with 'yellow henbane', a variety of tobacco that he thought originated in Brazil and was now widespread in England. He knew what it looked like, and where it grew. He described the saffron juice derived from the leaves as an effective expectorant for 'tough phlegm'. He also later noted in one of his medical books that the bruised leaves 'applied to the place aggrieved by the king's evil' would alleviate discomfort. 'Indeed,' he added, 'a man might fill a whole volume with the virtues of it.'[49] Given the context, this must surely have been a mischievous reference to royal disapproval of the domestic weed.[50] In 1619, James, under pressure from the settlers in Virginia and enticed by the prospect of greater revenues, issued a proclamation banning the cultivation of tobacco in England (which, being domestically grown, was free of excise duties and impositions). His grounds were that the 'Inland plantation' had allowed tobacco to 'become promiscuous, and begun to be taken in every mean Village even amongst the basest people', and because 'divers persons of skill and experience' had told him that the English variety was 'more crude, poisonous and dangerous' than the Virginian. The same disapproving policy continued into the reign of Charles I, who took further measures to monopolize its importation and to license its sale, on the grounds that it was 'taken for wantonness and excess'.[51]

Nicholas evidently saw smoking as a badge of the anti-authoritarianism that was to define his career, and it seems the two were combined into an intoxicating mix in his Cambridge days. However, it was another act of rebellion that was to have the most decisive influence on his forthcoming career.

The story is related in the most melodramatic style in a short, anonymous memoir concerning Nicholas that appeared in the introduction to a posthumous edition of one of his works:

> One of the first Diversions that he had amongst some other smaller transactions and changes, none of his Life proving more unfortunate, was that he had engaged himself in the Love of a Beautiful Lady; I shall not name her for some reasons; her Father was reported to be one of the noblest and wealthiest in Sussex.[52]

The identity of the lady remains a mystery. She had a personal estate worth £2,000 and a private income of £500 a year, according to the memoir, figures consistent with the wealth of, say, the daughter of a rich baronet, such as Sir John Shurley (1569–1631). Sir John was the owner of the manor of Isfield, and had an extended family that included a few possible candidates.[53] If the lady belonged to the Shurley clan, it is easy to see why Nicholas kept the love affair secret. Sir John was William Attersoll's patron. Attersoll dedicated two of his books to Sir John, and became a beneficiary of the baronet's will in 1631 – the time that the adolescent intensities of Nicholas's illicit love affair presumably came into flower in the woodlands around Isfield, and just before they were interrupted by his departure for Cambridge.

Nicholas was no match for a rich member of one of the most ancient and respected families in the county. He may have been a Culpeper, but he was from an inferior branch. The very suggestion of such a relationship would have caused his grandfather great embarrassment. 'Parents have often too severe eyes over their

Children', as the memoir observed, and Nicholas knew only too well that Attersoll would bring down the wrath of an Old Testament God upon such a union. So the couple decided upon their 'Martyrdoms' – an elopement. 'By letters and otherwise' they plotted to meet in Lewes, where they were to be married in secret 'and afterwards for a season . . . live privately till the incensed parents were pacified'.

On the appointed day, probably some time in 1633 or early 1634, the lady and one of her maids hid among their skirts 'such Rich Jewels and other necessaries as might best appertain to a Journey', while Nicholas pocketed the £200 left over from the money his mother had given him for his education at Cambridge. The Romeo set off by coach, the Juliet by foot, to rendezvous at the chapel in Lewes, where a priest waited to perform their secret nuptials.

As he approached his destination, news reached Nicholas of a providential intervention. As his bride-to-be and her companion were making their way across the Downs they were 'suddenly surprised with a dreadful storm, with fearful claps of Thunder surrounded with flames of Fire and flashes of Lightning, with some of which Mr Culpeper's fair Mistress was so stricken, that she immediately fell down dead'. A family friend passed by Nicholas's coach as he received the news and took the distraught young man to the rectory at Isfield. The unexpected appearance of her son filled Nicholas's mother with joy, until she became aware of the circumstances that had brought him there. The shock, according to the memoir, struck her down with an illness from which she would never recover.[54]

Nicholas's relationship with Attersoll was also terminally injured. It was yet more evidence of the young man's irredeemable rebelliousness. 'If we have warned them, and they would not be warned,' Attersoll thundered in one of his biblical commentaries, 'if we taught and trained them up in the fear of God, which is the beginning of wisdom, and they have broken the bands asunder, and cast the cords of duty and discipline from them, we may comfort our selves as the Minister doth, when he seeth his labour is spent in vain.'[55] Attersoll disinherited his ward, and gave up on his religious education.

Nicholas left Cambridge in a state of 'deep melancholy'. He could not stay in Sussex either; so, like many others who find themselves in need of a fresh start and a new life, he set off for that refuge of the dispossessed: London, where for a while he disappears from the historical record and our story, as others take centre stage.

BORAGE

Borago officinalis

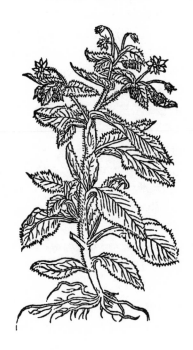

These are very Cordial. The Leaves or Roots are to very
good purpose used in putrid and Pestilential Fevers, to
defend the Heart, and help to resist and expel the Poison,
or the Venom of other Creatures.

The Flowers candied, or made into a Conserve are . . .
good for those that are weak with long sickness, and to consumptions, or troubled with often swoonings or passions of
the Heart: The Distilled Water is no less effectual to all the
purposes aforesaid, and helpeth the redness and inflamations

of the Eyes being washed therewith: The dried Herb is never used, but the green; yet the Ashes therof boiled in Mead, or Honeyed Water is available against Inflammations and Ulcers in the Mouth or Throat, to wash and gargle it therewith. The Roots are effectual being made into a licking Electuary, for the Cough, and to condensate thin phlegm, and Rheumatic Distillations upon the Lungs.

The Seed is of the like effect; and the Seed and Leaves are good to encrease Milk in Women's Breasts: The Leaves, Flowers and Seed, all, or any of them are good to expel Pensiveness and Melancholy. It helpeth to clarify the Blood, and mitigate heat in Fevers. The Juice made into a Syrup prevaileth much to all the purposes aforesaid, and is put with other cooling, opening, cleansing Herbs, to open obstructions, and help the yellow-Jaundice, and mixed with Fumitory, to cool, cleans, and temper the Blood, thereby it helpeth the Itch, Ringworms, and Tetters, or other spreading Scabs or Sores.

They are both Herbs of Jupiter, and under Leo, both great Cordials, great strengtheners of Nature.

Borage is covered with a soft down, and has round, 'succulent' stems about 1½ feet tall. The leaves are large, wrinkled, and deep green. It produces a froth of brilliant blue flowers. The fresh herb tastes of cucumber and is cooling, hence the association with staying the passions of the heart. Mixed with lemon and sugar in wine, it makes a refreshing summer drink which, according to the Victorian naturalist Richard Jefferies, used to be doled out to thirsty travellers at London railway stations.[1] 'A modern conceit,' writes Richard Mabey, 'is to freeze the blue flowers in ice-cubes.'[2] The leaves mixed in salad are also said to fend off despondency.

In many herbals, Bugloss was considered to be the same plant, though Culpeper recognized them as different herbs with similar medicinal effects.

According to some authorities, the name is a corruption of *corago*, from the Latin *cor*, the heart, and *ago*, I bring.

In 1512, soon after the succession of Henry VIII, an act was passed by Parliament complaining about the 'Science and Cunning of Physic and Surgery (to the perfect knowledge whereof be requisite both great Learning and ripe Experience)' being 'exercised by a great multitude of ignorant persons, of whom the greater part have no manner of insight in the same, nor in any other kind of learning'. Some of these ignorant persons were illiterate, others no better than 'common Artificers, as Smiths, Weavers, and Women' who 'boldly and accustomably take upon them great Cures, and things of great Difficulty; in the which they partly use Sorcery and Witchcraft, partly apply such Medicines unto the disease as be very no[x]ious, and nothing meet therefore, to the high displeasure of God, great infamy to the Faculty, and the grievous Hurt, Damage, and Destruction of many of the King's liege People, most especially of them that cannot discern the cunning from the uncunning'. The act therefore ruled that anyone wanting to practise medicine or 'physic' within seven miles of London must first submit themselves to examination by the Bishop of London or Dean of St Paul's Cathedral, 'calling to him or them [bishop and dean] four doctors of physic . . . as they thought convenient'.[3] The religious authorities were to police the system because it was still widely accepted that the Church was primarily responsible for personal welfare, body as well as soul.

However, in September 1518, Henry VIII himself intervened by issuing a Charter that took the power to regulate medicine in London out of the hands of the Church and gave it to a new body, the 'College of Physicians'. This would issue licences to those

considered learned and skilled enough to practise, and impose fines
of up to £5 per month upon those who practised without a licence.
The College was to be financed by these fines, as well as fees for
conducting examinations and issuing licences.

In London at the time, nearly all forms of commercial activity
were controlled by guilds. These organizations were responsible for
the apprenticeship system that trained new entrants into each trade,
trainees being 'bound' to a master for a period typically of seven
or eight years during which they would learn their craft. Once they
had reached a sufficient standard of skill, they were 'freed' to practise
in their own right. As freemen, they acquired a high degree of
political influence, at least by the standards of the time. They could
vote in elections for the Common Council, the City's parliament,
and through their guilds controlled the City's administration: the
Court of Aldermen and the Lord Mayor.

The guilds were concerned with social as well as political status,
and were preoccupied with matters of rank and dress. Each had its
own uniform and liked to parade their colours on special occasions,
which was why the guilds came to be known as livery companies.
They fought ferociously over matters of precedence, jockeying for
position in the official list of the twelve 'chief' companies, from
whose membership the Lord Mayor was chosen annually. The most
powerful was the Company of Mercers (cloth merchants), followed
by the Grocers (originally known as the 'Pepperers'), the Drapers,
the Fishmongers, the Goldsmiths, the Skinners, and so on.

The College of Physicians did not fit comfortably into this delicately arranged system. It was small – its membership was capped
at twenty to thirty members or 'Fellows' compared to a thousand
or so in the larger livery companies – yet its influence was enormous
as it served not only most members of the Privy Council but the
royal household itself, a fifth of the Fellows being officially engaged
in attending the monarch. It exercised a monopoly over practice,
and set standards, yet had no responsibility for training. In 1525, in
an attempt to regularize the position, the Common Council passed

an act accepting the College's monopoly of medical practice but banned Fellows from dispensing medicines. This was to protect the Grocers, among whose ranks were the apothecaries, specialists in medicinal supplies and the preparation of prescriptions.[4]

These arrangements laid the foundations for a medical system overrun with anomalies and riven with rivalries. It was a mess that got messier with every successive attempt to rationalize it. In the 1540s, an act was passed 'for the enlarging of their [the College's] privileges, with the addition of many new ones', as the College's first official history put it. Among the privileges so enlarged was the control the College exercised over the apothecaries. Henceforth, its officials were to have 'full authority and power, as often as they shall think meet and convenient, to enter into the house or houses of all and every Apothecary . . . to search, view and see such Apothecary wares, drugs and stuffs as the Apothecaries or any of them have'. Any stuffs found 'defective, corrupted and not meet nor convenient' the doctors could order to be immediately destroyed on the offender's doorstep.[5]

The same year, another act amalgamated the Company of Barbers and the Guild of Surgeons, perversely in order to separate the two crafts. Surgery – or 'chirurgery', as it was then known, derived from the Greek for handiwork – was a manual occupation, learned like any other craft through apprenticeship. Its role in healing was to deal with external operations: amputating limbs, cauterizing wounds, resetting dislocations, removing tumours, letting blood, extracting teeth, and – the area that produced the most common demarcation disputes with the physicians – treating skin conditions, including diseases such as plague and pox. Since many members of the Barbers' Company also offered such services, the aim of bringing them together with the surgeons was to ensure that they did so according to common standards. Surgeons who 'oftentimes meddle and take into their cure and houses such sick and diseased persons as [have] been infected with the Pestilence, great Pox, and such other contagious infirmities' were forbidden to 'use or exercise Barbery, as washing or shaving, and other feats thereunto belonging', and barbers were likewise forbidden from performing 'any Surgery, letting of blood, or any other thing belonging to Surgery (drawing of teeth only excepted)'. To encourage the development of surgical skills, the act pledged an annual entitlement of four fresh corpses from the gallows, for use in anatomical lectures.[6]

Having established surgery as a separate craft, another act was passed in 1543, just two years later, which threatened to destroy it. Dubbed the 'Quacks' Charter', its preamble launched a blistering attack on the surgeons for their 'small cunning'. 'They will take great sums of money and do little therefore, and by reason thereof they do oftentimes impair and hurt their patients,' it objected. Because of this, the act ruled that 'every person being the King's subject, having knowledge and experience of the nature of herbs, roots and waters or of the operation of the same' should be allowed 'to practise, use and minister in and to any outward sore, uncome [attack of disease], wound, apostemations [abcess], outward swelling or disease, any herb or herbs, ointment, baths, poultices and plasters, according to their cunning, experience and knowledge'.[7] This effectively allowed more or less anyone to perform any surgical operation that did not require a scalpel.

The identity of those who initiated the Quacks' Charter is unclear, but the physicians must be among the suspects. They were concerned that the Barber Surgeons Act had given the surgeons too much power and were eager to undermine their privileges. The act may also have been a response to Henry VIII's religious reforms. In the late 1530s, the process had begun of closing the Catholic monasteries, which until then had run the hospitals. This created a crisis in public healthcare that the act could help alleviate. Whatever prompted it, the effect was chaos, as it did not specify who was to determine the 'knowledge and experience' of those that it allowed to practise.

The College lobbied both monarch and Parliament for further acts and charters reinforcing its own position. It also produced its

own 'statutes', setting out in meticulous detail its rules and procedures. The earliest that survive date from 1555. They were
written by Dr John Caius, one of the College's most influential
sixteenth-century presidents. His name was originally 'Keys', but,
following a practice popular among intellectuals wanting to add
gravitas to their names, he Latinized it to 'Caius', but kept the
original pronunciation.

Dr Caius' statutes specified that there should be quarterly meetings, 'Comitia', attended by all the Fellows. At the Michaelmas
Comitia (held on 30 September), the College selected from among
its number a president and eight seniors or 'Elects'. The Elects
would then choose the 'censores literarum, morum et medicina-
rum', censors of letters, morality, and medicine – effectively the
custodians of the physicians' monopoly. They were to exercise these
roles, not with the 'rod of iron' of olden times, Caius declared, but
with a caduceus, the mythical wand entwined with two serpents
carried by the Greek god Hermes, representing gentleness, clem-
ency, and prudence, which has since become a symbol of medical
practice. Caius personally donated a silver caduceus to remind the
Censors of this responsibility. It was one they would often forget.[8]

Their first role as censors of 'letters', or medical literature, was
aspirational. They may have wanted to control the licensing of
medical books, but this responsibility belonged to another livery
company, the Stationers', working under the supervision of the
Church. As censors of morals they were primarily concerned with
enhancing the physicians' professional image. The Fellows were
touchy about their social status. Since antiquity, physicians had
aroused mixed feelings in society. 'The physician is more dangerous
than the disease,' went the proverb.[9] In the prologue of the *Canterbury Tales*, Chaucer introduced a 'Doctor of Physic' as a figure of
learning, knowledgeable in 'magic natural' and well read in the
medical classics, but 'His study was but little on the Bible'. This
was a reference to the old saying *ubi tres medici, duo athei*: 'where
there are three physicians, there are two atheists', the suspicion of

atheism arising from their devotion to classical (i.e. pagan) knowledge. The slur rankled – the 'general scandal of my profession', the physician, essayist, and Honorary Fellow of the College Sir Thomas Browne called it in his masterwork *Religio Medici* (1642). Chaucer had also alluded to another accusation, that doctors were greedy, making money out of the misery of others by prescribing expensive medicines and charging exorbitant fees: 'For gold in physic is a cordial;/Therefore he loved gold in special'.[10] The sentiment was echoed by Christopher Marlowe in his play *Dr Faustus* (published 1604), when the eponymous hero contemplates his prospects:

> Bid Economy farewell, and Galen come:
> Be a physician, Faustus; heap up gold.[11]

But, as every physician knew, in a medical emergency, attitudes were different. When a child sickens, when boils erupt, when fever grips, when plague knocks on the door, then the physician is 'God's second', as the playwright and satirist Thomas Dekker put it, lampooning the public response to plague. 'Love thy physician,' he advised, adding that 'a good physician comes to thee in the shape of an *Angel*', unable to resist the common play on a word that then referred both to a divine messenger and a gold coin.[12]

The Censors' moral role was aimed at counteracting this image by imposing a strict code of conduct. This code was not concerned with issues such as behaviour towards patients, the level of fees, or charitable obligations. It was about insisting that Fellows dressed in scarlet and silk caps on public occasions and addressed the College President always as 'your excellency'. It was about prohibiting College members from accusing one another of ignorance or malpractice, intervening in a colleague's case unless invited, questioning a colleague's diagnosis, employing apothecaries who practised medicine, or disclosing the recipes of medicines.[13]

The College's *Annals* show that most Fellows observed these 'moral' strictures to the letter. When it came to internal discipline,

the only matter the President and Censors had to concern themselves with on a regular basis was absenteeism, which was rife.
The primary concern was external discipline, the policing not of
colleagues, but competitors.

As censors of medicine, the College was entitled to control the
practice of medicine in London or within a seven-mile radius of
its walls. Anyone reported to be practising without a licence faced
a summons from the College beadle and the threat of a fine or
imprisonment. And what an apparently motley bunch the beadle
brought in, with names, as the medical historian Margaret Pelling
has noted, worthy of a Jacobean comedy: Gyle, Welmet, Wisdom,
Blackcoller, Lumkin, Doleberry, Sleep, Buggs, Hogfish, Mrs Pock,
Mrs Paine and Mother Cat Flap.[14] Those who voluntarily presented
themselves to the Censors, seeking a licence, tended to appear under
more respectable names, usually Latinized, like that of the College
luminary Dr Caius: Angelinus, Balsamus, Fluctibus. They had to
prove to the Censors that they had a firm grasp of medical theory.
To establish whether or not this was the case, they were examined,
not on their knowledge of the latest anatomical theories or diagnostic techniques, the revolutionary findings of the great Renaissance medics and anatomists such as Jean Fernel of Paris or Gabriele
Falloppia of Padua, but on their understanding of the works of a
physician and philosopher who had lived a millennium and a half
earlier.

No other field of knowledge has been dominated by a single
thinker as medicine was by Galen. Born in AD 129 in Pergamon
(modern Turkey) to wealthy parents, Galen was, in many respects,
a model physician: studious, clever, and arrogant. In his youth,
he studied at the Library of Alexandria, the great repository of
classical knowledge, and travelled to India and Africa, learning
about the drugs used there. He became a skilful anatomist who
could expertly cut up an animal living or dead, and, though the
dissection of humans was taboo, he had attained a grasp of human
physiology thanks to a spell as physician to the gladiators. He also

had an astute understanding of patient psychology and was very good at attracting prestigious clients, including the Roman Emperor Marcus Aurelius, an endorsement he never lost an opportunity to advertise.

As well as being a brilliant practitioner, Galen gave medicine academic respectability. Basing his ideas on those of Hippocrates, the semi-mythical Greek physician immortalized as the author of the Hippocratic Oath, he created a comprehensive theoretical system that seemed to provide a sound basis for understanding and treating disease. Underlying this system was a view of the body as a system of fluids in a state of constant flux. There were four such fluids or 'humours': blood, phlegm, choler (yellow bile), and melancholy (black bile). The relative proportions of these humours in different parts of the body determined its temperament, and an imbalance produced illness. A runny nose was a result of excess phlegm, diarrhoea of choler, a nosebleed or menstruation of blood, particles of black material in vomit or stools of melancholy (the most elusive of the humours). The identification of these four humours provided a convenient way of tying the workings of the body in with the prevailing view of how the universe worked. Everything in the cosmos was understood to have a character defined by its place in a quadrilateral scheme: the four seasons, the four ages of man (infancy, youth, middle age, old age), the four points of the compass, the four 'elements' that make up all matter (fire, air, water, and earth), the four 'qualities' that determine their character (hot, dry, moist, cold). Each humour had its place in this scheme: phlegm was cold and moist, combining the character of winter, frozen by northerly winds, and the wet weather of the westerlies that blew in spring, which explained why so many people suffered runny noses during those seasons; choler was hot and dry, excessive during summer and autumn, the seasons of stomach disorders, when it would flow most copiously.

The treatment of disease involved trying to rebalance the humours, achieved through diet or eliminating the surplus humour. A fever,

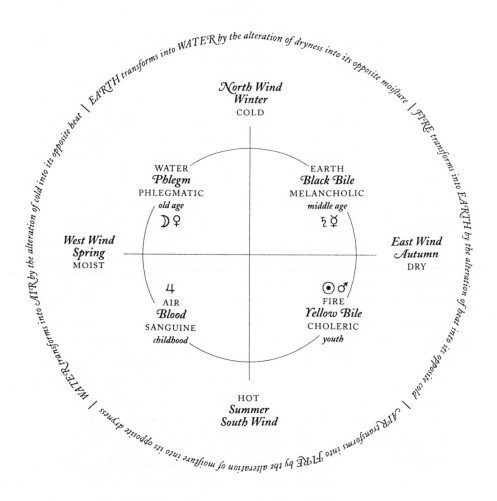

4 Jupiter is hot and moist like AIR and Blood

⊙ Sun
♂ Mars } are hot and dry like FIRE and Yellow Bile

♄ Saturn
☿ Mercury } are cold and moist like WATER and Phlegm

☽ Moon
♀ Venus } are cold and dry like EARTH and Black Bile

for example, might be caused by an excess of blood in a particular part of the body, which, unable to escape, putrefies, producing heat (just as organic material in a compost heap becomes warm as it rots). The solution, therefore, was to drain off the superfluity by such methods as blood-letting or, in the case of other humours, prescribing 'purgatives', medicines that provoke the evacuation of bile through vomiting or diarrhoea, or herbs that produce a runny nose.

Galen's understanding of disease was supplemented by an equally systematic understanding of the body, derived from his own dissection and vivisection experiments, as well as prevailing philosophical ideas. He saw the body as a system for extracting from the environment the life force or *pneuma*, an 'airy substance, very subtle and quick', and modifying it into three spirits or 'virtues': vital, which vivified the body; natural, which fed it; and animal, which produced sensation and movement. According to this view, 'chyle', a milky substance derived from the digestion of food in the intestine, is carried to the liver via the portal vein, where it is manufactured into blood imbued with natural spirit. This dark nutritive blood passes through the veins into the body, where it is consumed, feeding the muscles and creating tissue. Some of this blood also reaches the right chamber or 'ventricle' of the heart, from where it either passes into the lungs, which filter and cool it, or seeps into the left ventricle via invisible pores in the septum, the membrane separating the heart's two chambers. Thus the heart 'snatches and, as it were, drinks up the inflowing material, receiving it rapidly in the hollows of its chambers. For [think if you will] of a smith's bellows drawing in the air when they are expanded [and you will find] that this action is above all characteristic of the heart; or if you think of the flame of a lamp drawing up the oil, then the heart does not lack this facility either, being, as it is, the source of the innate heat, or if you think of the Herculean stone [a loadstone or magnet] attracting iron by the affinity of its quality, then what would have a stronger affinity for the heart than air for its refriger-

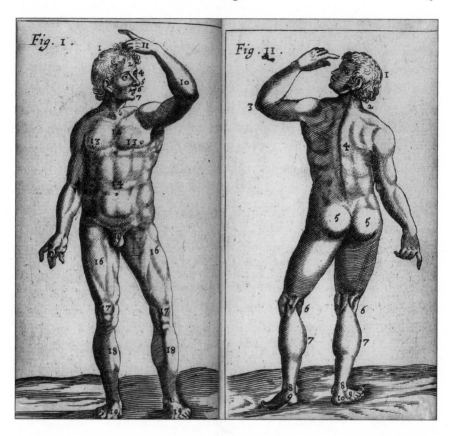

ation? Or what would be more useful than blood to nourish it?'[15]
Like nutritive blood in the veins, the bright red blood vitalized by
the heart ebbs and flows through the pulsing arteries, like tidal
water through rivers and streams, irrigating the body. The brain
produces the animal virtue, which is distributed through the body
via the nerves, producing feeling and movement. In addition to
these three virtues, the male body also produces procreative spirit
in the testicles that is distributed as sperm through the 'spermatic
vessels' to the woman's womb (whether the ovaries produced procreative material in a similar manner was to remain a matter of
controversy for centuries to come).[16]

Galen was very pleased with this theory, and considered it definitive.

'I have done as much for medicine as Trajan did for the Roman Empire, when he built bridges and roads through Italy,' he wrote. 'It is I, and I alone, who have revealed the true path of medicine. It must be admitted that Hippocrates already staked out this path . . . he prepared the way, but I have made it passable.'[17]

Galen underestimated his influence. His ideas survived not only Trajan's Rome, but the sacking of the great Library of Alexandria, the birth and spread of Christianity and Islam, the Black Death, the invention of printing, and the Reformation – a millennium and a half of history – with barely any adjustment. As late as 1665, one medical reformer was complaining that 'an Extreme Affection to Antiquity [has] kept Physic, till of late years as well as other Sciences, low, at a stay and very heartless, without any notable Growth or Advancement'. Galenism held sway over the College of Physicians from the day it was founded. Everyone who wanted to practise medicine in London had to conform to its principles. This was still the case on 4 May 1603 when the twenty-five-year-old William Harvey presented himself to the Censors of the College of Physicians to apply for a licence to practise.[18]

Little did the Censors appreciate what the young man who sat before them would do for their profession. William Harvey went on to become a colossus of the medical world, hailed as one of the world's greatest anatomists and England's first true scientist. Sir Geoffrey Keynes, author of the definitive 1967 biography of Harvey, was so overcome with admiration for his subject, he concluded that 'even if we wished to do so, it would be difficult, from the evidence in our possession, to find any serious flaw in Harvey's character'. One contemporary wrote that his 'Sharpness of Wit and brightness of mind, as a light darted from Heaven, has illuminated the whole learned world'.[19]

Harvey was born on 1 April 1578 to Joan, 'a Godly harmless Woman . . . a careful tender-hearted Mother', and Thomas Harvey, mayor of Folkestone in Kent, a rich landowner with properties not far from Isfield.[20] After attending King's School in Canterbury, he was sent to Gonville and Caius College Cambridge, where its bene-factor Dr Caius was Master. Caius had made medicine a core part of his college's curriculum, securing a royal charter allowing two bodies of criminals executed in Cambridge to be used for anatomical demonstrations. Harvey's own education benefited from this arrangement as he later recalled seeing 'a frightened person hanged on a ladder' at Cambridge, and presumably witnessed the sub-sequent dissection.[21] The variety of medicine taught was, of course, devoutly Galenic. Caius had studied at Padua with Andreas Vesalius, the father of modern anatomy, whose discoveries based on human dissections had challenged many of Galen's, which had relied upon animals. Despite this, when Vesalius later suggested to Caius that an obsolete passage should be dropped from a collection of Galen's writings Caius was editing, Caius refused on the grounds it would be too dangerous to tamper with such an ancient work.

In 1600, Harvey himself went to Padua and studied anatomy under one of Vesalius' successors, Hieronymus Fabricius. Fabricius had designed the first modern anatomy theatre, a wooden structure set up in the university's precincts, which featured a stone pit surrounded by five concentric oval terraces. Harvey gazed from those terraces and into that blood-spattered pit on many anatomi-cal, and in particular venereal, marvels that he would later memor-ably recall in his lectures, including syphilitic ulcers that had gnawed into the stomach of a prostitute, a boy whose genitals had been bitten off by a dog, and a man without a penis who was apparently still capable of sex.[22]

Harvey may also have witnessed Fabricius' work on one small but important area of anatomical controversy: valves in the veins. These were shown by dissection to block the passage of blood through the veins into parts of the body such as the legs. Though working in the shadow of Vesalius, Fabricius was a Galenist such as Caius would have been proud of and was concerned that the valves conflicted with Galen's view that the veins carried blood from the liver into the body. His ingenious solution was to argue that the valves were there to act like sluice gates, preventing the legs becoming engorged with blood, and ensuring an even distribution of nutritive spirit to other parts.

Harvey received his Doctorate in Medicine (MD) in Padua after just two years and was back in London by 1603, living in a modest house near Ludgate, under the shadow of St Paul's Cathedral. Eager to start work, he approached the College of Physicians, perhaps with an introduction from Caius, seeking the all-important licence he needed to practise. He arrived at the College for his first examination at a nervous time. The previous week, Queen Elizabeth had been buried at Westminster Abbey after forty-four years on the throne. Her legacy to her Scottish cousin and successor James was not the settled stability of patriotic memory but seismic tensions produced by her refusal in her final years to deal with pressing issues of political and religious reform. London also faced the onset of plague, one of the worst epidemics for a generation. 'He that durst . . . have been so valiant, as to have walked through the still and melancholy streets, what think you should have been his music?' wrote Thomas Dekker in his review of the year. 'Surely the loud groans of raving sick men, the struggling pangs of souls departing, in every house grief striking up an alarum, servants crying out for masters, wives for husbands, parents for children, children for mothers; here he should have met some frantically running to knock up Sextons; there, others fearfully sweating with coffins, to steal forth bodies, least the fatal handwriting of death should seal up their doors.'[23] It was through such streets that Harvey walked as he made his way to the small stone house in Knightrider Street then occupied by the College.

Harvey's credentials assured him a sympathetic reception. For his first examination he faced an interview board of four rather than

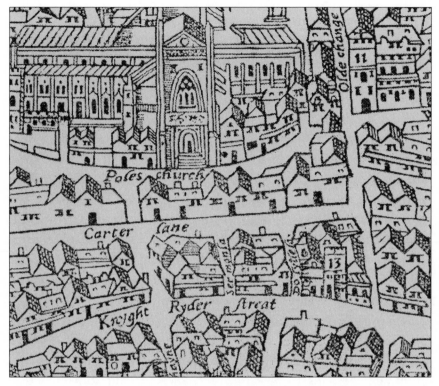

Knightrider Street, South of St Paul's Cathedral ('Poles church'), as shown on late 16th century 'Agas' map of London.

the usual five Fellows, the absentee presumably being one of the many physicians who had fled the capital during the epidemic. The young man the assembled doctors beheld was short, with raven-black hair and small dark eyes 'full of spirit'. He was, as a contemporary put it, 'choleric', referring to the Galenic tradition that associated an individual's character with his or her 'complexion', the natural balance of their humours – choleric, melancholic, sanguine, phlegmatic. Choleric people had an excess of choler, which made them, as Nicholas Culpeper later put it in his guide to Galen's medicine, 'quick witted, bold, no way shame-fac'd, furious, hasty, quarrelsome, fraudulent, eloquent, courageous, stout-hearted Creatures'.[24] In some respects at least, this appears to be an accurate portrait of Harvey, who was certainly quick-tempered. According to one gossip, as a youth he carried a dagger with him, and was apt to draw it 'upon every slight occasion'.[25]

He presumably turned up at the College unarmed, and, being a stickler for decorum, dressed respectfully (but not fashionably – he disliked fashion, considering it a 'redundant covering, a fantastic arrangement').[26] He was the only candidate to be interviewed that day, leaving plenty of time for a rigorous examination. There were four parts, usually conducted over three or four separate sessions, all based on the works of Galen. They covered physiology, pathology (the symptoms, 'signs' and causes of disease), methods of treatment, and 'materia medica' (pharmacy). Examinees were then given three questions chosen at random by the President, and asked to cite passages in the works of Galen that answered them. The entire proceedings were conducted orally in Latin.[27]

Being his first appearance, Harvey was probably examined on physiology and, thanks to his time at Padua, was likely to have acquitted himself well. It would be nearly a year before he was next examined, perhaps to give him a chance to gain some practical experience and bone up on the seventeen Galenic treatises on the College's reading list. He faced the Censors three times in 1604: on 2 April, 11 May, and finally on 7 August, when he was elected a candidate. This meant he was free to practise and, after four years, would become a full Fellow.

Harvey climbed London's monumental medical hierarchy with the deftness of a steeplejack. Four months after becoming a candidate, he married Elizabeth, the daughter of a former College Censor and royal physician, Dr Lancelot Browne. Very little is known about Elizabeth, not even the year of her death, which was some time between 1645 and 1652. She apparently bore no children, and contemporaries who wrote about Harvey do not even mention her. Thomas Fuller, in his *Worthies of England*, published five years after Harvey's death, described him as 'living a Batchelor'.[28] Harvey never wrote about Elizabeth, except in connection with her pet parrot.

He evidently spent hours resentfully scrutinizing the creature, 'which was long her delight', noting how it had 'grown so familiar that he was permitted to walk at liberty through the whole house'.

> Where he missed his Mistress, he would search her out, and when he had found her, he would court her with cheerful congratulation. If she had called him, he would make answer, and flying to her, he would grasp her garments with his claws and bill, till by degrees he had scaled her shoulder . . . Many times he was sportive and wanton, he would sit in her lap, where he loved to have her scratch his head, and stroke his back, and then testify his contentment, by kind mutterings and shaking of his wings.

The flirtations finally ceased when the bird 'which had lived many years, grew sick, and being much oppressed by many convulsive motions, did at length deposit his much lamented spirit in his Mistress's bosom, where he had so often sported'. Harvey exacted his revenge on the pampered pet by performing a prompt dissection. Perhaps because of its adoring relationship with his wife, he had assumed it to be a cock, so was surprised to discover a nearly fully formed egg in its 'womb'.[29]

Elizabeth's influential father wasted no time in trying to advance his new son-in-law's career. In 1605, he heard that the post of physician at the Tower of London was about to come vacant and wrote at least twice on Harvey's behalf to the King's secretary of state, Robert Cecil, the Earl of Salisbury, once in haste from an apothecary's shop in Fenchurch Street, where he was presumably ordering up prescriptions. The application failed, but by 1609, his son-in-law was sufficiently well placed with the royal household to receive a letter of recommendation from the King proposing Harvey for the post of hospital physician at St Bartholomew's Hospital in Spitalfields. St Bart's (as it was and still is known) was one of only two general hospitals in London that survived the Reformation, the other being St Thomas's in Southwark (Bethlehem Hospital, or

'Bedlam', north of Bishopsgate, was a lunatic asylum). Its role was to offer hospitality, including free medical care, to London's poor 'in their extremes and sickness'. This was an immense task at a time when London's population was ravaged by some of the highest mortality rates in the country, and swelled by influxes of migrants. St Bart's had around two hundred beds, cared for by a 'hospitaler' (a cleric, who also acted as gatekeeper), a matron, twelve nursing sisters, and three full-time surgeons. The physician's job was to visit the hospital at least one day a week, usually a Monday, when a crowd of patients would await him in the cloister, ready to be assessed and treated when necessary. In return, he was provided with lodgings, a salary of £25 a year (approximately four times the annual living costs of a tradesman such as a miller or blacksmith) plus 40s. for the all-important livery of office.[30]

Harvey was offered the job in October 1609. At around the same time he was admitted as a full Fellow of the College of Physicians, confirmed with the publication in the College *Annals* of the list of Fellows according to 'seniority and position', which placed him twenty-third.[31]

As well as providing a regular salary, the position at St Bart's proved fruitful in introducing new clients, as influential courtiers often found it convenient to call upon the hospital's medical staff when they were ill. In early 1612, the most powerful politician of them all, Robert Cecil, was laid low 'by reason of the weakness of his body', a reference to a deformity described unflatteringly by one enemy as a 'wry neck, a crooked back and a splay foot'. According to the courtier John Chamberlain, 'a whole college of physicians' eagerly crowded around Cecil's sick-bed, Sir Theodore de Mayerne, James I's personal physician, being 'very confident' of success, 'though he failed as often in judgement as any of the rest'. Treatment was hampered by a disagreement over diagnosis, which within a fortnight changed 'twice or thrice, for first it was held the scorbut [scurvy], then the dropsy, and now it hath got another Greek name that I have forgotten'. Harvey and his surgeon, Joseph Fenton, were then summoned from St Bart's and were deemed to have done 'most good' in treating the condition, Fenton particularly, though neither managed a cure, as Cecil died two months later – probably of the disease originally diagnosed, scurvy.[32]

In 1613, Harvey took a further step towards the summit of his profession by offering himself for election as a Censor, one of the key positions in the College hierarchy. He attended his first session on 19 October and made an immediate impact. He and his three colleagues, Mark Ridley, Thomas Davies, and Richard Andrews, examined the case of one Edward Clarke, who had given 'some mercury pills to a certain man named Becket, which caused his throat to become inflamed and even spitting ensued'. Dr Ridley, a veteran Fellow and serving his sixth term as a Censor, demanded a fine of £8, much higher than usual (apothecaries and other medical tradesmen were typically fined around forty shillings; fines of £5 or more were usually reserved for foreign physicians who set up practice in London without a licence). The distinguished scholarly physician Dr Davies, less active in College affairs and serving his third term as a Censor, objected that this was too severe a punishment for a first offence. Then Harvey, uninhibited by his lack of experience, intervened. He backed Ridley, arguing that such 'ill practice' demanded an exemplary punishment. However, he conceded Clarke's fine should be 'remitted', reduced, on account of his 'submission' to the College, though he should be imprisoned if he failed to pay it. In November, Harvey further demonstrated his zest for discipline and standards by apparently insisting that an applicant for a licence to practise be examined three times on the same day.

And so the meetings continued, week after week, considering case after case, imposing fine upon fine. In December, a Mr Clapham, an apothecary of Fenchurch Street, was brought before the Censors, charged with, among other things, selling an unauthorized medicine 'for the stone'. Kidney stones were one of the most common complaints physicians had to deal with, and many doctors, including Harvey, had their own secret and lucrative remedies for treating them. Mr Clapham omitted to mention that he sold his own formula and, being 'reminded' of it by the Censors, 'confessed that he often accepted five shillings for this'. In response to questions about its recipe, he was oddly specific about the absence of 'distilled goats' milk', possibly because this would reveal the origin of his recipe and open him to further charges. As well as Mr Clapham, another apothecary, Peter Watson of St John's Street, was asked to produce copies of four prescriptions he had made up, two of which had not been written by a physician.

The records are sketchy but suggest that, in the year Harvey served his first term as a Censor, he enthusiastically enforced, if he did not actually initiate, one of the most comprehensive crackdowns on unlicensed practitioners to date. The main target was the apothecaries, whose combination of medical experience and knowledge of medicines made them a particularly potent threat to the physicians' monopoly. During this period, as many as one in ten of the capital's hundred and twenty or so practising apothecaries were summoned before the Censors, to receive a reprimand if they were lucky, a heavy fine and threat of imprisonment if they were not.[33] They seemed to lurk everywhere, down every alley, on every corner, in every backroom. The Censors heard their mocking laughter at the College's impotence echo through the streets.

As well as threatening the health of the capital's citizens, these insolent quacks undermined the dignity of the College, at a time when it was preparing to move from its cramped rooms in Knightrider Street to prestigious headquarters next to St Paul's Cathedral, at Amen Corner – a fitting address for an institution that considered itself the last word in medical expertise. From their grand new premises, they decided it was time to step up their campaign by making a direct appeal to the sovereign.

Harvey was still too junior a member of the King's household to take on this role, so it was entrusted to a more senior royal physician, Dr Henry Atkins. In early 1614 Atkins was enlisted to whisper the College's grievances into King James's ear during one of their routine consultations. On 23 May 1614, the College called an emergency Comitia so that Atkins 'might inform them what he had done on our behalf before the most serene King'. He 'reported much' about his discussions, but did not want to have his words recorded in the *Annals*, presumably because he felt it might compromise royal confidentiality. His unrecorded remarks encouraged the Fellows, Harvey among them, to draft a letter to the King, entreating James, 'the founder of the health of the citizens', to 'cure this distress of ours, and deign to understand the paroxysms and symptoms of this our infirmity'. The letter reminded the King that under 'royal edicts ... the audacity of the quacks, and the wickedness of the degraded were committed to our senate for correction and punishment'. But the writ of the College was now routinely flouted. 'They fling scorn and all things are condemned', particularly by the apothecaries, who 'ought to be corrected: for as we minister to the universe so they are the attendants of the physicians'.[34]

Their proposed remedy was to support a move to separate the apothecaries from the Grocers' Company – the reverse of the manoeuvre used to control the surgeons. The College had little influence over the Grocers, but might have over a company of apothecaries, as long as its founding charter established the physicians' superiority, which existing legislation only ambiguously supported. Their wish was to be granted, despite the protests of the grocers themselves and of the City authorities, who feared the new apothecaries' company would, like the College, fall outside their influence.

The new Society of Apothecaries was granted its charter on 6 December 1617, after a great deal of wrangling between the College, the Grocers, the City, and the royal court's law officers. As a sop to the City, it was agreed that the Society should operate as a guild, with the same organization as other livery companies, having powers to bind apprentices to masters, and free them once they had completed their apprenticeship, and to police the practice of its trade. The doctors also agreed to observe the Society's monopoly by refraining from making and selling medicines themselves. However, unlike the other guilds, it was not to be regulated by the City fathers. Instead, it fell under the supervision of the College, which was given powers to intervene in crucial aspects of the Society's business: the passing of by-laws, the 'freeing' of apprentices when they completed their term, and the searching of shops.

Another important provision was that apothecaries would have to make their medicines according to a standard set of recipes set out in a 'London Antidotary' or dispensatory, drawn up by the College: a bible of medicine.

Bergamo in Italy and Nuremberg in Germany had long used official dispensatories that prescribed exactly how medicines were to be made by apothecaries trading within their borders. Now that the apothecaries of London were to be constituted as a separate body, the College of Physicians decided it was time, after years of discussion, to introduce one of its own.

They did not do a very good job of it. In 1614, a group of Fellows were appointed to produce a draft. Two years later, on 14 September 1616, a meeting was called to review progress. It turned out that very little work had been done. Papers were missing, and there were complaints that the Fellows given the task 'went away leaving the matter unfinished'.[35] After bouts of recrimination, another committee, with Harvey probably among its members, was set up to complete the project. A year later, it was sufficiently advanced for a draft to be handed to a delegation of apothecaries for consultation – a rare moment of cooperation between the two bodies. In January 1618, the publisher John Marriot was given permission to register the title with the Stationers' Company, giving him an exclusive right to sell the work on the College's behalf. Marriot would go on to publish the likes of John Donne, but at the time of his appointment by the College, he had only recently set up shop at the sign of the White Flower de Luce, in St Dunstan's Churchyard. The College presumably hoped that commercial dependence would make such a callow operator more tractable. They were wrong.

On 26 April 1618, a royal proclamation was circulated ordering all apothecaries, who were then in the throes of forming their Society, to buy the new book, to be published in Latin under the title *Pharmacopoeia Londinensis*.[36] In May, the more eager and obedient queued up at the sign of the White Flower de Luce to buy copies. Some of these early copies were discovered to have a blank page where the King's Proclamation should have been and so had to be withdrawn. The Proclamation that appeared in the amended editions was the only section of the book in English, to ensure its message was understood. The King, it announced verbosely, did 'command all and singular Apothecaries, within this our Realm of ENGLAND or the dominions thereof, that they and every of them, immediately after the said Pharmacopoeia Londin: shall be printed and published: do not compound, or make any Medicine, or medicinal receipt, or praescription; or distil any Oil, or Waters, or other extractions . . . after the ways or means praescribed or directed, by any other books or Dispensatories whatsoever, but after the only manner and form that hereby is, or shall be directed, praescribed, and set down by the said book, and according to the weights and measures that are or shall be therein limited, and not otherwise &c. upon pain of our high displeasure, and to incur such penalties and punishment as may be inflicted upon Offenders herein for their contempt or neglect of this our royal commandment'.[37]

The book was, compared with the continental dispensatories upon which it was modelled, concise and simple. Unfortunately, its 'manner and form' was, according to its own authors, defective. The College claimed that Marriot had 'hurled it into the light' prematurely. Dr Henry Atkins, the royal physician who had first approached the King about the apothecaries and was now the

College's President, had returned from a trip to the country to find, 'with indignation', that the work to which he and the College had 'devoted so much care . . . had crept into publicity defiled with so many faults and errors, incomplete and mutilated because of lost and cut off members'.[38] A meeting was hastily convened at Atkins's house, and it was decided that the book should be withdrawn from publication and a new edition issued.

Marriot published this 'second endeavour' in early 1619 (though the publication date remained 1618, to obscure the first endeavour's existence). The fact that Marriot, rather than another publisher, was selected to do the job seems to contradict the College's claim, in a new epilogue, that he was to blame for the premature release of the defective first edition. So did the news, reported at a Comitia on 25 September 1618, that Marriot was still awaiting material from the College and that he had been promised a further payment 'when the corrected book appeared'.[39]

An examination of the differences between the two editions confirms that the need for a reissue had little or nothing to do with printing mistakes or the publisher. The second edition is a substantially different work, containing over a third more recipes. And far from eliminating errors, it introduced several of its own. The real reason for the reissue appears to have been an editorial dispute within the College over the contents. The bulk of the recipes it contained were Galenicals – medicines based on Galen's writings and drawn from ancient Greek, Roman, and Arabic pharmacopoeias, most dating back to the early centuries AD. However, ten pages of novel 'chemical' medicines were also included. Some of the traditionalists in the College probably objected to this and tried to have them removed, in the process provoking a review of the book's entire contents. When the College, in a metaphorical frenzy, accused the printer of snatching away the manuscript 'as a blaze flares up from a fire and in a greedy famine deprives the stomach of its still unprepared food', it was using him to draw the heat from disputes within its own profession.[40]

Harvey's involvement in the drafting of the dispensatory is undocumented. However, he is listed as one of its authors, bearing the title *Medicus Regis juratus*, which shows that by 1618, aged forty, he had become a member of King James's medical retinue, placing him near the peak of his profession. However, posterity would remember him not for his dazzling rise, nor for his contribution to the botched *Pharmacopoeia*, but for another achievement made over this period.

In 1615, Harvey was appointed the College's Lumleian Lecturer in Anatomy, succeeding his fellow Censor Dr Thomas Davies, who had held the post since 1607. The lectureship had been founded in 1582 by Lord Lumley to advance England's 'knowledge of physic'.[41] Attendance for College Fellows was mandatory, twice a week for an hour through the year, though they came reluctantly, the College at one stage being forced to more than double the fine for non-attendance to 2*s*. 6*d*.

Harvey was well qualified for the post. Unlike many of his colleagues, he was an enthusiastic and unflinching anatomist. At various stages in his career he performed or witnessed dissections of cats, deer, chickens, guinea-pigs, seals, snakes, moles, rats, frogs, fish, pigeons, an ostrich, his wife's parrot, a pet monkey, a human foetus, his father, and his sister. It has been estimated that he cut up 128 species of animal as well as numerous humans. His autopsies revealed the size of his father's 'huge' colon, his sister's 'large' spleen (which weighed five pounds), and the condition of the genitalia of a man who was claimed to have died at the age of a hundred and fifty-two, which, as Harvey reported to the King, was entirely consistent with a prosecution for fornication the subject had received after turning a hundred.[42]

Harvey looked upon anything that moved as potential material, complaining during a journey to the Continent in 1630 that he 'could scarce see a dog, crow, kite, raven or any bird, or anything to anatomise, only some few miserable people'.[43] London in the early seventeenth century would provide a richer source of specimens, both human and animal. The aviary in St James's Park had ostriches and parrots; merchants arrived from the East Indies with monkeys and snakes; and the streets were packed with a ready supply of feral dogs and cats. He and his colleagues also had access to a supply of human specimens taken from the scaffolds at Tyburn and Newgate, the traditional places of execution. Examining bodies freshly taken down, and noting how they were soaked in urine, he opened them up while the noose was still tight, in the hope of examining the organs before the final signs of life were extinguished.[44]

Harvey's Lumleian lectures began in December 1616, and they were masterpieces. His lecture notes have, unlike most of his other papers, survived, proudly introduced by a title-page upon which he inscribed in red ink, in Latin, 'Lectures on the Whole of Anatomy by me William Harvey, Doctor of London, Professor of Anatomy and Surgery, Anno Domini 1616, aged 37'. Presumably to guard against casual perusal, the notes that follow are written in the barely legible scrawl for which future generations of physicians were notorious. Though the bulk are in Latin (not very good Latin), they are peppered with fascinating case studies and bawdy asides, all in the vulgar tongue. He poked fun at 'saints' – Puritans like William Attersoll – for their calloused knees, the stigmata of their overearnest piety.[45] He told the story of Sir William Rigdon, whose stomach filled with yellow bile, as a result of which he died hiccoughing. He noted that 'in [men with] effeminate constitution the breasts [may be enlarged]; and in some milk', citing as an example Sir Robert Shurley (*c*.1518–1628), envoy to the Shah of Persia and a kinsman of William Attersoll's patron. Commenting on the anatomy of the penis, he noted that Lord Carey, presumably another aristocratic client, had a 'pretty bauble, a whale', and that a man who lived

'behind Covent Garden' to the west of the City had one 'bigger
than his belly . . . as if for a buffalo'.[46] He observed how 'fecund'
the penis is in 'giving birth to so many names for itself': twenty in
Greek, sixteen in Latin. He dwelt on the nature of sexual urges,
estimating that a healthy man can achieve up to eight copulations
a night, though 'some lusty Laurence will crack . . . 12 times'. 'Few
pass 3 in one night,' he added, more realistically.[47] He also asserted
that males 'woo, allure, make love; female[s] yield, condescend,
suffer – the contrary preposterous'. There were not, of course, any
women in Harvey's audience to challenge these assertions.[48]

The lectures were broken into three 'courses' performed 'according to the [hour]glass', in other words to a strict schedule: '1st lower
venter [belly], nasty yet recompensed by admirable variety. 2nd the
parlour [thorax or chest]. 3rd divine Banquet of the brain.'[49] The
first course was completed in December 1616, the second in January
1618, the third, the 'divine Banquet of the brain', in February 1619.
The exact date of the lectures depended on the availability of specimens and the weather, which had to be cold enough to prevent
the body from decomposing before the dissection was complete.[50]
Harvey reckoned that in the right conditions he had three days to
complete a lecture before the body would start to 'annoy'.[51]

The proceedings would have been conducted with ceremony and
decorum. Harvey was no foppish 'gallant' and disliked fancy clothes
– 'the best fashion to leap, to run, to do anything [is] strip[ped]
to ye skin,' he would tell his audience during the section on the
epidermis.[52] Nevertheless, he would have felt obliged to wear a
purple gown and silk cap, the College livery for such occasions. He
also carried a magnificent whalebone probe tipped with silver, which
he used to point out parts of the body.

His lectures would begin with a few philosophical observations.
Harvey adopted the strictly scholastic view of anatomy, that it was
first philosophical (concerned with revealing universal truths about
nature and the cosmos), then medical (demonstrating medical
theory), and finally mechanical (showing how the body worked).

When it came to the philosophy, Harvey's authority was Aristotle, his intellectual hero. Aristotle taught that knowledge was derived from observation and experimentation. He also taught that the cosmos had an order and unity. Every physical entity, including every organ of the body, had its place and purpose in this greater scheme, which he called nature. 'The body as a whole and its several parts individually have definite operations for which they are made,' he wrote in *On the Parts of Animals*.[53] Time and again in his lectures, Harvey would remind his audience of this. 'Nature rummages as she can best stow' in the way she arranges the organs, 'as in ships', adding that this arrangement was upset during pregnancy by 'young girls . . . lacing' their girdles too tight, which was why they should be told to 'cut their laces'. Nature had also created 'divers offices and divers instruments' in the digestive tract, so that it could act like a chemical still, with 'divers Heats [temperatures], vessels, furnaces to draw away the phlegm, raise the spirit, extract oil, ferment and prepare, circulate and perfect'. Considering genitalia, he noted that nature made sex pleasurable, even though it was 'per se *loathsome*'. This was so that humans could produce 'a kind of eternity by generating [offspring] similar to themselves through the ages'. Harvey, whose marriage produced no children, added in a strikingly poetical aside that we are 'by the string [umbilical cord] tied to eternity'.[54]

Having covered the philosophical issues, he would move on to the medical ones. His lecture on the thorax would thus begin with some general and orthodox remarks about its function and anatomy, quoting Galen's observation that the chest provides for the heart, lungs, respiration, and voice. Before it was cut open, he would invite the audience to note the flatness of the human thorax compared to that of the ape and dog, which protrude like a ship's keel.

Then he threw out a question to his audience: What is the connection between the width of the chest and the 'heat' or vital spirit of the animal? 'Wherefore [do] butterflies in the summer flourish on a drop of blood?' Because, would come the answer, the heart and lungs act like a furnace, heating the blood that suffuses energy through the body. The potency of that blood is demonstrated by its effect on the cold-blooded butterfly. 'Especially in the summer the newt is hotter than the fish,' he added, gnomically.

The shape of the chest also revealed important truths about rank. Roman emperors, Harvey noted, were distinguished by having broad chests, which explained their exceptional 'heat, animation [and] boldness'. His authority for this claim was the Roman biographer Gaius Suetonius Tranquillus, though the only broad chest mentioned in Suetonius' *On the Lives of the Caesars* was that of the 'well chested' Tiberius, better known for his hot pursuit of young boys than political or military objectives.[55]

With the medical remarks concluded, it was the time to open up the body, and reveal the mechanics. Traditionally, physicians did not perform the actual dissection, leaving that job to a surgeon. But Harvey believed in getting his hands dirty. His method was to start with the general and work towards the specific, 'shew as much in one observation as can be ... then subdivide according to sites and connections'. Speed and dexterity were essential, not just to complete the course before the body began to putrefy, but to prevent the audience from losing the thread of the argument. There was no time to 'dispute [or] confute'. 'Cut up as much as may be,' he commanded, 'so that skill may illustrate narrative.'[56]

Harvey evidently enjoyed playing on the squeamishness of his audience. As a waft of flatus permeated the room, he would recall for the assembled physicians, many of whom had no practical experience of dissections, how cutting up parts of the body, particularly of abscessed livers, provoked 'nausea and loathing and stench'. The interior of the chest would prove less noxious than the liver, however. Cutting through the 'skin, epidermis, membrana carnosa', penetrating 'sternum, cartilages, ribs', piercing 'breasts, nipples, emunctory [lymphatic] glands',[57] touching upon respiration, ingestion, hiccoughs, and laughter – prompting a digression on Aristotle's observation 'that when men in battle are wounded anywhere

near the midriff, they are seen to laugh' – he would finally come
to the pericardium. This was the 'capsule' surrounding the heart.[58]
He would make some remarks about the structure and use of the
pericardium, and respectfully correct errors made by Vesalius relating to the mediastinum (the compartment between the lungs). He
discussed the humour or fluid which 'abounds' within the percardial
sac, a liquid like 'serum or urine', which is 'provided by nature lest
the heart become dry; therefore water rather than blood [issued]
from Christ's wounds', adding that it was 'wasted away ... in
persons hanged in the sun'. Then he revealed the organ within.

The heart prompted Harvey into raptures. Other organs were
usually described with clinical detachment, but not this one. The
'empire of the heart' was 'the principle part of all ... the citadel
and home of heat, lar [household god] of the edifice[; the] fountain,
conduit, head' of life: 'All things are united in the heart.' Then his
notes contain what appears to be an innocuous observation,
scribbled next to his initials: 'Query regarding the origin of the
veins. I believe from the heart.' It was the first sign of the intellectual
convulsion to come.[59]

Fundamental to Galen's physiology was the belief that the veins
originate in the liver. Harvey's dissection showed that this was not
the case, but was 'an error held now for 2000 years'. He did not
say this lightly. 'I have given attention to it,' he added, 'because [it
is] so ancient and accepted by such great men.'[60] His notes are
ambiguous, but suggest that at some point a live animal was brought
into the room, probably stunned with a blow to the head, and
strapped to the table for vivisection.[61] Only by such means could
Harvey show the audience what he wanted them to see: the beat
of a living heart lying in the watery reservoir of pericardial humour.
The movements of this glistening organ were complex. He had
gazed upon it 'whole hours at a time'. Initially he had been 'unable
to discern easily by sight or touch' how it worked, but, by watching
the heart as the animal gradually expired, as the muscles began to
slacken and the heartbeat slowed, he beheld a revelation, which he

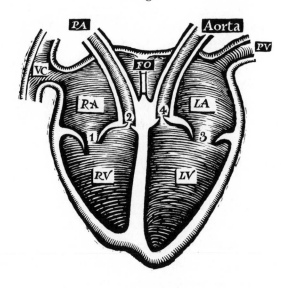

THE STRUCTURE OF THE HEART

VC	Vena Cava		LA	Left Atrium
RA	Right Atrium		PV	Pulmonary Vein
RV	Right Ventricle		1	Tricuspid Valve
PA	Pulmonary Artery		2	Pulmonary Valve
FO	Foramen Ovale (open in foetus but closed after birth)		3	Bicuspid (mitral) Valve
			4	Aortic Valve
LV	Left Ventricle			

now wanted to share with his audience in the most compelling fashion possible. 'Observe and note,' he instructed. 'It seems to me that what is called diastole is rather contraction of the heart and therefore badly defined . . . or at least diastole [is] distension of the fleshiness of the heart and compression of the ventricles.'[62]

Galen saw 'diastole', the phase of the heart's beat when it expands, as the active phase, when it mixes *pneuma,* or vital spirit, from the lungs with blood to vivify it. Systole, the phase when the heart contracts, was when it relaxed. Galen further concluded that, since the pulse of the arteries did not synchronize with the diastole phase, they must pulse of their own accord, in a manner similar to the 'pulse' of the intestine passing food through the digestive system.

Harvey turned this idea upside down. He argued that the active phase was systole, when the heart contracted, pushing out the blood that had flowed into the heart's chambers, or ventricles, during diastole. The pulse was thus not 'from an innate faculty of the arteries, as according to Galen', but the pressure wave produced by the heart pumping blood at high pressure into the arteries, which explained why they had walls thicker than those of veins.[63] 'From the structure of the heart it is clear that the blood is constantly carried through the lungs into the aorta as by two clacks of a water bellows to raise water,' Harvey concluded. He was referring to the system of valves used to fill a pair of bellows with water, which is then squirted out under pressure.

He used another experiment to show where the blood goes to once it has left the heart. Physicians were familiar with applying 'bandages' (tourniquets) to the upper arm for blood-letting. They would know how a tourniquet applied very tightly would cut off both veins (which run just beneath the surface of the skin) and arteries (which are deeper in the arm), while a looser tourniquet would restore the flow of the arteries (indicated by the return of the pulse in the wrist) but not of the veins. Harvey noted that when the tourniquet is applied at its tightest, the hand would turn cold, but when it was loosened sufficiently to restore flow through the arteries it would become flushed and swollen, with the veins standing out. The hand would remain in that state while the tourniquet remained in place, with no sign of the engorgement dispersing, which is what would have been expected if the venal blood was consumed. But when flow was restored to the veins by releasing the tourniquet altogether, the swelling would disappear instantly. Thus, 'by [application of] a bandage it is clear that there is a transit of blood from the arteries into the veins, whereof the beat of the heart produces a perpetual circular motion of the blood'. In other words, blood did not seep out into the extremities of the body to be turned into living tissue, but circulated around, pumped by the heart. This meant that Galen was wrong, not only about the heart, but about the liver also, and it raised serious questions about the role of blood. If it was not the fuel that fed as well as animated the body, what was it for? On this, Harvey for the time being held to the Galenic belief that it was something to do with delivering 'natural heat', the vital spirit that animated the body. The heart's two chambers were 'two cisterns of blood and spirit', as he put it, and the role of the circulation was to ensure the even distribution of these products through the body.[64]

Charles Darwin wrote to a friend that to publish his theory of evolution by natural selection was 'like confessing to a murder'.[65] Harvey's confession was no less dangerous. According to the dating evidence of his lecture notes, he first explained his theory in January 1618. This was eight years after Galileo, who had held the chair of mathematics at Padua at the time Harvey had studied there, had used a telescope to confirm Copernicus' theory that the earth went round the sun, and just three years after the Catholic Inquisition had formally declared Copernicanism to be heretical. And it was only eighteen years after the philosopher and mystic Giordano Bruno was burned at the stake in Rome for suggesting, among other speculations, that the blood must go round the body as the planets go round the sun.

Harvey faced no such extreme reaction to his theory. In fact, there was barely any reaction at all, merely a respectful hush. This was partly because, though the lectures were in public, no one reported on them, and their content would not be published by Harvey himself for another decade. But, given the College's commitment to Galen, and its harsh treatment of anyone who failed to follow his principles, some sort of expression of shock might have been expected from his colleagues. There was none. There is not a single mention of the idea in the College *Annals* for the period, merely lengthy discussions about the chaotic publication of the *Pharmacopoeia*, the discovery of yet more 'impure' medicines during searches of the apothecaries' shops, and arrangements for the College's annual feast.

This silence may have been because so few of the Fellows bothered to come to the lectures, or because so few understood them. More likely, it was because Harvey realized from the beginning the political as well as medical implications of his ideas. He did not at this stage spell them out, but they are evident in his discussions about the relative importance of the heart versus the brain.

Despite references to bellows and cisterns, Harvey was emphatic that the heart was no mere mechanical pump. He kept to the principle that it was the body's most important organ, the 'source of all heat', that the 'vital spirits are manufactured in the heart', invigorating the blood to keep the body alive.[66] However, when he came to his final lecture, the 'banquet of the Brain', he ran into difficulties sustaining this position. The cerebrum, he pronounced, was 'the highest body in a very well-protected tower; hair, skin &c., as safeguards, so that nature [protects] no part more'. Having reached this conclusion, he paused for thought, as though realizing too late that he had compromised the primacy of the heart. This prompted the assertion that the brain was 'not to be compared with the heart'. But he could not resist trying, provoking a Herculean struggle to reconcile the importance of one with the ingenuity of the other:

> The empire of the heart extends more widely in those [creatures] in which [there is] no brain. Perhaps more worthy than the heart, but the heart is necessarily prior . . . All animals have one most perfect part; man [has] this, excelling all the rest; and through this the rest are dominated; it is dominated by the stars wherefore the head [is] the most divine, and to swear by the head; sacrosanct; to eat [the brain is] execrable.[67]

Why did he expend so much effort deliberating on this anatomically trivial rivalry? The reason partly revealed itself in some subsequent remarks about the relative sizes of organs in different animals. The human body, he noted, was like a 'commonwealth', with different organs being the different branches of state, each having its function, each having its divinely ordained place. 'Politicians,' he added, can acquire 'many examples from our art', in other words from anatomy.[68] And with this, he left the matter tantalizingly suspended.

As the body politic began to disintegrate, he would return to this issue. And he would argue that his revelations about the heart, far from overturning the existing order, reinforced it.

ANGELICA

Angelica archangelica

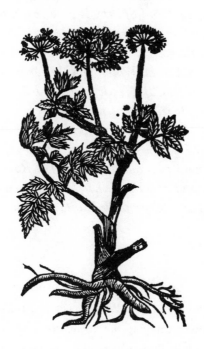

*In times of Heathenism when men had found out any
excellent Herb &c. they dedicated it to their gods, As the
Bay-tree to Apollo, the Oak to Jupiter, the Vine to Bacchus,
the Poplar to Hercules: These the Papists following as their
Patriarchs, they dedicate them to their Saints, as our Ladies
Thistle to the Blessed Virgin, St. Johns Wort to St. John,
and another Wort to St. Peter, &c.*

*Our Physitians must imitate like Apes, (though they can-
not come off half so cleverly) for they Blasphemously call*

*Pansies, or Hartseas, an Herb of the Trinity, because it is
of three colours: and a certain Ointment, an Ointment of
the Apostles, because it consisteth of twelve Ingredients; Alas
poor Fools, I am sorry for their folly, and grieved at their
Blasphemy . . .*

    *[Angelica] resists Poison, by defending and comforting
the Heart, Blood, and Spirits, it doth the like against the
Plague, and all Epidemical Diseases if the Root be taken
in powder to the weight of half a dram at a time with some
good Treacle in Cardus Water, and the party thereupon laid
to sweat in his Bed. If Treacle be not at hand, take it alone
in Cardus or Angelica Water.*

    *The Stalks or Roots candied and eaten fasting are good
Preservatives in time of Infection; and at other times to
warm and comfort a cold Stomach. The Root also steeped
in Vinegar, and a little of that Vinegar taken sometimes
fasting, and the Root smelled unto is good for the same
purpose . . .*

According to Grieve, in early summer-time, peasants living around the
lakelands of Pomerania and East Prussia, where Angelica grew plentifully,
marched into the towns carrying the flower-stems chanting songs 'so antiquated as to be unintelligible even to the singers themselves', the relic of
some pagan festival. According to Christian legend, the plant's ability to
cure the plague was revealed in a dream by an angel. Another explanation
of the name of this plant is that it blooms on 8 May (Old Style), the day
associated with an apparition of Michael the Archangel at Monte Gargano
in Italy.

    The candied stems are used as cake decorations.

n the spring 1625, King James, approaching his sixtieth birthday, 'retired for fresh air and quietness to his manor at Theobald's', his country retreat in Hertford-shire, built by Elizabeth's chief minister William Cecil. In March, he fell ill with a 'tertian fever', malaria, and was confined to a sickroom at the house, which later was formally dubbed his 'Chamber of Sorrows'. As he lay there, he was attended by a busy swarm of courtiers, servants, and medics, bringing documents, linen, and medicines, taking messages, bedpans, and pulses.

Throughout, James's team of physicians stood by, conferring. They included at least two loyal Scots doctors he had brought with him from Edinburgh when he succeeded to the English throne in 1603, Drs Craig and Ramsay. There was also a sizeable portion of London's medical élite, including Sir William Paddy, erstwhile President of the College of Physicians, and Dr Henry Atkins, the current President, together with Drs Lister, Chambers, and William Harvey, whose role in the unfolding drama was to be as central as it was obscure.

At this stage, James's condition gave no cause for alarm, as mal-arial attacks were common, and in the past the King had managed to fight them off without too much difficulty. As the Venetian ambassador put it in a note to the Doge, 'His majesty's tertian fever continues but as the last attack diminished the mischief the physicians consider that he will soon be completely recovered. His impatience and irregularities do him more harm than the sickness.'[1] James was a notoriously difficult patient.

However, on Monday, 21 March his condition took an abrupt

turn for the worse. In the afternoon he anticipated a seizure, telling his doctors he felt a 'heaviness in his heart'. The physicians appear to have been undecided on what to do. At about 4 p.m., the royal surgeon, one Hayes, arrived with a strip of soft leather and a box containing a thick syrup. Watched by Harvey, Hayes soaked the leather with the syrup and lay the impregnated 'plaster' upon the King's abdomen. Soon after, the King suffered a series of fits, as many as eight according to one report.[2] The plaster was removed. However, later in the evening it was put back, whereupon the King started 'panting, raving', and his pulse became irregular. The following day, Tuesday, he went into dangerous decline, and it began to dawn on his medical team that the illness might prove fatal. He was given a soothing drink or 'posset' made with gillyflower together with some of the same syrup used to impregnate the plaster, but he complained that it made him 'burn and roast'. Despite this, he apparently asked for more. Harvey left for London, perhaps to brief officials there. On the road he met John Williams, Bishop of Lincoln and recently made Lord Keeper of the Great Seal, the seal used to ratify documents of state. Harvey informed Williams of the King's grave state.

On Wednesday night, James suffered another violent fit. Blood was let in the hope of bringing relief. On Friday the plaster was apparently applied again, and in the evening another symptom reportedly appeared: his tongue swelled up to such a size that he could no longer speak clearly. On Saturday the physicians held a crisis meeting, but could not agree on the nature of the King's illness or how to proceed. The following day, James died.[3]

Within forty-eight hours, his body was back in London and subjected to a post-mortem. A witness described the procedure:

> The King's body was about the 29th of March disbowelled, and his heart was found to be great but soft, his liver fresh as a young man's; one of his kidneys very good, but the other shrunk so little as they could hardly find yt, wherein there was two stones; his lights [lungs] and gall black, judged to proceed of

melancholy; the semyture of his head [skull] so strong as that they could hardly break it open with a chisel and a saw, and so full of brains as they could not, upon the opening, keep them from spilling, a great mark of his infinite judgement. His bowels were presently put into a leaden vessel and buried; his body embalmed.[4]

The autopsy confirmed the King's known problems with recurring urinary infections, kidney stones, and, as the blackened lungs and gall particularly indicated, the predominance of melancholia in his complexion. The surplus of grey matter that burst out of his brain case also provided the King's subjects with reassuring physiological evidence of his intelligence. But nothing was revealed about the cause of death. Rumours soon began to circulate that he had been poisoned.

Such suspicions were stimulated by widespread anxieties about the state of the court. Many believed it had become rife with corruption and Catholicism, nurtured by James's favouritism. One man more than any other was seen as the embodiment of such concerns: George Villiers, James's favourite, whispered to be his lover, 'raised from the bottom of Fortune's wheel to the top'.[5] Villiers had benefited more than anyone else from royal favours. The son of a sheriff and a 'servant woman', Villiers had been elevated by James to Duke of Buckingham in 1623. The last duke in England had been Thomas Howard, Duke of Norfolk, executed in 1572 for his plan to marry Mary Queen of Scots and found a Catholic dynasty to replace Elizabeth's. Elizabeth, as parsimonious with titles as James was extravagant, and disturbed by having to order the execution of a close kinsman, had thenceforth refused to raise even her closest favourites to a rank traditionally reserved for those with royal blood, and now tainted with treasonous associations.

Such a high position provided the perfect stage for Villiers to play out his political ambitions, which now included arranging the future of James's son and heir, Prince Charles. The sickly, shy, stammering prince was initially jealous of Villiers' closeness to the

King. When he was sixteen, he had lost one of Villiers' rings, prompting James to summon his son and use 'such bitter language to him as forced His Highness to shed tears'. A few months later, during a walk in Greenwich Park, James boxed the boy's ears for squirting water from a fountain into Villiers' face.[6] But by the later years of James's reign, loyalties began to shift. Villiers began to lavish his attentions on Charles, who responded by declaring himself Villiers' 'true, constant, loving friend', trusted enough to take charge of his marriage negotiations. Villiers promoted matches first with the Infanta Maria, the daughter of the King of Spain, then Henrietta Maria of France, both Catholic royals. The Puritans, a body with growing influence in the House of Commons, sensed danger, which intensified in May 1625, just two months after Charles had succeeded to the throne, when he married Henrietta Maria by proxy (she was still in France at that stage, Villiers having been dispatched immediately after James's funeral to fetch her). Fears spread that with her arrival would come a Catholic dispensation and, as the MP John Pym put it melodramatically: 'If the papists once obtain a connivance, they will press for a toleration; from thence to an equality; from an equality to a superiority; from a superiority to an extirpation of all contrary religions.'[7] Thus, when the charges that James had been poisoned first emerged, there were many ready to identify Villiers as the chief suspect, working to hasten the succession of his new best friend.

Suspicions were first voiced by John Craig. Being a Scottish doctor, he had initially practised in London without a licence but had agreed to submit himself to examination by the College of Physicians, appearing before the Censors on 2 April 1604 alongside Harvey, who was receiving his second examination that day. Unlike Harvey, Craig was admitted immediately, despite being a Scot and therefore according to the College's own statutes ineligible for membership. Craig had very little to do with the College thereafter, devoting himself almost exclusively to the King.

It was in the early days of James's final illness that Craig's suspicions were aroused. Villiers' mother, the Countess of Buckingham, had taken it upon herself to nurse the King, and, Craig claimed, it was she who first applied a plaster to the King's stomach without the permission of James's attending physicians. Her intervention 'occasioned so much discontent in Dr Craig, that he uttered some plain speeches, for which he was commanded out of court'. He was escorted from Theobalds and banned from returning to James's side, and from further contact with Charles.[8] Soon after, he accused the Countess and her son the Duke of poisoning the King.

Aspects of Craig's story were confirmed by others who were present in the 'Chamber of Sorrows'. Thomas Erskine, Earl of Kellie, a Villiers supporter who was at Theobalds throughout, wrote in a letter dated 22 March 1625 to his kinsman John Erskine, Earl of Mar: 'There is something fallen out here much disliked, and I for myself think much mistaken, and that is this. My Lord of Buckingham, wishing much the King's health caused a plaster to be applied to the King's breast, after which his Majesty was extremely sick, and with all did give him a drink or syrup to drink; and this was done without the consent or knowledge of any of the doctors; which has spread such a business here and discontent as you would wonder.'[9]

The accusation became public some months later in a pamphlet by George Eglisham (or Eglington), doctor to James Hamilton, the Earl of Abercorn. Eglisham also claimed to have treated the King on various occasions over the previous ten years. He was not apparently in attendance during the King's final days, though he may have been at Theobalds in mid-March. He alleged that Villiers, having seen that 'the King's mind was beginning to alter towards him', decided it was time for James to 'be at rest' so his son could inherit. When the King fell sick 'of a certain ague, and in that spring [infection], was of itself never found deadly, the Duke took his opportunity when all the king's Doctors of Physic were at dinner, upon the Monday before the King died, without their knowledge and consent, offered him a white powder to take: the which he a long time refused; but overcome with his flattering importunity at length took it in wine, and immediately became worse and worse, falling into many swoonings and pains, and violent fluxes of the belly so tormented, that his Majesty cried out aloud of this white powder, would to God I had never taken it, it will cost me my life'. The following Friday, Villiers' mother was involved in 'applying a plaster to the King's heart and breast, whereupon he grew faint, short breathed, and in a great agony'. The smell of the plaster attracted the attention of the physicians, who, returning to the King's chamber, found 'something to be about him hurtful unto him and searched what it should be, found it out, and exclaimed that the King was poisoned'. Buckingham himself then intervened, threatening all the physicians with exile from the court 'if they kept not good tongues in their heads'. 'But in the mean time,' Eglisham added, 'the King's body and head swelled above measure, his hair with the skin of his head stuck to the pillow, his nails became loose upon his fingers and toes' – signs, perhaps, of poisoning by white arsenic or sublimate of mercury, substances implicated in another courtly scandal fresh in the public mind, the murder of Sir Thomas Overbury in 1613. As to the source of the poison, Eglisham's finger pointed straight at Buckingham's astrologer, 'Dr' John Lambe. Lambe had become a figure almost as hated as his master, accused of performing 'diabolical and execrable arts called Witchcrafts, Enchantments, Charmers and Sorcerers', and in 1623 of raping an eleven-year-old girl. He also practised medicine, which in 1627 led to him being referred to the College of Physicians by the Bishop of Durham.[10]

The poisoning allegations were ignored by the new king and his ministers, but taken up by a number of the Duke's enemies in Parliament. Relations between Charles and Parliament soured within weeks of his accession, as the matter of his subsidy, the amount of tax revenue to be paid into the royal exchequer, was debated. Villiers' influence over the new king became one of the main points of contention, and it soon emerged that a number of

MPs were planning to bring charges against the Duke for his role in instigating a number of extravagant and disastrous policies. The primary role of Parliament was supposed to be debating laws and raising taxes, not sitting in judgement over the court, and the King was outraged by its presumption.

Meanwhile, a terrible epidemic of the plague had broken out in London, forcing the King to take refuge at Hampton Court. Charles wanted Parliament to continue sitting, to ensure it voted the subsidy he desperately needed, so he forced both houses to reconvene in Oxford – a precursor of the government in exile that Charles set up during the Civil War. The reassembled MPs were in no mood to be compliant, and after an angry debate one of them, Sir George Goring, demanded that Villiers be summoned 'to clear himself' – in other words, account for the policies he had advised the King to adopt. This produced a furious response from Charles. He summoned his Council and, according to the snippets picked up by the Venetian ambassador, told his ministers he could not tolerate his 'servants to be molested' in this manner. 'All deliberations were made by his command and consent, notably convoking Parliament; he exculpated the Duke of Buckingham; complained that Parliament had wished to touch his own sovereignty; his condition would be too miserable if he could not command and be obeyed.' These complaints, made within six months of his succession, would set the tone of his entire reign.[11]

Parliament, however, continued to touch the King's sovereignty, which became increasingly tender. In the spring of 1626, as Charles still impatiently awaited a settlement on his subsidy, the Commons passed a motion that it would 'proceed in the business in hand concerning the Duke of Buckingham, forenoon and afternoon, setting all other businesses aside till that be done'. As part of this business, a select committee was appointed to hear the evidence that the Duke had poisoned James.

Only a garbled account of the proceedings survives.[12] Several, but not all, of the King's physicians were called to give evidence. Craig was notably absent, as was Sir William Paddy, the most senior member of the College to have attended the King, and Sir Theodore de Mayerne, James's principal physician, who had been abroad since 1624. Those who did attend include Dr Alexander Ramsay, one of James's Scottish doctors; Dr John Moore, a licentiate of the College (i.e. granted a licence to practise) but never admitted as a Fellow because he was publicly identified as a Catholic; Dr Henry Atkins, the current President of the College; Dr David Beton, another Scottish physician; a Dr Chambers, a 'sworn' royal physician but not a Fellow of the College; Dr Edward Lister, a veteran of the College and a Censor at the time of Harvey's admission; and William Harvey. The King's surgeon Hayes was also called, together with Thomas Howard, Earl of Arundel, a courtier who was in attendance throughout most of the King's illness.

All agreed that the Duke had persuaded the King to take a medicine in the form of a posset and a plaster. They also admitted that, soon after the King's death, they had been asked to endorse a 'bill' that was purported to contain the recipe for that medicine. Thereafter, confusion and obfuscation abounded. No one could recall what was in the bill presented to them after the King's death, or confirm that the recipe was for the medicine given to the King, which implied that they did not know what was in the medicine. Various justifications were offered as to why they allowed an unknown substance to be given to a patient under their care: that they were absent when it was administered, that the King had ordered it to be administered, that they believed it to be safe because it smelt of a theriac or 'treacle', specifically Mithridate, an elaborate but familiar medicinal compound which, the doctors reassured the committee, would not have caused any harm in this case.

As to who prepared the medicine, there was little agreement. Some said it was the Duke himself, some that it was the King's apothecary, one Woolfe. When asked who had been present when the medicine was given, fingers started pointing in many directions, but mostly towards the royal surgeon, Hayes, and the physician in closest attendance at the crucial stages of the King's illness, William Harvey.

Dr Moore claimed that Harvey had been in attendance when the plaster was first brought in and should have prevented it from being applied. Moore had been identified from the beginning of the inquiry as a Catholic and, as Dr Atkins put it, 'not sworn', in other words not officially recognized as a royal physician. He was also forced to admit that it was he who presented the physicians with the supposed recipe for the medicine for their endorsement after the King's death. This made him more vulnerable than any of the other doctors, and probably explains why he tried to deflect blame in the direction of Harvey.[13]

Harvey, however, was serene. He admitted to being present when the plaster was applied, the surgeon Hayes performing the operation. He 'gave way' to the procedure because it was 'commended by [the] Duke as good for [the King]'. Furthermore, since it was an external treatment, he could safely monitor its effects from the King's bedside. Trying to spread the responsibility a little, he pointed out that Dr Lister had been there at the time the plaster was first applied, a claim Dr Lister later denied. As for the posset, Harvey had allowed it to be administered as 'the King desired it, because the Duke and [Earl of] Warwick had used it'. The select committee notes also add the words 'He commended the posset', though whether the commendation was Harvey's or the King's is unclear. Harvey confirmed that a recipe had been presented to the physicians soon after James's death, brought in by Sir William Paddy. However, alone of all the physicians questioned, he suggested that the physicians had 'approved' it. Unlike some of his colleagues, Harvey appears not to have questioned whether the recipe was the same as that used to make the medicine. As to its origin, all he would say was that it was a 'secret of a man of Essex', referring to a John Remington of Dunmow.[14]

The question that remained unanswered throughout the proceedings was why a plaster should have been applied at all. Harvey gave a hint – not to the parliamentary select committee, but to Bishop Williams, the Lord Keeper of the Great Seal, when the two met on the road from London to Theobalds on the Tuesday before the King's death. Williams later recalled Harvey describing the illness suffered by the King in these terms: 'That the King used to have a Beneficial Evacuation of Nature, a sweating in his left Arm, as helpful to him as any Fontanel could be; which of late had failed.' In other words, there was an area probably around the upper left ribs, where he would sweat copiously, allowing the release of surplus humours that would otherwise accumulate and putrefy in that part of the body. This outlet, Harvey claimed, had become blocked, causing a dangerous build-up of those humours. It was a puzzling diagnosis, as James's underarm fontanel is mentioned nowhere else. Theodore de Mayerne left detailed medical notes on his patient which record, for example, that the King 'often swells out with wind' and suffered from legs 'not strong enough to sustain the weight of the body'; but the only 'Beneficial Evacuation' Mayerne mentions was the King's almost daily 'haemorrhoidal flow', which, if blocked, made him 'very irascible, melancholy, jaundiced'.[15]

Williams, too, was puzzled by Harvey's diagnosis. 'This symptom of the King's weakness I never heard from any else,' he commented, 'yet I believed it upon so learned a Doctor's observation.' He even attempted to deduce his own theory on how the disease developed, suggesting that the 'ague' had become 'Mortal' because the infection or 'Spring' had entered so far that it had been able 'to make a commotion in the Humours of the Body' that could no longer be expelled with 'accustomed vapouration'.[16] It would also explain why a hot plaster applied to the King's stomach might help, for, by provoking sweat, or even blisters, it might encourage 'vapouration' of the offending humours and so restore the body to a state of healthy balance.

The effect of Harvey's testimony to the select committee and to Bishop Williams was to deflate the poisoning case. It did not exonerate the Duke, nor did it reveal the all-important recipe for the medicine; but it strongly suggested that Villiers' intervention was no more than inconvenient, and that it had been insisted upon by James himself, who was an exasperating patient (one fact upon which nearly everyone seemed to agree). The King, Harvey told the select committee, 'took divers things' regardless of his medical team's advice, on account of his 'undervaluing physicians'.

In its report to the House of Commons, the select committee concluded that 'when the King [was] in declination', the Duke had 'made [the posset and plaster] be applied and given, whereupon great distempers and evil symptoms appeared, and physicians did after advise Duke to do so no more, which is by us resolved a transcendent presumption of dangerous consequence'. On the basis of this, it resolved that the charges should be annexed to the others levelled against the Duke.

When the report was presented to the House, Sir Richard Weston, Charles's Chancellor of the Exchequer, led a rearguard action on the King's behalf to defend the Duke, claiming that there was no evidence of a crime being committed. Despite this intervention, the MPs backed the select committee's report and added the charge to their list of grievances.

But Charles would not sacrifice Villiers. Days after his submission to the select committee, the King sent the Earl of Arundel to the Tower of London. His pretext was that the Earl had allowed his son to marry a royal ward, but everyone knew it was for supporting the anti-Buckingham faction in the House of Lords. After repeated commands to the Commons to drop the charges, Charles eventually dissolved Parliament, thus bringing the impeachment proceedings to a peremptory close. He still did not have the subsidy he needed, at a time when he was having to pay for a disastrous military adventure launched by Villiers against Spain. Facing bankruptcy, he turned over royal lands to the value of around £350,000 to the City in return for the liquidation of his debts, which amounted to £230,000. He also decided to impose a 'forced loan', the menacing term for an interest-free, non-refundable levy extracted from tax-payers, claimed as a royal prerogative at times of national emergency. Charles's predecessors had used this technique, but the levies had generally been small, few had to pay, and many were let off – William Harvey, for example, had managed to avoid a loan of £6. 13s. 4d. imposed by James I in 1604 when a group of influential friends petitioned on his behalf.[17] This time, all rateable taxpayers were expected to contribute, and five separate payments were demanded. A series of high-profile protests resulted. Seventy-six members of the gentry were imprisoned and several peers were dismissed from their offices for refusing to pay. Pondering on the ancient common-law principle of *habeas corpus*, judges considered whether the royal prerogative extended to imprisoning without charge individuals who represented no threat to national safety; but they could not bring themselves to rule definitively on such a sensitive matter.

The poisoning charges against Villiers were lost in the midst of these epic struggles, and became irrelevant when John Felton, a naval lieutenant, stabbed the Duke to death at Portsmouth in 1628. As to the truth of the charges, they were widely believed at the time, and historians have debated the matter ever since, on the basis of evidence that can never be decisive. Villiers was probably capable of hatching such a plot, and Charles, who had suffered many humiliations at the hands of his father and who was impatient to take the reins of government, may even have connived. But James was already ill before the Duke's interventions. In addition to malaria, he was suffering from a variety of chronic ailments, including gout and possibly the royal malady porphyria (the 'madness' of King George III, a non-fatal but debilitating intermittent disease that got its name from the Greek for purple, the colour of the sufferer's urine). Poisoning is one possible reason why a condition originally considered to be non-threatening turned lethal, but there are plenty of others.

No censures were brought against the physicians. They could have been accused of negligence, but the committee was only interested in attacking Villiers and seemed to accept the difficulties of managing a royal patient. However, the episode left a mark on their profession, barely noticeable in the mid-1620s but soon to become as obvious to its enemies as the most unsightly wart. In 1624, an Oxford scholar called John Gee had published *The Foot out of the Snare*, a list of all Catholics known or suspected of living in London. In addition to naming priests and 'Jesuits', it had a section devoted entirely to 'Popish Physicians now practising about London'. Dr Moore was the first to be listed, but there were many others, including Thomas Cadyman, Robert Fludd, John Giffard, and Francis Prujean, all of them prominent members of the College. Many had, Gee pointed out, been to 'Popish Universities beyond the seas' such as Padua, 'and it is vehemently suspected that some of these have a private faculty and power from the See of Rome' to administer the last rites to their patients. Harvey was not among those listed, and never would be. Though disliking Puritans, he steered clear of religious controversy. Protestants in Parliament, however, demanded, in 1626 and again in 1628, that the College identify any practising physicians who were 'recusant' (Catholics who refused to attend Anglican services). Lists were duly drawn up that identified Moore and Cadyman among others. No action was taken against them, either by Parliament or by the College. Many, in particular Prujean, went on to prosper; but the poisoning episode served to reinforce further the feeling among some Protestant radicals that the College had the same papist leanings and corrupt attitudes as the court it served.[18]

William Harvey came out best from the whole controversy. Within a few weeks of the select committee inquiry drawing to a close he received a 'free gift' of £100 from Charles I 'for his pains and attendance about the person of his Majesty's late dear father, of happy memory, in time of his sickness'. There is also a reference among the College's papers to Harvey receiving a 'general pardon' from Charles in early 1627, at the time when the parliamentary impeachment of Villiers was launched. The pardon appears to have

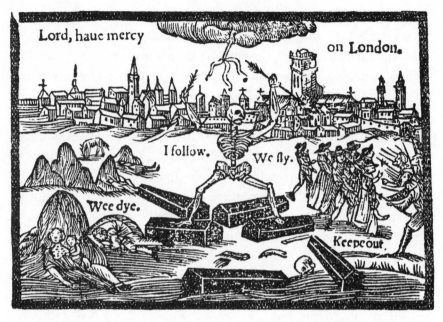

A visitation of plague to London as depicted in Thomas Dekker's A Rod for Run-Aways, *1625.*

been designed to provide retrospective immunity from any charges relating to Harvey's time as one of James's physicians. Such immunity was not routinely provided to royal physicians, so the fact that it was granted suggests a specific charge was anticipated – for example that Harvey was somehow complicit in James's death.[19] Whatever the significance of the new king's generosity, it confirmed Harvey's special position at Charles's side, where he would remain the most loyal and devoted of royal servants, unshakeable in his attachment to the King during one of the roughest reigns in English history.

In the summer months of 1625, while Parliament and the court were at Oxford debating Buckingham's impeachment, the scholar and poet John Taylor chaperoned Queen Henrietta Maria, just arrived from France, on a trip up the Thames from Hampton Court to Oxford. Gliding on the royal barge through the lush countryside, past Runnymede, where the Magna Carta was signed, and the towers of Windsor Castle, the royal party found the gentle pleasures of a summer cruise transformed into a 'miserable & cold entertainment'. Crowds of starving, homeless people lined the banks. They were Londoners, desperately trying to escape one of the deadliest outbreaks of the plague in the city's history – at least as severe as the more famous Great Plague of 1665. Having reached the country, these refugees had faced what Taylor described as a 'bitter wormwood welcome' from the country folk. Greeted as wealthy tourists in better times, they were shunned for fear that they carried the contagion. 'For a man to say that he came from Hell would yield him better welcome without money, than one would give to his own father and mother that come from London,' Taylor observed.[20]

Back in London, a stray visitor would not at first have beheld the apocalypse, just empty streets deodorized with oak and juniper smoke, musket fumes, rosemary garlands and frankincense, and peals of bells. They would pass dormant houses, the staring eyes of their inhabitants glimpsed through windows thrown open to let in the fragranced air and the clarions. They would spot stray dogs who had lost their masters, ditches left undredged for fear of stirring up pestilential airs, lone pedestrians chewing angelica or gentian or wearing arsenic amulets to ward off infection, some coming to a sudden halt and holding out their arms in curious positions, as though carrying invisible pails of water – signs of the first twinges of the characteristic plague sores or 'buboes' that appear under the arms.[21]

'The walks in [St] Paul's are empty,' observed Thomas Dekker, who having written about the last plague outbreak in 1603 found his fascination revived along with the contagion. Not a 'rapier or feather [was] worn in London'. The rich were gone, the rest unable to bear the inflating cost of a ticket out. 'Coachmen ride a cockhorse,' Dekker wrote, 'and are so full of jadish tricks, that you cannot be jolted six miles from London [for] under thirty or forty shillings.' Shops were shut, businesses closed, 'few woollen drapers sell any cloth, but every churchyard is every day full of linen-drapers'. Cheapside, London's main market, was empty, 'a comfortable Garden, where all Physic Herbs grow'.[22]

Physic herbs may have been plentiful, but not physicians. More Fellows of the College were in attendance to minister to James I during his final illness than in all of London during that deadly spring and summer of 1625. On 21 April, less than a month after the royal medical retinue had returned to the capital, the entire membership of the College was summoned to Amen Corner to undertake a solemn selection procedure to decide who should remain in the capital to deal with the epidemic. They filed into the Comitia room one by one and, before the President, Dr Atkins, named those they thought should stay to represent the College. The names that emerged were Sir William Paddy, John Argent (an 'Elect' or senior member of the College and soon to become its president), Simeon Foxe (another future president), and William Harvey. All the others were relieved of their collegiate duties, and most presumably fled.

The official College line for dealing with the plague was set out in a treatise entitled *Certaine Rules, Directions, or Advertisements for this Time of Pestilential Contagion*, first published in 1603 at the time of the last 'visitation', and reissued to deal with the current one. Written by Francis Herring, a College Elect, and dedicated to the King, its first words defined the plague in terms of a Latin dictum taken from the Bible, which translated as: 'The stroke of God's wrath for the sins of mankind'. This view of plague as a punishment, in particular for pride, was backed up by ministers like William Attersoll, who pointed out that God sent the first plague to strike the Israelites for 'rebelliously contending against the high Priest, and the chiefest Magistrate to whom God committed the oversight of all'. 'This is not only the opinion of Divines,' Herring continued, 'but of all learned Physicians ... Therefore his [the physician's] appropriate and special Antidote is *Seria paeniten-tia, & conversio ad Deum*: unfeigned and hearty repentance, and conversion to God.'[23]

The doctors did have some medical advice to offer. 'Eschew all perturbations of the mind, especially anger and fear' Herring wrote. 'Let your exercise be moderate . . . an hour before dinner or supper, not in the heat of the day, or when the stomach is full. Use seldom familiarity with *Venus*, for she enfeebleth the body.' As for remedies, they were various, in particular 'theriacs' or treacles of the sort used to treat James in his final illness. Herring did not provide recipes for these – it would break the College statutes to do so, and in any case he expected those educated and rich enough to read his treatise to consult a physician. However, he did provide a set of basic remedies for treating those too poor to afford medical fees. The aim of these was to produce beneficial sweating at various intervals in the illness's development. They could be made at home and included ingredients that were relatively easy to get hold of, such as radish, caraway seeds, and 'middle or six-shilling beer'.

Herring also provided advice to the city authorities, in particular relating to the matter of hygiene in public spaces. The College had a low opinion of urban health standards, noting the multitude of 'annoyances' that had been allowed to develop and which now aided the epidemic's spread. Rampant development had produced overcrowding, 'by which means the air is much offended and provision is made more scarce which are the two prime means of begetting or increasing the plague'; there was 'neglect of cleansing of Common Sewers and town ditches and the permitting of standing ponds in diverse Inns which are very offensive to the near inhabiting neighbours'. More offensive still were the 'laystalls' or dumping and burial grounds accumulating beyond the city's northern limit. Over the city wall at Bishopsgate or Moorgate lay an unsavoury landscape of fens, shacks, kilns, compost heaps, plantations, ruined abbeys, rubbish piles, firing ranges, laundries, dog houses, and pig stalls. This was the world of Bedlam, the famous hospital for mental patients, and the Finsbury windmills, built atop a vast heap of human remains excavated from a charnel house next to Amen Corner. This would also become the setting for Nicholas Culpeper's practice, and where he and his comrades would muster for the future fight against the sovereign the physicians now served. As far as the physicians were concerned, the whole area was the brewery of infection. From this wasteland the 'South Sun' drew 'ill vapours cross the City', polluting the north wind, 'which should be the best cleanser and purifier of the City'. It was upon these dumps of 'well rotted' waste that the city gardens were gorged, 'making thereby our cabbages and many of our herbs unwholesome'.[24]

In response to such complaints, the authorities drew up a series of emergency 'Orders to be used in the time of the infection of the plague within the City and Liberties of London'. The aim was to deal with the situation 'till further charitable provision may be had for places of receipt for the visited with infection' – in other words, in anticipation of an evacuation of plague victims to surrounding pest hospitals, a monumental undertaking which the authorities were not prepared to pay for out of city funds. The orders focused primarily on identifying sites of infection and sealing them off. Any house or shop in which a resident had died of, or become infected with, the plague was to be shut up for twenty-eight days, and over the door 'in a place notorious and plain for them that pass to see it, the Clerk or sexton of the parish shall cause to be set on Paper printed with these words: "Lord have mercy upon us", in such large form as shall be appointed'. One person appointed by official parish 'surveyors' would be allowed out to 'go abroad' to buy provisions for the incarcerated residents, at all times carrying 'in their hand openly upright in the plainest manner to be seen, one red wand of the length iii foot ... without carrying it closely, or covering any part of it with their cloak or garment, or otherwise'. They were further required to always walk next to the gutter, 'shunning as much as may be, the meeting and usual way of other people'.

Those who failed to do this faced eight days locked up in a cage set beside their home.

As to the 'annoyances' pointed out by the physicians, the orders called for the streets to be cleaned daily by the parish Scavenger and Raker, for dunghills to be cleared, for pavements to be mended 'where any holes be wherein any water or filth may stand to increase corruption', and for the owners of pumps and wells to draw each night between 8 p.m. and 6 a.m. at least ten pails of water to sluice out the street gutters. On the matter of treating the sick, the orders were much less specific. They simply mentioned that a 'treaty' should be agreed with the College 'that some certain and convenient number of physicians and surgeons be appointed and notified to attend for the counsel and cure of persons infected'.[25]

The Mayor and Aldermen published a further set of orders, hard to date, but probably in the summer of 1625. These show that the College was no longer involved in the city's increasingly desperate measures to control the crisis. Only surgeons are mentioned, six to accompany the searchers and identify cases of plague, there having been 'heretofore great abuse in misreporting the diseases, to the further spreading of the infection'. These new orders were more draconian than the previous ones. The surgeons were offered 12*d.* per body examined, 'to be paid out of the goods of the party searched, if he be able, or otherwise by the parish'. Infected properties were to be identified, not just with a sign, but with a large red cross painted in the middle of the front door – the first appearance of what became the universal mark of contamination. No longer were appointed residents allowed out to buy necessities. Instead, everyone was to be confined indoors for a month, with a day- and a night-watchman to stand guard and fetch provisions as required, locking up the house and taking the key while away from his post.[26]

The physicians were left out of these orders because they had fallen out with the city authorities. This is confirmed by a meeting held at the College in 1630 to discuss a less serious outbreak, during which Harvey pointed out that there was no point in selecting a team of practitioners to advise and help city officials because during 1625 he and his colleagues had been ignored. The exact cause of the dispute is unknown, but the very fact that it had come at a time of such intense medical need shows that, on the streets at least, the physicians had become an irrelevance. Those who had disappeared became resentfully numbered among the rich 'run-aways' attacked by Dekker, so much so that when they returned many stopped wearing their official robes in public to prevent being identified, despite reprimands from the College President. Harvey and the three lone colleagues who remained presumably treated their own patients, but they had no documented involvement in dealing with the escalating number of cases that arose among the mass of the population, which produced 593 deaths in the first week of July, 1,004 in the second, 1,819 in the third, 2,471 in the fourth, peaking at 4,463 in the third week of August.[27] Throughout these desperate months, Amen Corner remained empty, the Censors inactive. The only meeting to be called was convened at the house of the President, Dr Atkins, to appoint his successor.

The inaction of the doctors left the market for medicine wide open, and the apothecaries, no longer mere Grocers but now enjoying the dignity of a Society of their own, stepped into the gaping breach. As the number of cases mounted, it was they who visited the sick and distributed the medicine. They began mass-producing Theriaca Andromache, Mithridate, and London Treacle, the physicians' favourite antidotes. One particularly industrious apothecary managed to produce 160 lb of Mithridate in one month, enough for 15,360 doses.[28] These medicines included an enormous number of ingredients: animal derivatives such as deer antler and viper flesh, spices such as nutmeg and saffron, flowers such as roses and marigolds, herbs such as dittany and St John's wort, anodynes such as opium and Malaga wine. By June, supplies of some key ingredients had run out. As required by its charter, the Society of Apothecaries consulted Harvey and his three colleagues, as the College's official representatives, on the use of substitutes. At other times, the College insisted on the recipes in the *Pharmacopoeia Londinensis* being rigidly followed, but on this occasion no resistance was offered.[29]

The physicians had in any case tacitly accepted that the apothecaries were in charge, as they had apparently let them prescribe as well as dispense medicines on a routine basis, breaking the cardinal rule of the College's as well as the Society's charter. It was impractical for a handful of physicians to write bills for the thousands of patients clamouring for medical help. In Harvey's tiny parish of St Martin's in Ludgate, one of the worst affected, there were over 250 deaths and an unrecorded number of infections, among a population unlikely to have been much more than a thousand.[30] No lone physician could be expected to cope with such levels of sickness, even if the victims were able to afford his fees.

The most obvious sign that the physicians had relinquished responsibility for dealing with the plague came in early 1626, when it had passed its height. Harvey had once more been elected a Censor, and at a meeting he attended in 1626 one John Antony appeared accused of having practised without a licence for over two years. A month later Antony returned with 8 lb of a medicine he was prescribing 'which he handed over to the President and asked that he might be allowed to practise and connived at: which was granted to him by those present' – an unprecedented display of tolerance.[31]

Nehemiah Wallington the wood turner had a small shop in Little Eastcheap, between Pudding Lane and Fish Street Hill. Standing upon the doorstep in early 1625, he surveyed 'this doleful city', listened to the 'bells tolling and ringing out continually', and wondered what would become of him and his family.[32]

If the courtiers, the physicians, the rich merchants with royal monopolies, the 'great Masters of Riches', as Dekker called them,

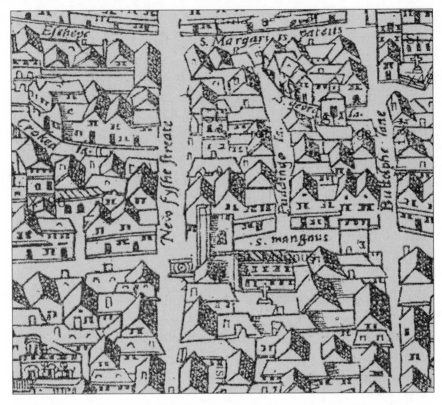

Nehemiah's neighbourhood. Little Eastcheap is the lane at the top of the map, here identified as 'St Margarets patens'.

were the runaways, Wallington was typical of those left behind.[33] Figures are imprecise, but by the 1620s crafts- and tradesmen like him made up the bulk of London's householders.[34] Their standard of living was modest, and for some barely distinguishable from poverty in bad years; but they had something few of their sort enjoyed outside London – political influence. The City could not be called democratic, but it was closer to that ideal than most other institutions of the era. Wallington and his 'middling sort' were 'freemen', citizens, with a say in the running of their livery companies (the Turners, in Wallington's case). These companies in turn not only ran London's government, but were bankrolling the debts

James, and now Charles, had run up in their attempts to avoid having to go cap-in-hand to Parliament.

Nehemiah Wallington shared another feature common to many Londoners of his class: he was a Puritan, and an avid reader of the Bible and biblical exegeses, such as William Attersoll's analysis of the Book of Numbers. But where Attersoll's rural congregation rejected theological innovation, that to which Wallington belonged thrived on it. They lapped up lectures on predestination, the role of Church government and the meaning of divine election.

Wallington also believed in divine providence – that events on earth somehow expressed God's will. From the moment he 'came forth polluted into this wicked world' in 1598, every event, from the tiniest domestic incident to the greatest international affairs, was to be investigated to see how it fitted in with God's plan. Most Puritans understood events in this way, but Wallington took it a step further: he wrote all his deliberations down, creating a journal of human struggle amounting to over two and a half thousand pages.

The plague of 1625 represented one of the first major episodes to be examined by Wallington in this way, and his account of it provides a vivid street-level view of what it was like for the ordinary citizens of London left behind and how they dealt with it – not just medically, but philosophically and emotionally.

Like the College of Physicians, Wallington assumed that the plague must have been sent by God. But where the College, taking its line from the religious establishment, saw it as a 'general humiliation of the people', Wallington believed it was a sign of how 'idolatry crept in by little and little' and how 'cunningly and craftily hath the enemies of God's free grace brought in superstition'.[35] In other words, it was a divine reaction to the established Church of England being drawn dangerously back towards the idolatrous rites and doctrinaire attitudes of Catholicism. Charles I had already revealed himself to be an enemy of Puritan reform, having chosen the controversial religious conservative Robert Montagu as his theological adviser. In a book ostentatiously dedicated to Charles that appeared in 1625, Montagu had attacked 'those Classical Puritans who were wont to pass all their Strange Determinations, Sabbatarian Paradoxes, and Apocalyptical Frenzies under the Name and Covert of the True Professors of Protestant Doctrine'.[36] Puritans such as Nehemiah Wallington would have found it hard not to see the distorted reflection of themselves in Montagu's caricature and to conclude that their beliefs were under threat.

Thus the plague could not have descended on London at a more significant or sensitive time: it was part of the unfolding struggle between the Puritan saints and the courtly sinners. Wallington had already noted, a few years before, a 'poor man of Buckinghamshire, that went all in black clothes, with his hat commonly under his arm' and who for the space of a year stood before the palace gates at Whitehall calling to the King 'for woe and vengeance on all Papists'. 'I myself have seen and heard him,' Wallington wrote, 'crying, Woe to London, woe to the inhabitants of London.'[37]

Woe indeed. In the summer months of 1625, the tolling of the bells was ceaseless, and 'could not but make us wonder at the hand of God to be so hot round about us'. Would even Nehemiah's godly family be touched? He certainly did not regard himself as immune. He was a sinner too, all his efforts at saintliness, set out in a list of seventy-seven articles drawn up on his twenty-first birthday, proving paltry in the face of temptation. 'I have many sorrows and am weak,' he admitted to his journal.[38]

Through the summer weeks of 1625, all he could do was study the Bills of Mortality nailed to the door of his local church, St Margaret's in New Fish Street: 5,205 dead in August, 43,265 in the year up to 27 October. He heard gossip about whole families – fifteen or sixteen in a single household – being wiped out, or perhaps leaving a lone survivor to endure a life of isolation, 'a torment which is not threatened in hell itself', as the poet and preacher John Donne observed at the time.[39]

There was no tale too terrible to go unrecorded; all had their place in Wallington's ledger of misery – the woman who had laid out eight sheets in the churchyard of St Mary's in Whitechapel as shrouds for her family, the sixty children who had died in one alley, the sixty pregnant women lost in Shoreditch. 'And thus would I meditate with myself alone: What if the sickness should come into this house; who would I willing spare? Then would I say, the maid. Who next? My son John. Who next? My daughter Elizabeth. Who next? Myself . . . Many tears I did shed with these thoughts, and I desired the Lord, if it might stand with His glory and my soul's good, that I might die first and never see that day.'

But he lived through those dreadful summer months, and so did his family. One Friday in October 1625, when the numbers reported in the Bills of Mortality were beginning to fall for the first time in months, Wallington, his pregnant wife Grace, his daughter Elizabeth, his son John, his half-sister Patience, and his maid Ruth decided upon a trip to Lewisham, a pleasant, rural suburb downstream of London on the opposite bank of the Thames. The object of the trip was 'refreshment', to celebrate the family's survival, and the third birthday of little Elizabeth.

After setting out, the boat they hired to carry them down the river became snagged with a ship's cable and nearly capsized, and the oarsman several times managed to run aground. The fact that they survived these mishaps unharmed and were safely delivered to Lewisham seemed to provide further evidence of the family's blessed deliverance. There, the wan group could breathe in the fresh, pure breeze running across the fields and look from a safe distance upon their city, its ravages now invisible beneath the canopy of spires, pinnacles, and towers, and the exhalation of wood smoke venting through the slits of narrow streets. 'We were all very merry together,' Wallington wrote. At Lewisham, the Puritan could forget the cares of daily life and picnic in the warmth of God's benefaction. 'And so we came all safe home again, the Lord's name be praised for evermore. Amen.'[40]

Not amen. The following afternoon, back at home, there was a change of humour. The maid told Wallington's wife Grace that she felt a pricking sensation in her neck. At eight that evening, while Grace was washing the dishes in the kitchen, little Elizabeth, 'being merry', toddled up to her and mimicked her father, asking 'What do you here, my wife?' That night, as Nehemiah tucked her up, Elizabeth said, 'Father, I go abroad tomorrow, and buy you a plum pie.' These were the last words that his 'sweet child' would speak to him. That night she was overcome by a series of agonizing spasms – 'the very pangs of death . . . which was very grievous unto us the beholders'. The pangs lasted until the following Tuesday, when at four in the morning she died. The city still being on a plague footing, the tiny body had to be disposed of quickly. It was wrapped in a sheet and buried the following night.

We reassure ourselves that our distant forebears tolerated such high levels of mortality because they put a lower value on life. This was not so in the instance of Nehemiah Wallington, nor is it borne out by other evidence. Dr Richard Napier was a vicar and physician based fifty miles north of London at Lindford in Buckinghamshire whose papers ended up in the hands of the astrologer William Lilly. Napier recorded over a hundred cases of melancholia, and of these nearly a half were linked to the sorrow of losing a child.[41]

The grief Nehemiah Wallington felt at the loss of Elizabeth 'was so great that I forgot myself . . . I did offend God in it; for I broke all my purposes, promises and covenants with my God . . . I was much distracted in my mind, and could not be comforted, although my friends speak so comfortably to me.' The resilient Grace struggled to bring her husband back from his distracted state. 'Consider how willingly Abraham went to offer up his only son Isaac, although he was to be his own executioner,' she scolded, hoping that a biblical allusion would bring him to his senses. 'Do you not grieve for [the] child?' Nehemiah asked. 'No, truly husband, if you will believe me, I do as freely give it again unto God, as I did receive it of him,' Grace replied.

Grace herself fell ill a few days later, and seemed close to death. Her recovery – or, in Nehemiah's eyes, deliverance – did not help overcome a rift growing between them. In the following weeks, 'what quarrellings, grievous reproaches, and slanders I and my wife had'. These were to be interrupted in December when Grace gave birth to an apparently healthy boy, whom they named Nehemiah after his father. Grace had difficulty feeding the infant, and so handed him over to a wet-nurse. Women of her class were unused to allowing others to nurse their children, and she was worried little Nehemiah might never be returned.

In late March, their son John, a little over two years old, fell ill. Though a 'merry' infant, 'full of play', within months of his birth he had suffered a series of epileptic seizures – the 'falling sickness', as epilepsy was then called. His parents looked into his cot and beheld the most violent fit yet. His eyes rolled, his little hands clenched, and his mouth foamed.

Only now did Wallington turn to the medical profession for help. People like him would normally have nothing to do with Fellows of the College, who remained aloof (quite literally, as many made their rounds on horseback) from the healthcare of ordinary citizens. But the situation was now so desperate that Wallington needed help, and he sought it from a Dr Sanders. The identity of this doctor is unclear. He may have been Patrick Saunders, who lived at Bishopsgate and was made a probationary member of the College in 1620. He may have been the 'Sanders' brought before the College Censors in 1613 who had been warned to desist from practising because it was claimed he had only been to university for two months.[42] If Wallington's Sanders was unlicensed, he would at least be cheaper. Nursing the sick was itself an unbearable cost to the humble and impecunious turner, what 'with fire and candles all night and day'. The 'great expenses' of a doctor, combined with the cost of paying an apothecary to mix up any medicines pre-scribed, could be devastating. But faced with the imminent death of his first son, he felt he had no choice.[43] Dr Sanders prescribed a cordial, but the boy continued 'very sick till the next Sabbath day when be broke forth in the measles'.

The appearance of measles would have been seen by both Wallington and Sanders as hopeful. They signalled the eruption of the noxious humours that had accumulated in the infant's body, and the expulsion of these humours would, with God's providence, restore balance and health.

This turned out to be the case, but the respite was temporary. A few months later, John started to refuse solid food, accepting nothing except sips of small beer, the virtually non-alcoholic brew that was likely to be the only potable liquid in the household. Clearly in great pain, and feeling cold down one side of his body, the boy kept crying out 'Mame, Oh, John's hand, Oh, John's foot'. On the night of 3 April 1626, his exhausted parents asked a Mrs Trotter to watch over their son as they tried to get some sleep. Mrs Trotter awoke them at three in the morning, and Grace found John in a state of delirium. Aware that his mother had come to him, he called 'Mame, John fall down, op-a-day; Mame, John fall down, op-a-day'. The following day he suffered a series of fits, asked for some more beer, said 'op-a-day', and died. 'So ended his miserable life,' his inconsolable father noted in his journal.[44]

By the following year the plague was long past, and Grace gave birth to another child, christened Samuel. But he did not thrive, suffering convulsions similar to those endured by John. Dr Sanders was called again, but admitted there was nothing he could do. In desperation, Wallington turned to a Mrs Mason for help. She was probably a cunning woman of the sort routinely reported to the College Censors, though one who used natural rather than magical methods: Wallington would never have tolerated the use of incantations or spells. Mrs Mason busied herself applying 'plasters unto his head, stomach, and his feet', hoping to draw out the displaced humours. There was a brief recovery but the child then continued to waste away, whereupon Mrs Mason advised that the boy be sent to a nurse in Peckham, on the south side of the River Thames, in the hope that the country air might strengthen his constitution. A few weeks later, Wallington set off to visit his convalescing son, crossing London Bridge and heading past the theatres, brothels, bear gardens, and palaces of Southwark. *En route*, news reached him that Samuel had died. The plague orders had now lapsed, so the Wallingtons could bury their child at a more leisurely pace, which they did with a mile and a half procession from their house to his grave on 'a very wet and doleful day' that soaked them all to the skin.[45]

Nehemiah Wallington's experiences were typical, even though his recording of them was exceptional. Tens of thousands of tradesfolk suffered as he did. And they could not but see their sufferings as somehow linked to current events, particularly to the political uncertainties and upheavals surrounding Charles I's succession. Thomas Dekker noted that, just as Queen Elizabeth's death had coincided with an outbreak of the plague, so had James's, summoning 'a second angel ... to turn over the Audit Books of Transgressions'. Dekker argued that the reason for the visitation was because 'we were too bad for them [Elizabeth and James] and were therefore then, at the decease of one, and now of the other ... deservedly punished'.[46]

Nehemiah Wallington chose a different interpretation, and continued to gather evidence in support of it. He saw signs of a deeper malaise, of transgressions not against monarchs, but against godly principles. Thus a hundred died in a house collapse in Blackfriars because they had gathered to hear Mr Drury, 'a Jesuit'. 'It was on the Lord's day,' Wallington grimly noted. A young man had fallen from a ship's mast and smashed his skull open because he and a friend had chosen to board the ship and play in the rigging on the Sabbath.[47] A house in Honey Lane burned down after a maid carelessly lit a candle because the family had been 'gadding forth' on the Sabbath.[48] A carter returning home late one night to the appropriately named Pickled Herring in Southwark had accidentally set light to fifty houses and seven horses because of the 'filthy swinish sin of drunkenness'. Wallington saw for himself a terrible blaze break out on London Bridge, 'vaunting itself over the tops of houses like a captain flourishing and displaying his banner'. It was a judgment on the city's sins, 'which are now grown to their height: as idolatry, superstition, woeful profaning of the names, titles, attributes, creatures, and of God himself, with the perfect language of hellish swearers in every child's mouth, whoredoms, adulteries' . . . he could not stop . . . 'fornication, murders, oppressions, drunkenness, cozening, lying, slandering, mocking, flouting, chiding, silencing and stopping the mouths of God's prophets and servants, and other gross secret sins'. But he also saw the failure of the fire to spread as evidence of God's mercy, noting that 'there was but little wind, for had the wind been as high as it was a week before, I think it would have endangered most of the City, for in Thames Street there is much pitch, tar, rosin, and oil in their houses'. 'We must as well look from what we have been delivered, as what we have endured, that our thankfulness may moderate our sorrows, and our joy in one may temper our griefs for the other.'[49] This was, to use the terminology of the time, a rare display of a more sanguine side to Wallington's otherwise melancholic complexion. His wife would have been proud of him.

One report was particularly disturbing. In 1628, a letter was sent by one John Hoskins of Wantage in Berkshire to a relative, Mr Dawson, a gunsmith in the Minories, near Aldgate. Dawson was a Puritan and circulated the letter among the brethren, including Wallington. 'The cause of my writing to you at this time is by reason of an accident that the Lord sent among us,' Hoskins had written. 'On Wednesday before Easter, being the ninth of April, about six of the clock, in the afternoon, there was such a noise in the air, and after such a strange manner, as the oldest man alive never heard the like. And it began as followeth: First, as it were, one piece of ordnance went off alone. Then after that, a little distance, two more, and then they went as thick as ever I heard a volley of shot in all my life; and after that, as if it were the sound of a drum, to the amazement of me, your mother, and a hundred more besides.' This spectral battle Hoskins took to be a warning of war. 'Let the Atheist ... stand amazed at this work of the Lord. But let it be to us, as Jonathan's arrows were to David, a warning to flee from the wrath to come.' 'The sword,' Wallington noted, 'is coming.'[50]

William Harvey stood upon 'a rugged and dangerous Clift' on Bass Rock, a barren island in the Firth of Forth, Scotland. Overhead, clouds of flocking birds swirled so thick that, he wrote, 'they darken and obscure the day'. Beneath, upon black rocks glazed white with bird excrement, perched multitudes more – none, he noted, 'Citizens of the place, but Foreigners all', who would disappear when their eggs were laid and their young hatched. Looking down upon the sea, 'as from a steep Tower', he saw it 'all spread over with several sort of fowl, swimming to and fro, in pursuit of their Prey, just at the rate as some ditches and lakes in the Spring time are paved with Frogs; and open Hills, and steep mountains, are stuck and embossed with flocks of sheep and Goats'.

Harvey's attention was particularly caught by the egg of the guillemot. It was laid upon the 'steep point of a sharp stone', with neither nest nor mother to protect it. Intrigued as to how such a delicate object could survive in so exposed a position, he picked it off, to discover that it was attached by a form of cement. Once removed from its station, 'no art nor cunning in the world can fasten it again, but it instantly falleth into the sea, as from a precipice, without redemption'.[51]

It was 1633, and Harvey had come to the island as a break from accompanying Charles I. The King was making his first visit to the country of his birth since departing in 1604, coming for his very belated coronation as King of the Scots. Harvey was now in constant attendance on Charles, having in December 1630 been promoted to the regular staff position of 'Physician-in-Ordinary' (most of the King's doctors were 'Physicians Extraordinary', which was more an honorific than a job title, indicating that they had served the King in a medical capacity and allowing them to advertise the fact to potential clients). To devote himself to his royal work, Harvey had announced that he must reduce his commitments at the College of Physicians (which had made him treasurer in 1628), marking the occasion in the traditional manner by throwing a sumptuous feast for the Fellows. He had also curtailed his duties as hospital physician at St Bartholomew's Hospital. This provoked protests from the staff, particularly the hard-pressed surgeons, and forced the hospital governors to appoint a deputy, though they hastened to reassure their royally endorsed employee that they did so without 'prejudice [to] Dr Harvey in his yearly fee'.[52]

For the trip to Scotland, Harvey had been put in charge of a medical retinue comprising two physicians (the other being Dr Beton, who had also been alongside Harvey during James I's final illness), three surgeons, a barber, eight servants, and as many horses. Their role was to support a large and lavish royal progress, and deal with any medical emergencies that arose along the way, such as the Lord High Treasurer's 'fit of the stone, not without some aguish Distemper', which overcame his lordship near Doncaster.[53]

The Scottish coronation came at a difficult time for Charles. In England, he had called and dissolved a succession of parliaments, all of which had impudently voted him inadequate subsidies entangled with long strings: demands for changes in his religious policies, protests about royal monopolies, and impeachments of his favourites. The latest target had been the Duke of Buckingham's chaplain, Roger Maynwaring, who, in a sermon published by order of Charles himself, had argued that Parliament should vote the King all the taxes he wanted because 'to Kings . . . nothing can be denied (without manifest and sinful Law and Conscience) that may answer their Royal state and Excellency: that may further the supply of their Urgent Necessities: that may be for the security of their Royal persons (whose lives are worth millions of others)'.[54]

By the spring of 1629, Charles had lost patience and published a proclamation. Proclamations were a favourite device for venting royal displeasure, appearing on an almost weekly basis and covering subjects such as 'the restraint of killing, dressing and eating flesh in Lent or on fish days', 'the speedy sending away of Irish beggars', and 'the making of Starch'. The 'proclamation for [the] suppressing of false rumours touching Parliament' was on weightier matters. The King, it announced, had proved his 'love to the use of Parliaments; yet the late abuse, having for the present driven us unwillingly out of that course, we shall account it presumption, for any to prescribe any time unto us for Parliaments, the Calling, Continuing, and Dissolving of which is always in our own power, and we shall be more inclinable to meet in Parliament again, when our People shall see more clearly into Our Intents and Actions'.[55] He would not become inclinable for another eleven years, the period that became known as 'Personal Rule'. To make up for the shortfall of tax revenues, Charles had to implement all sorts of fiscal novelties, unpopular if not always swingeing, such as a fine of between £10 and £70 levied on all landowners with an income greater than £40 per year who were not knighted (the ingenious logic being that in feudal times landowners were supposed to pledge military service by presenting themselves at the time of the King's coronation to be knighted, those who failed to do so paying a fine to compensate).

In many respects, Charles faced the same problems in his neglected northern kingdom as in England, only worse. His rule had been marked by what one historian has described as 'clumsy authoritarianism'. One of his first acts was to introduce an 'act of revocation', an instrument originally designed to protect the property of royal minors vulnerable to having their lands seized by unscrupulous regents. Since Charles had succeeded to the Scottish throne as an adult (the first to do so since Robert III in 1390), the act was widely seen as an attempt, not to protect his own lands, but to get his hands on those of the Scots nobles.[56] Having thus unnerved the nobility, he had upset much of the remainder of the population with his religious policies. The Scottish Kirk was predominantly Presbyterian, governed by 'sessions' or councils of elders and ministers rather than royally-appointed bishops, the model many Puritans wanted adopted in England. This made the Kirk virtually independent of the Scottish monarchy, and an often vocal critic of its religious policies. The Church of England, by contrast, was under direct royal control, as Charles's father James discovered to his delight when he inherited the English throne in 1603. So James had set about trying to anglicize the Kirk, a policy Charles had intensified by appointing bishops to his Scottish Privy Council and giving them a level of influence over the country's secular as well as religious affairs not seen since Catholic times.

Thus, when Charles and his huge retinue rolled into Edinburgh for his coronation, five years and several postponements after it had first been announced, he was greeted by nervous subjects in need of reassurance.

They were not to get it. The coronation ceremony was conducted according to Anglican rites, the King surrounded by bishops extravagantly attired in blue and gold. If that were not enough to demonstrate Charles's religious intentions, the following day he invoked another royal rite designed to show his spiritual supremacy, one that would have directly involved Harvey: the laying on of the Royal Touch.

There was an ancient belief that the touch of a monarch would cure a disease known as the King's Evil (scrofula, an infection of the lymph glands that causes a painful and disfiguring swelling of the neck). Monarchs had practised the Royal Touch since at least the reign of Henry II, but it had fallen out of use. Then Elizabeth revived it, partly to show that, despite excommunication from the Roman Catholic Church by the Pope, her rule was still divinely endorsed.

The ritual developed by Elizabeth involved royal physicians and surgeons picking a hundred or so diseased and desperate paupers to be presented to the monarch. As prayers were recited she would 'lay her hands on each side of them that are . . . diseased with the evil, on the jaws, or the throat, of the affected part, and touches the sore places with her bare hands, and forthwith heals them'. They were then given a specially-minted angel, a gold coin worth ten shillings, which hung from a ribbon placed around their neck.[57]

James continued the tradition, anxious to demonstrate his divine election. 'Kings are justly called Gods,' he had told the English Parliament in 1609, 'for that they exercise a manner or resemblance of divine power on earth.' The Royal Touch was a demonstration of this.[58] Charles was keener still, perhaps because he felt he had more to prove, perhaps because of the influence of his wife Henrietta Maria, who would have seen the rite performed regularly at the French court. He commanded the minting of a new series of 'healing angels', bearing the unconsciously ominous legend 'The Love of his People is the King's safeguard'. Charles's angels were made of silver – ''twas not a golden age for him', as one contemporary noted.[59]

Charles's healing angels may have been less precious than those of his father, but as the number that survive shows, he doled out plenty of them. In a proclamation 'for the better ordering of those who repair to the Court for their cure of the disease called the King's Evil', he boasted that his 'sacred touch and invocation . . . hath had good success', so much so that he would have to limit access to Easter and Michaelmas and to those carrying certificates of proof that they had not received the Royal Touch before.[60]

Thus on 24 June 1633 one hundred scrofulous Scots were duly lined up in the great hall at Holyrood, the royal palace in Edinburgh. Charles did not perform the ritual as Elizabeth had done. Following a practice first introduced by his father, it appears he laid a hand upon the victim, but not upon the diseased part of the body. The order of prayer for the ceremony specifies only that the monarch 'shall lay their hand on the sick, and they shall recover'.

Not all sufferers recovered as commanded, of course, but it was considered their fault, not the King's. 'Some think, that if they have but a Touch from the King, they are presently made whole,' wrote the physician and College Fellow Thomas Allen. But it depended on the attitude of the sufferer. 'Indifferency' or mendacity would 'mar the Success', as Allen put it. Nevertheless, with Harvey there to select cases that were moderate enough to be amenable to the royal cure, a high rate of success could probably be assured.

It is hard to tell if Harvey believed such a supernatural rite had real medical benefits. On the issue of magic in general he appears to have been a sceptic. Soon after the Scottish coronation, he and the surgeon Alexander Read had, on the King's orders, inspected four women accused of witchcraft. He found during a 'diligent' examination of one, conducted in the presence of several midwives, 'two things [that] may be called teats, the one between her secrets and the fundament on the edge thereof, the other on the middle of her left buttock'. Witches were believed to have a callus on their bodies with which they would suckle their demonic accomplice or 'familiar', which traditionally took the form of a black cat. However, having found such suspect features, Harvey argued that one was likely to be scarring left by 'piles or application of leeches', the other a skin blemish, as there was no 'hollowness or issue for any blood or juice to come from thence'. The women were later pardoned.

At St Bart's, Harvey had seen a number of similar cases. In at least one, he diagnosed, not demonic possession, but a 'strange Distemper ... chiefly Uterine' – hysteria, in other words, 'and curable only by Hymeneal Exercises', sexual intercourse. He evidently did not discount supernatural explanations for such puzzling medical phenomena but preferred natural ones, and this attitude may have extended to his attitude to the Royal Touch.[61]

While the King was in Scotland, an event was proposed in London to greet his return. An ambitious young lawyer, Bulstrode Whitelocke, son of a judge, suggested that the legal profession lay on a welcome of such spectacular sycophancy as would befit a monarch now crowned in two kingdoms. He proposed a masque, a favourite royal entertainment which would be, Whitelocke wrote in his diary, 'very well taken by their Majesties, & held the more seasonable in shewing [the lawyers'] difference of opinion from Mr Prynne's new book of Histriomastickes against interludes'.[62]

The book to which he referred – *Histriomastix: The Players Scourge, or, Actors tragoedie* by the Puritan pamphleteer and fellow lawyer William Prynne – had just been published. It was an attack on theatres as dens of immorality, and included in its table of contents an entry which read: 'Women actors notorious whores'. Since Queen Henrietta Maria was an enthusiastic participant in masques, the thought was planted in her head by the Bishop of London and Puritan scourge William Laud that Prynne was referring to her. For this libel, Prynne was sentenced to be fined £5,000, expelled from Lincoln's Inn (depriving him of his living as a lawyer), locked in a pillory, imprisoned for life and have his ears lopped.

A lavish pageant of the sort the Puritanical Prynne had condemned would demonstrate the lawyers' loyalty to the monarchy. So a committee was formed to organize it. Inigo Jones, the greatest architect of the age, was appointed to design the scenery and costumes, the popular playwright James Shirley was hired to write a drama entitled 'The triumph of peace', and Whitelocke engineered to take 'whole care & charge' of the music. He busied himself appointing masters and players, including four members of the Queen's Chapel 'the more to please her Majesty', and invited them all to his house in Salisbury Court, off Fleet Street, to practise. There he listened with satisfaction to '40 lutes, besides other instruments & voices, in consort together', performing music of his own composition, including a piece he had entitled 'Whitelocke's Coranto', which he claimed was later 'played by all the musicians in the Town, & afterwards all England'.

The date for the event was set for the evening of 2 February 1634 – a further provocation to Prynne and the Puritans, as it was Candlemas, a Catholic feast day celebrating the purification of the Virgin Mary. The venue was the Banqueting House in Whitehall, the spectacular venue for state receptions designed by Inigo Jones. It would provide a setting fit for a king to receive his faithful subjects – and, fifteen years later, his executioner.

A spat broke out between Whitelocke and Sir Henry Vane, the royal controller, over precedence. Sir Henry, who had a 'scornful, slighting way of expressing himself', considered lawyers too lowly to be given a viewing gallery of their own in the Banqueting House. This provoked Whitelocke to deliver a lecture on the dignity of his profession and the honour due the Inns of Court, the legal world's equivalent of the College of Physicians. It took the intervention of the Lord Chamberlain, the Earl of Pembroke, to settle the dispute, with Whitelocke apparently the beneficiary.

Harvey returned with the King from Scotland in the autumn of 1633, and attended Comitia meetings at the College in October and December, the latter to discuss the selling of 'purging ales' in taverns, which were suspected of violating the physicians' prescribing monopoly. He was in London the following February, endorsing for one of his patients a licence to eat meat during Lent (in one of his proclamations Charles had prohibited the consumption of animal foods during Lent, except on grounds of illness, which required a note from the doctor).[63] On the third of that month, Whitelocke's masque was held before the King, Queen and members of their household.

The royal party watched through the windows of the Banqueting Hall overlooking the wide boulevard of Whitehall, running from Charing Cross to the Holbein Gate, Henry VIII's magnificent portico to Whitehall Palace. The first sign that the procession had begun was the shimmer of hundreds of torches approaching. They illuminated the way for four great chariots driven abreast, 'after the manner of the Roman Tryumphant chariots', bedecked in silver and 'several colours', drawn by horses carrying 'great plumes on their heads and buttocks', attended by a train of coachmen and assorted lackeys. Each chariot carried four leading lawyers selected from one of the Inns of Court to be the 'Grand Masquers'. They bounced up and down upon seats set in 'an Ovall forme to prevent questions about precedence', bedecked in 'very rich' fancy dress.

In the wake of this great cavalcade, announced by whistles and pipes, clanking tongs and keys, followed the 'antimasquers'. There was a tradition in royal pageantry of representing the dark side of civic life to throw the glitter of regal authority into more brilliant relief. It also provided an opportunity to satirize, even criticize the current regime, though in a manner so heavily disguised as to avoid causing offence to the royal audience.

Thus the King was presented with a great procession of beggars and cripples, mounted on emaciated old nags borrowed from rag and bone men. This obvious reference to the poverty suffered by so many of his subjects would not have upset Charles, as it could easily be interpreted as a pious reminder of his charitable obligations rather than an attack on his policies. But thereafter, the issues became more sensitive, and the symbolism more obscure. Boys danced by dressed as birds fluttering around a great owl in an ivy bush. A man appeared wearing a horse's bridle and biting on an oversized bit, another holding a chicken in his hand and with carrots sprouting from his head. References to oppressive monopolies, perhaps, or overbearing royal privileges?

Whatever the meaning of these strange burlesques, they delighted the King, and he sent the Marshal of the Horse outside to command the cavalcade to loop round the tiltyard opposite the Banqueting House and return, 'that they might have a double view of the show'.

Once the parade had come to an end, the masquers dismounted, and entered the Banqueting Hall 'so crowded with Lords Ladies & gentlemen all richly clothed, & the Ladies glistering with rich garments & richer Jewe[l]s, & the room so full, that they scarce left room for the King and Queen'. With the masquers settled in the gallery so reluctantly reserved for them by the King's controller, Whitelocke now presented the royal entourage, and sat with the Privy Councillors as the masque itself began. Entitled *Triumph of Peace*, it comprised a series of dances, mimes, songs and recitations, with the antimasquers occasionally erupting into the action, poking fun at the Puritans.

The entire show, which Whitelocke later estimated cost around £20,000, 'was incomparably performed, & the Queen did the honour to some of the Masquers to dance with them'. The revelries continued into the early morning, when the King and Queen retired, and the lawyers and players 'were brought to a great banquet, after which they all dispersed'. So a great day came to a close, '& thus this worldly pomp & glory, if not vanity[,] was soon gone & past over as if it had never been'.

Queen Henrietta Maria was not prepared to let it go quite so easily. Concerned that its anti-Puritan message be heard by as wide an audience as possible, she ordered the masque to be restaged at the Merchant Tailors' Hall, in the heart of the City. This, she thought, was where a witty royalist rejoinder to Prynne's impertinence might have its most useful effect, among London's citizenry, 'especially the younger sort of them'.[64]

One of those 'younger sort' was a new arrival from the country, approaching eighteen years, with £50 in his pocket and a future in the balance: Nicholas Culpeper.

BALM

Melissa officinalis

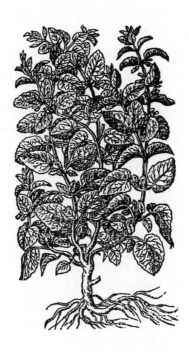

The Arabian Physicians have extolled the Virtues hereof to the Skies, although the Greeks thought it not worth mentioning. Serapio saith, It causeth the Mind and Heart to become merry, and reviveth the Heart fainting into foundlings, especially of such who are over taken in their sleep, and driveth away all troublesome cares and thoughts out of the mind arising from Melancholy, or black Choler; which Avicenna also confirmeth.

It is very good to help Digestion, and open Obstructions

of the Brain; and hath so much purging quality in it (saith Avicenna) as to expel those Melancholy vapours from the Spirits & Blood which are in the Heart and Arteries although it cannot do so in other parts of the Body.

A Tansy [omelette] or Caudle [hot drink] made with Eggs and the Juice thereof while it is young, putting to it some Sugar and Rosewater is good for Women in Childbed when the After-birth is not thoroughly avoided, and for their faintings upon, or after their sore travel. The Herb bruised and boiled in a little Wine and Oil and laid warm on a Boil, will ripen and break it.

The Leaves also with a little Nitre [saltpetre] taken in Drink helps the griping pains of the Belly and being made into an Electuary is good for them that cannot fetch their breath: Used with Salt it takes away Wens [warts], Kernels, or hard Swellings in the Flesh or Throat; it cleanseth foul Sores and easeth pains of the Gout: It is good for the Liver and Spleen.

Let a Syrup made with the Juice of it and Sugar, be kept in every Gentlewoman's house, to relieve the weak stomachs and sick Bodies of their poor sickly Neighbours; as also the Herb kept dry in the House that so with other convenient Simples you may make it into an Electuary with Honey according as the Disease is.

Balm 'cheers the heart, refresheth the mind, takes away grief, sorrow and care, instead of which it produceth joy and mirth', according to Culpeper in his translation of the *Pharmacopoeia Londinensis*.[1] Its name is a contraction of 'balsam', an aromatic oil. This refers to its sweet, restorative smell, which is why the term has since become the general expression for any 'healing, soothing, or softly restorative, agency or influence'.[2]

he young man we find wandering the fringes of London's great political pageant was a striking individual, 'somewhat of spare lean body ... eyes quick and piercing ... full of agility, very active and nimble'. He was described by his friends as being of 'choleric-melancholic' temperament, which meant that choler and melancholy predominated in his makeup, and shaped both his appearance and character. According Nicholas himself, such people were 'by natural inclination ... quick Witted, excellent Students' who will 'begin many businesses ere they finish one'. 'They are bold, furious, quarrelsome, something fraudulent, prodigal and eloquent ... and dream of falling from high places.' In many ways, he could have been (and possibly was) writing of himself, though as a self-portrait, the description understates his capacity for irreverence and fun: 'He was an excellent companion, and for the most part of a merry temper', wrote a friend, a good drinking companion who preferred taverns to palaces, as critics and friends alike acknowledged. With 'things of most serious concernment, he would mingle matters of Levity, and extremely please himself in so doing'.[3]

Now, however, was no time for enjoyment. He had lost a lover, abandoned his vocation and left his home. In those bewildering streets, jostling among the crowds of players, chancers, vagabonds and hawkers, Nicholas needed to find a new direction. He found it in an apprenticeship to a craft, under the tutelage of a 'master'.

In literature, the popular imagination, even city by-laws and livery company regulations, a master was expected to act as a surrogate father to his apprentice son. As well as providing food, clothing, shelter, and education, he was also to offer religious instruction and moral guidance, to help country lads like Nicholas find their way in the big city, avoid its temptations, and embrace its opportunities. It was the best substitute for his own brand of Puritanical paternalism that Attersoll could hope for. Nicholas, who had never felt a father's guiding hand upon his shoulder, only his grandfather's stranglehold, may have felt the same way.

The craft chosen was that of an apothecary. It is not known why, but medical and religious careers were considered by many to be parallel occupations. One of the most popular (and eccentric) medical books of the early seventeenth century, *The Anatomy of Melancholy* (1621), was inspired by this theme.[4] Its author, Robert Burton (1577–1640), was a minister based in Oxford who seems to have suffered personally from bouts of the sickness he anatomized. In the late 1590s, a 'Robart Burton', suffering 'much pain [in the] head & much wind & melancholy', paid several visits to the physician and astrologer Simon Foreman, who made regular appearances before the College of Physicians' Censors for unlicensed practice.[5]

Burton considered medicine to be a calling, like the priesthood. Pre-empting the criticism that he was not qualified to write about medical matters, he argued that 'A good Divine is or ought to be a good Physician'. Matters of spiritual and physical health, he maintained, are connected, and melancholy demonstrated this because it was a malady of both body and soul. It went beyond even that: it was a disease of the whole body politic. 'Kingdoms, provinces, and politic bodies are likewise sensible and subject to this disease,' he wrote, and 'tumults, discords, contentions, law-suits . . . excess in apparel, diet, decay of tillage' were its symptoms. Burton argued that the treatment for such a condition was radical political and medical reform, which must include the election of magistrates and free healthcare, with physicians 'to be maintained out of the common treasure, no fees to be given or taken, upon pain of losing their places'.

Wider still, Burton could see the pattern of melancholy in the cosmos. For this reason, he considered astrology to be important to medical understanding. 'Paracelsus is of the opinion, that a physician, without the knowledge of stars, can neither understand the cause, or cure of any disease, either of this, or gout, no not so much as toothache,' he wrote. The reference was to Philippus Aureolus Theophrastus Bombastus von Hohenheim (1493–1541), a Swiss physician and controversialist who adopted the name 'Paracelsus' because he considered himself to be 'above Celsus', the great Roman medical philosopher and forerunner of Galen. While teaching at the University of Basel, he had launched one of the first serious challenges to Galenic authority, publicly burning Galen's works and offering as an alternative an obscure, semi-mystical theory of alchemical and astrological medicine based around the use of 'chemical' (metal and mineral) rather than just herbal remedies. Though slow to take off in England, his work had produced a number of practical improvements, notably in the treatment of new diseases such as syphilis, which was thought to have come from the New World.

Nicholas would later echo some of Burton's revolutionary views almost word for word, and it is certainly possible that he first encountered them in a copy of *The Anatomy of Melancholy* in William Attersoll's library. It was an irresistible title for a young man struggling with his own emotional turmoils, and the utopian, redemptive message to be found in the pages of Burton's book provided a poignant contrast to Attersoll's dead-end predestinarianism.[6]

Nicholas's first step into the world of medicine was through the door of Simon White's shop at Temple Bar. White was an apothecary, and the Society of Apothecaries had arranged for Nicholas to become his apprentice.

In terms of discovering the London of Charles I's reign, Nicholas

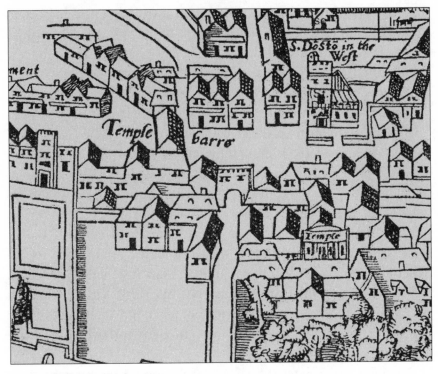

Temple Bar: where Westminster met London.

could not have been better placed. White's front window provided
a proscenium arch through which political pageant, urban development, and social change could be observed. Temple Bar was the
gate marking the western limit of the City of London's jurisdiction.
According to tradition, whenever the monarch entered the City the
royal cortège would come to a halt outside White's shop to be
received by the Lord Mayor. The monarch would then ask permission to enter, and the Lord Mayor would signify his acceptance
by offering his sword – a piece of political theatre that acknowledged
the City's ancient privileges and the sovereign's dependency upon
its wealth.

Temple Bar also marked the border between the old, tightly
packed tenements of Fleet Street and the notorious Fleet Prison to

the east, and the new, airy opulence of the Strand to the west, recently developed as part of Charles I's attempt to refine and 'beautify' his capital. The Strand, which connected the City to Westminster, the seat of Parliament, had once been lined with the palaces of nobles and bishops, many recently parcelled up into apartments for the burgeoning merchant classes. Covent Garden to the north, formerly the gardens of Westminster Abbey, was now being turned by Inigo Jones into a housing estate 'fit for the habitations of Gentlemen and men of ability'. When Nicholas arrived, building work was still underway. A tourist noted 'many good structures cloistered underneath some of them, with a large Piazza'. Next to a maypole a few yards from Simon White's door stood the capital's first hackney carriage rank with cabs waiting to carry curious tourists to Hyde Park, just then opened to the public, or to the menagerie at St James's, where exotic animals imported from the New World could be seen, or to the huge and magnificent new portico of St Paul's Cathedral, one of London's first neoclassical structures, its elegant and rational geometry standing in startling contrast to the cathedral's backdrop of Gothic filigree. These were the landmarks of a flourishing conurbation spanning the Thames, spilling over the city walls, stretching into the countryside, and encompassing, according to one overawed visitor, half a million homes and three million citizens.[7]

Simon White's clientele would have included the merchants and professionals who were making the area their own, people like Gilbert Wright who lived a few doors up from White's shop in the 'Corner House' at the top of Strand Lane. Wright, like his address, straddled the divide between Westminster politics and City commerce. He was a merchant and a senior member of the Company of Salters in the City, and also a civil servant at Westminster, working for Sir John Puckering, Lord Keeper of Privy Seal and Speaker of the House. He died in 1627, and his former footman William Lilly stepped deftly into his shoes, marrying Wright's widow and eventually taking possession of his estate. Lilly, like Nicholas and so many thousands of others, was a migrant from the country, having come to London from Leicestershire in 1620 with 7s. 6d, in his pocket. At around the time of Nicholas's arrival, he was setting up an astrological and medical practice at his old master's corner house, and may well have used White's neighbouring shop for supplies. He would later become bracketed with Nicholas as one of the capital's most prolific political and popular writers.[8]

Competition among apothecaries for clients was tough, and they would attract passing trade by decorating their windows with botanical curiosa and marvels. It was here that many Londoners first saw the exotic fruits of the New World. For example, Thomas Johnson, one of the most successful apothecaries in the capital, had drawn crowds to his shop window in Snow Hill near Newgate with a large bunch of bananas. It had been presented to him by Dr John Argent, President of the College of Physicians, who in turn had received it from a merchant returning from Bermuda. Johnson was at the time working on a new edition of Gerard's famous and massive *Herball* (1597), then the primary English botanical textbook (there were only two others of any note: William Turner's *Newe Herball* of 1551 and Henry Lyte's *Nievve Herbal* of 1578, a translation from the French of a Dutch original). Johnson added a detailed description of these tropical curiosities to Gerard's less exotic selection:

> The length of the stalk was some two foot; the thickness thereof some seven inches about, being crested, and full of a soft pith, so that one might easily with a knife cut it asunder. It was crooked a little, or indented, so that each two or three inches space it put forth a knot of some half inch thickness, and some inch in length, which incompassed it more than half about; and upon each of these joints or knots, in two ranks one above another, grew the fruit ... The fruit which I received was not ripe, but green, each of them was about the bigness of a large Bean; the length of them some five inches, and the breadth some inch and half: they all hang their heads downwards, have rough or uneven ends, and are five cornered; and if you turn

the upper side downward, they somewhat resemble a boat, as you may see by one of them exprest by it self: the husk is as thick as a Bean's, and will easily shell off it: the pulp is white and soft: the stalk whereby it is fastened to the knot is very short, and almost as thick as ones little finger.

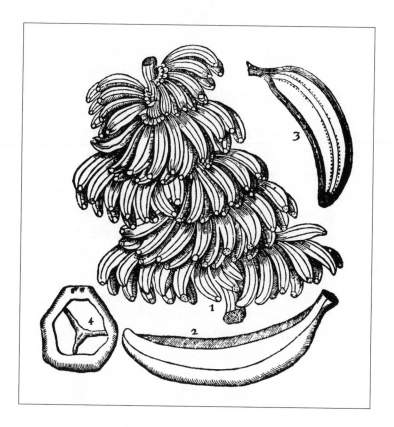

Johnson was so proud of his prize that he hung it in his window for nearly two months, at the end of which the 'very soft and tender' pulp tasted, he decided, of 'Musk-Melon'.[9]

No such marvels would have been found in Mr White's window, perhaps an adder's skin or a fragment of ivory, a pomegranate or a potato. White was in a much lower league than Johnson. He had very little to do with the Society of Apothecaries, never serving on any of its committees, or participating in its functions, and his business was not prospering. His property would not have shared the opulence on display in the Strand, more the meanness of the Fleet Street tenements to the east. In his 1612 survey of London, Ralph Treswell described such a tenement on Fleet Lane, a few hundred yards away, which included an apothecary shop probably similar to White's, built up against the walls of the Fleet Prison. It had a front room 24 feet long and 8 feet deep that would have acted as the shop, and, to the rear, a kitchen/workshop with two ovens next to a tiny triangular yard, no more than ten feet on each side. Tightly packed around were other cramped properties, 'a chamber . . . with the chimney, 15½' x 14½' with a little house of office [lavatory] over the Fleet ditch, in which dwelleth George Priest . . . a chamber adjoining the aforementioned chamber and in a little tenement wherein dwelleth one Thomas Brookes 14' x 9½' with the chimney', and so on, chamber adjoining chamber, tenement upon tenement, garrets heaped above, cellars below, roof-top 'leads' (lead-lined balconies and walkways), and low passages providing access to suffocating inner courtyards. Into such smoky stews Nicholas now found himself immersed.[10]

The life of the humbler apothecaries was not an easy one, particularly at the time of Nicholas's arrival in London. Most were, like White, quite poor, their standard of living similar to craftsmen such as the wood turner Nehemiah Wallington, and precariously linked to the fortunes of the city. In the early 1630s, despite outward extravagances, these fortunes were in decline. The decade had begun with one of the worst harvests in living memory, and its effects were made worse by the deteriorating political situation. The Venetian ambassador wrote home regularly with sombre news of the 'shortness of money, which increases daily', and of the unpopularity of the 'devices and subtleties' invented by Charles's government to raise money without recourse to Parliament. In the medical world, tensions were sharpened by the College of Physicians' jealousy of the Society of Apothecaries' growing self-sufficiency. In 1632, the Society had left its temporary home at the Painters-Stainers' Hall and moved into its own premises, a modest affair built on the site of the old Priory at Blackfriars. Despite the shortage of money, it had also managed to acquire its own seal, charter, book of ordinances, set of gold weights, pewter 'Standish' (inkstand), 'four covered leather stools', twelve green cushions, 'long table carpet', hammer, and hour glass.[11] The physicians shuddered to see a fledgling organization that was supposed to be dependent on them flaunt such trappings.

The College Censors began to roam the streets in vindictive mood. They turned up unannounced at apothecary shops to inspect paperwork and search storerooms and even the apothecaries' private rooms, looking for evidence of illicit trade. In popular culture, the apothecary was often portrayed as a disreputable figure on the edge of criminality, the sort of character Romeo found as he stalked the streets in search of a toxic draught with which to do away with himself:

> Meagre were his looks.
> Sharp misery had worn him to the bones,
> And in his needy shop a tortoise hung,
> An alligator stuffed, and other skins
> Of ill-shaped fishes; and about his shelves
> A beggarly account of empty boxes,
> Green earthen pots, bladders and musty seeds,
> Remnants of packthread, and old cakes of roses
> Were thinly scattered, to make up a show.[12]

Despite all the Society of Apothecaries' airs and fineries, the College Censors were convinced that such figures were still at large throughout the city, and it was determined to root them out. An opportunity arose with a high-profile case that first came to the College's attention in 1632 and culminated at exactly the time Nicholas arrived at White's shop.

On 2 April of that year, Joseph Lane, a prosperous businessman, fell ill with a bout of a recurring stomach complaint. Lane sent his servant Cromwell to the shop of the apothecary Christopher Matthewes for a purgative, a potion designed to cleanse the body of poisons by provoking the evacuation of the bowels. Matthewes made up a medicine previously prescribed by Lane's physician, Dr Leonard Poe, who had died the year before. The treatment did not work, and a week later another doctor was called, a 'Dr Gifford' (perhaps John Giffard, the College treasurer). Gifford found Lane vomiting frequently, 'his mouth black, especially on the right side and about his gums'. The doctor wrote out a prescription for a large pill or 'bolus' containing laudanum, the opium-based medicine commonly prescribed for stomach complaints. He departed just before Lane's father-in-law, Francis Banister, arrived from Bedford to help care for his ailing son-in-law. Finding the prescription left by Gifford, Banister gave it to Cromwell to take immediately to Matthewes.

Banister apparently possessed some medical expertise, and noted that the bolus Cromwell brought back was unusually large. Furthermore, the tamper-proof 'gilding' applied to the outside of the pill was damaged. His suspicions aroused, Banister tasted the bolus and found it 'sharp; offending his tongue'. He sent Cromwell back to Matthewes's shop to get another, but kept the first. The following morning, Dr Gifford was summoned, and Banister shared with the doctor his suspicions that Lane had the symptoms of mercury poisoning, 'for his evacuations are bloody, his torsions [twisting of the body] great, his mouth black; exulcerated, stinking and withal he had Convulsions'. Lane expired soon afterwards.

Lane had friends in high places, and suspected enemies in lower ones. Perhaps on the instigation of Banister, the servant Cromwell was arrested for poisoning his master. A preliminary investigation of the bolus with the tampered gilding retained by Banister revealed that it contained a white powder, possibly the toxic preparation mercury sublimate. It was then discovered that Cromwell had bought a quantity of the substance from the shop of a Mrs Bacon.

On 28 May 1632, an already serious case escalated to a new level with the intervention of the King himself. At an extraordinary meeting at Amen Corner, President John Argent read out a letter from Charles at Greenwich asking the College to investigate the case. The royal interest sent the physicians into a frenzy of activity. Two Fellows were swiftly deputed to perform an autopsy. Watched by two other physicians and four surgeons, they found some 'inflammation and mortification' in the body, but no indication of poisoning, by mercury or any other substance.

There followed a fierce debate at the College, after which the President forced a series of votes. Four senior Fellows abstained, but eighteen, including William Harvey, supported the conclusion that Lane had died of mercury poisoning. The possibility of death by natural causes was not discussed, nor was the fact that the bolus apparently poisoned with mercury had never been consumed by the victim.

The report, written in Latin and presented to the King by the College President at Greenwich on 1 June 1632, was to prove fatal, not just for Cromwell, who faced execution, but also for the College's relationship with the apothecaries. The physicians insisted that, in the light of this case, the sale of eight toxic substances stocked by apothecaries should henceforth be controlled by the College: arsenic, orpiment (a bright yellow mineral, containing arsenic), mercury sublimate and precipitate (two forms of refined mercury), opium, colocynth (derived from a melon-like plant also called bitter apple, native to Turkey), scammony (derived from a type of bindweed, found in the Middle East), and hellebore (an English herb, used with poison-tipped arrows and daggers).

William Harvey was chosen to go to the Privy Council in person to reinforce the call for tighter regulation. No apothecary should be allowed to make any medicine without a 'living Doctor's bill', he said. Furthermore, they should take an oath to make only those medicines set out in the official *Pharmacopoeia Londinensis* (to prevent them selling compounds of their own), which should be sold for prices fixed by the College. While he was there, Harvey also set about the surgeons, whom the College wanted to be prevented from performing a 'trepan' (drilling through the skull) or any other operation without first consulting a physician.

It was a devastating attack, and provoked a furious response from the Society of Apothecaries targeted directly at Harvey. Leaving the prescription of medicines to the sole discretion of the doctors could cause 'much harm', the apothecaries argued, citing as evidence the experience of Richard Glover, the apothecary at St Bartholomew's Hospital. He claimed to have made up a prescription for colocynth, one of the poisons listed by the College, under the direction of the hospital physician (i.e. Harvey) that had led to a patient's death. Colocynth is a 'drastic hydragogue cathartic', the most powerful form of purgative, which provokes the evacuation not just of stools but of fluids through the bowel. It was used as a medicine, but only in tiny quantities, usually no more than five grains (a few hundredths of an ounce). Glover and his apprentice, Nathaniel Ridd, claimed that the prescription or 'bill' drawn up by the 'Rational physician' – they dared not identify Harvey by name – contained a dram (sixty grains, an eighth of an ounce) of colocynth mixed in with four ounces of wine. This was a hefty dose, half a fatal dose for a healthy individual.[13]

The protection of his royal appointment meant Harvey was not seriously threatened by such a charge. Nevertheless, it unnerved the College. At the following 'Ordinarius Maius Collegium', the main meeting of Fellows, held in June 1633, a mood of paranoia prevailed. The apothecaries were said to 'consult daily, how they may wrong or cross the Physicians'. It was suggested that the physicians should secrete a substance in every medicine they prescribed so that they could identify preparations that had not been made under their authority, as well as draw up a blacklist of apothecaries who refused to be 'conformable to the College'.

The matter continued to be debated at College meetings throughout the winter and spring of 1633–4. Example after example of indiscipline was cited in a rising tone of outrage: the sale of tainted drugs, the displays of insolence, the failure to dress properly. And it was not just the apothecaries. The whole city seemed to be disrespecting the doctors. A long-running dispute with the City aldermen over the College's right to attach a 'quill' or pipe to the public water supply flared up after plumbers sent by the authorities showed 'incivility' towards the Fellows. The plumbers had 'cut off our cock under pretence to mind their pipes', the President complained, 'and having cut off our quill, scoff us, willing us to [stop them] when we could'.[14]

Affronted by these constant challenges to their authority, the doctors decided to step up their offensive. They began by summoning the Society of Apothecaries to Amen Corner, where they were to be given a dressing down. The man chosen to do the job was William Harvey, in the hope that his medical reputation and status as royal physician would instil some respect.

On 4 July 1634, Harvey arrived for the meeting carrying the hide of a 'man tanned', which he intended to donate to the College's collection of medical curiosa. This bizarre gift duly presented, he stood before the apothecaries and told them that they needed to attend more closely to their obligations. They must accept 'conformity', and demonstrate 'sufficiency for the well understanding of their art . . . honesty in the right and well preparing of their medicines, and conscience in rating [i.e. pricing] them so that they may not be burdensome to the poor'. Coming from the physician accused of poisoning his patients, who was notorious for conducting his rounds literally on his high horse, in a plush coat, this message was not well received.

Anger turned to fear when the apothecaries discovered that the College, once again drawing on its connections with the royal court, had made an application for the Society's affairs to be investigated by a legal device known as a *Quo Warranto*. This was political colocynth. A *Quo Warranto* (meaning 'By what authority?') gave the Privy Council power to investigate the rights granted to the Society under its charter. Since it was conducted under the royal prerogative, the investigation was virtually unlimited in scope and subject to neither parliamentary nor judicial checks.[15]

To add yet more pressure, in November 1634 the College also petitioned for its grievances to be heard by the Court of the Star Chamber. This was another instrument of the royal prerogative, the cases set before the court being heard by a panel of Privy Councillors rather than a judge and jury.[16] No fewer than thirty-two apothecaries and several apprentices were summoned to appear before the Star Chamber over the coming months. Three were singled out by the College as the leading trouble makers: Thomas Hicks, the Society's Master; Edward Cooke, one of the Society's wardens; and Richard Edwards, a former Master. They were accused of inciting other apothecaries against the College 'by scandalous speeches' and of esteeming 'the worst brother of their Company more than the best of the College'.

The catalogue of complaints put forward by the College against these three was a long one, dating back to the start of Charles's reign. They had, the College's lawyer declared without pausing for breath, 'by oaths, promises, & suits, bound themselves each to [the] other to shake off the government of them & their trade by the said College, & to make their medicines as they please, & to free themselves & other Apothec[aries] from the search & Censure of their Medicines, & from all dependency upon the College, And in execution thereof have ever since the publishing of the phar[maco-poeia] contrary to their oaths & the duty of their profession, & to the said proclamation, made & vended in London & 7 miles thereof several Corrupt unwholesome & adulterated Medicines'.

The College also had more specific grievances: that Hicks had fomented rebellion among the apothecaries by claiming the 'actions of the physicians were against [the] Magna Charta & diverse other statutes'; that Edwards was openly practising physic; that Cooke 'hath pills, called Cook's pills, & a Medicine called Cook's golden

Egg, And Edwards a water called Edward's Cordial Water'. Perhaps the biggest bone of contention concerned one particular medicine, lac sulphuris or milk of sulphur, a form of precipitated sulphur used to treat asthma, coughs, and catarrh. Though it was not one of the permitted medicines listed in the *Pharmacopoeia*, it had become a fashionable treatment in London in the 1630s and doctors were eager to prescribe it: one senior physician told the Star Chamber that it was a 'Magistral medicine'. It was, however, extremely difficult to prepare, requiring 'about a month's time, & the charge and trouble about it is very great', as one apothecary put it. It was also easy to get wrong, particularly if a metal container was used during preparation, as the ingredients, which included powerful acids, would react with the surface of the vessel producing a corrosive medicine with an irritant effect. There was also some terminological confusion among the doctors as to what they were prescribing, with several apparently expecting another form of sulphur altogether. As a result of all these factors, some patients had apparently been harmed by taking the medicine, and, since it was not in the *Pharmacopoeia*, the College had felt it was reasonable to lay the blame for this at the apothecaries' door and to demand that they submit samples to the Censors for examination. But the apothecaries, provoked by Edward Cooke, had refused to cooperate.

For the physicians, this behaviour was an example of a more general issue: the failure of the apothecaries to accept their subordinate status. This attitude was causing serious problems, and was quite at odds with the way their counterparts behaved in Germany, Bohemia, and Italy – countries acknowledged to have superior health systems. The College now called upon William Harvey, who as royal physician had travelled extensively on the King's behalf, to give the evidence to the Star Chamber. According to a record of his testimony, he claimed:

> In all the places where he hath travelled, as at Cologne, Frankfurt, Nuremberg, Vienna, Prague, Venice, Sienna, Florence,

Rome, Naples, the Apothecar[ies] are in reference & dependency
upon the Physicians . . . their numbers limited, their medicines
taxed, & tied to make only such medicines for common sale as
are appointed by the dispensatories of every several place, And
their Medicines searched & corrected by the physicians in all
places.

The apothecaries responded to these complaints with several of
their own. They resented the College's power to examine its own
apprentices. They regarded the College's right both to search their
shops and test their medicines intrusive. They also pointed out that
the physicians were not necessarily well qualified to test medicines.
Many did not know how to make medicines, which several of the
physicians attending the trial reluctantly confirmed. Furthermore,
they pointed out that the physicians themselves prescribed medicines such as lac sulphuris that were not in the *Pharmacopoeia*, and
expected the apothecaries to make them up when there was no
standard procedure for doing so.

As to the issue of the apothecaries' status, Edward Cooke called
witnesses to show that he at least was as important as any doctor.
He made 'as good Medicines as any Apothecary in London', said
one, '& his shop continually furnished therewith. And sells them
in London, into the Country, & to sea, as cheap as any can or doth
do.' Furthermore, he 'hath for 7 or 8 years served the Emperor of
Muscovia [Moscow] & divers of his peers and nobles'. Then, as a
final flourish, he called the physician to the Emperor of Russia
himself, Dr Arthur Dee.

Dr Dee was the son of Elizabeth I's magus, Dr John Dee. He had
appeared several times before the Censors of the College of Physicians for practising without a licence and had been ordered to
stop, even though he had presented to the Censors (as the College
clerk was forced to admit) 'beautifully written letters patent from the
University of Basle' proving that he held a doctorate in medicine.[17]
Despite these rebuffs, in 1627 Charles had himself recommended
Dee to the court of the Emperor of Russia in Moscow, where he

had lived until the death of his wife, returning to England around the time Cooke asked him to act as a witness. Dr Dee's statement to the Star Chamber was brief, confirming Cooke's status as an apothecary of international standing whose medical supplies were used by the Emperor and considered of the highest quality.[18]

The Star Chamber proceedings rumbled on, and became so entangled with the College's other actions against the Society that they appear not to have reached a conclusion. Meanwhile, the inflammation festered, bursting in late 1634 when a delegation of three physicians, dressed in their formal robes, set off for Apothecaries' Hall to examine apprentices. The meeting, attended by at least sixteen leading members of the Society, including Edward Cooke and Thomas Hicks, was the first that the physicians had attended for some time, and the apothecaries resented the intrusion, still more the presence, of Simeon Foxe, an aggressive Censor during the recent hostilities.

When Foxe and his two companions entered the Hall, several officials of the Society sitting at high table rose from their seats to offer them to the new arrivals. But Thomas Hicks, the Society's Master, ordered them to sit down again. Hicks ordered that three stools (perhaps the leather-covered ones listed in the Society's inventory) be brought for the doctors, upon which they were forced to perch as the examinations of the apprentices began. Riled by the humiliation, the doctors challenged the quality of the questions being put by the examiners, whereupon Richard Glover, the apothecary at St Bartholomew's Hospital who had accused Harvey of poisoning a patient, stood up and started to examine Simeon Foxe on his knowledge of medicines. The doctors were outraged. They rose from their stools and, gathering up their robes and remaining dignity, walked out.

As the Society's minutes record, Simon White presented his eighteen-year-old apprentice Nicholas Culpeper to receive his indentures from Master Thomas Hicks and Warden Edward Cooke just a few weeks after the physicians walked out. White may even

have taken Nicholas to Amen Corner. Soon after his visit to Apothecaries' Hall, Foxe had issued an ultimatum demanding that the
apothecaries' apprentices or 'servants' should henceforth be presented at the College, as the Fellows were no longer prepared to
submit themselves to the sort of treatment they had received at the
Apothecaries' Hall. Whether or not this happened, Nicholas would
certainly have been aware of what was going on, for three days
after his induction Hicks and other leading members of the Society
were summoned to the Star Chamber, where the College was presenting its case against the apothecaries to the Lords of the Privy
Council. None of this set a very good example. The induction of
an apprentice was supposed to be about submission, a ceremony
at which he formally accepted being 'bound' to a master and under-
took to abide by the rules set out in royal charters and company
by-laws. But could apprentices be expected to accept such under-
takings with meek humility if their masters could not?[19]

MELANCHOLY THISTLE

Carduus heterophyllus

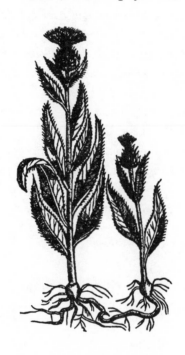

This riseth up with a tender single hoary green Stalk, bearing thereon four or five long hoary green Leaves, dented about the edges, the points whereof are little or nothing prickly, and at the top usually but one Head, yet sometimes from the bosom of the upper most Leaf there shooteth forth another smaller Head, scaly and somewhat prickly; with many reddish Purple Thrums or Threads in the middle, which being gathered fresh will keep the colour a long time, and fadeth not from the Stalk in a long time, while it

perfecteth the Seed, which is of a mean bigness lying in the Down: The Root hath many long Strings fastened to the Head, or upper part, which is blackish and perisheth not.

Their Virtues are but a few, but those not to be despised, for the Decoction of the Thistles in Wine being drunk, expels superfluous Melancholy out of the Body, and make a man as merry as a Cricket. Superfluous Melancholy causeth care, fear, sadness, despair, envy, and many evils more besides, but Religion teacheth to wait upon God's Providence, and cast our care upon Him, who careth for us; what a fine thing were it if men and women could live so? and yet seven year's care and fear makes a man never the wiser, nor a farthing the richer.

Dioscorides saith, the Root born about one doth the like, and removes all diseases of Melancholy. Modern Writers laugh at him, let them laugh that wins, my Opinion is, that 'tis the best Remedy against all Melancholy Diseases that grow, they that please may use it.

This was said to have been the thistle used in the original insignia of the Royal House of Stuart, to which James I and Charles I belonged.

icholas had now accepted a solemn binding to his master. Before the officers of the Society of Apothecaries, he had promised to serve Simon White faithfully, obediently, exclusively, not working for any other, nor marrying, nor becoming betrothed. He had promised to do this for at least seven years, living in his master's house, doing his master's bidding, paying for his own board and lodging. After all this, he could become a 'free man'.

Having undertaken to fulfil these requirements, Nicholas was ready to be initiated into the 'mystery' of the apothecaries' craft. The term was derived from the Latin *ministerium*, meaning employment, and had nothing to do with occult knowledge. Nevertheless, the word's esoteric connotations were particularly appropriate to the arcane, complex, and exotic world Nicholas was about to discover.

To begin with, Nicholas would have begun to uncover this mystery in the back room of Simon White's shop, where the medicines were prepared. The atmosphere was hot, humid, and often noxious. Whorls of steam and smoke rose continuously from a large fire or furnace that was the centrepiece of the room. Surrounding it was an array of equipment: giant brass mortars and iron pestles (the apothecaries' emblem, used for crushing ingredients into pastes and powders); spatulas, slotted spoons, copper pans, galley pots, pipkins (tubs), rasps, presses, a 'refrigatory' (parts of a still, for condensing liquids), sieves made of hair, a smooth porphyry stone with a 'mule' for grinding fine powders, a grooved ruler for making tablets, bains-marie and sand baths for the gentle heating of glass vessels, crucibles for the fierce reduction or 'calcination' of liquids to solid deposits;

ceramic and metal vessels for coagulating (thickening), decocting (boiling), and infusing (soaking) ingredients; piles of blankets, towels and strainers made of wool called 'Hippocrates' Sleeves' for sieving out solids; filters made of brown paper for clarifying and purifying liquids.[1]

There were also scales and cups used to measure weights and volumes. All apothecaries were required to own a set of standard 'Troy' weights and measures, which were to be used in the preparation of all medical recipes. Apprentices had to chant measures like times tables: twenty grains to a scruple, three scruples to a dram, eight drams to an ounce, twelve ounces to a pound. To confuse matters, the Latin names of some measuring vessels were often used as terms for the quantities they held: the cochlearium (which held half an ounce of syrup or three drams of distilled water), the cyathus (an ounce and a half), the hemina or cotyla (nine ounces), the libra (twelve ounces), the sextary (eighteen ounces, about a pint) and the congy (six sextaries, about a gallon).

Beside the weights and measures rested a book, the *Pharmaco- poeia Londinensis*. Nicholas would have seen such large folio volumes with similar lavish leather bindings in his grandfather's study at Isfield and in his college library in Cambridge. Simon White, on the other hand, would have owned nothing else like it, the rest of his library probably consisting of only one or two other books, including perhaps one of the pocket editions of the Bible that had recently come onto the market.

With the exception of the Royal Proclamation ordering all apothecaries to follow the *Pharmacopoeia*, the tome was written entirely in Latin, including the introductory letter addressed to the '*Candido Lectori*', or honest reader. Few of the book's honest readers, however, would have been able to read the text. Though some apothecaries attended grammar school, where basic Latin was taught, very few had gone to university – such levels of education were not expected of craftsmen. Most, therefore, probably referred to the list of ingredients given for the most common recipes and left it at that. Few would find it necessary even to refer to the terse instructions on how the ingredients should be combined, as such information was part of the 'mystery' passed on from master to apprentice. Having gone to university, Nicholas was good at Latin – at least as good as any physician, including William Harvey.[2] Perhaps he was the first to acquaint his new master with the meaning of some of the *Pharmacopoeia*'s more complex passages, such as the section warning of a 'dangerous plague which our book will counteract, namely the very noxious fraud or deceit of those people who are allowed to sell most filthy concoctions, and even mud, under the name and title of medicaments for the sake of profit'.[3]

The title-page of the *Pharmacopoeia* was the literary equivalent of Inigo Jones's portico for St Paul's: a Classical entrance to a Gothic world. It depicted a Classical temple dominated on either side by two statues, one of Hippocrates, the other of Galen, both gesturing towards the title of the book: *Pharmacopoeia Londinensis in qua Medicamenta Antiqua et Nova usitatissima sedulo collecta accuratissime examinata quotidiana experientia confirmata describuntur*. Then came an inscription proclaiming the book to be *Opera Medicorum Collegij Londinensis. Ex Serenissimi Regis Mandato cum R. M. Privilegio* – the work of the College of Physicians of London, published by the royal mandate of his Serene Highness the King.[4]

Inside, following the dedication to '*Serenissimo Principi Iacobo, Magnae Britanniae*' and the introductory letter, there followed a list of 'simples', basic medicinal ingredients – 1,190 of them. Nicholas would already be familiar with several: roots such as levistica (lovage) and rhaphani (radish), barks such as cinnamomum (cinnamon), herbs such as acetosa (sorrel) and solanum (nightshade). But there were also exotic flowers and fruits that a country boy from Sussex was unlikely to have encountered, such as pomegranates, still rare in England and extremely expensive – a few years later, the physician John Ward would be introduced to them by an apothecary who described them as being 'about as big as a good large apple;

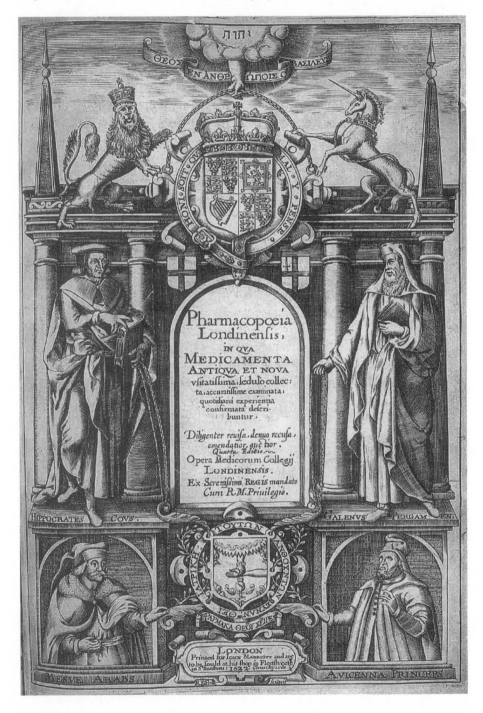

worth from 2 shillings a piece' when they were available, around Christmas time.[5]

As the list progressed, so the ingredients became more outlandish. After a page cataloguing 'tears, liquors and rozins' came a list of animals: capons, crayfish, ants, swallows, 'intestines of the earth' (earthworms), millipedes, frogs, scorpions, snakes, foxes, silkworms, whelks, castrated dogs, young swans, grasshoppers, leeches, badgers, lizards, moles, moths, and 'tenches, the physicians of the fishes', all to be cooked or dried, pounded or sliced, and used as ingredients. Over another page, there was a list of animal parts and 'excrements': '*Cornu Unicorni, Monocerotis, Rhinocerotis Capre*' – horn of unicorn, that of the monoceros (narwhal) or rhinoceros being permitted substitutes; mussel shells; the grease of duck, heron, and ram; the fat of vulture; the suet of cows and badgers; the marrow of cow's shin-bones; the bile of bull, cow, hawk, kite, hog, hare; the milk of goat, ass, sheep, cow, and woman; the excrements (i.e. dungs) of man, wolves, mice, sheep, pigeons, horses, hens, swallows, cows, and dogs. There was unsalted butter, fish glue, bozoar stone (in two varieties: oriental, taken from intestines of the Persian wild goat, and occidental, from Peruvian llamas), musk, civet; '*Mumia Sepulchrorum, Pissaphaltum*' (a mummy taken from a tomb, '*pissaphaltum*', asphalt or pitch, being a substitute), human blood, frog spawn, rooster testicles, beaver glands, wax, crayfish eyes, stag ankles, sparrow brains; human skulls 'containing triangular bone', boar teeth, duck livers, wolf intestines, cheese, the stomach membrane of a hen, sweat, saliva, honey (including 'virgin', i.e. from young bees, white-yellow in colour); bee glue from cracks in hives ... The term 'apothecary' was derived from the Greek for storehouse, and the enormous variety of ingredients they were expected to stock shows why.

Following the simples came the compounds. These were the medicines the physicians prescribed, and it was the apothecaries' job to prepare them. Simple versions of some of them were used in home remedies, but most of the recipes were known only to the medical trade and would have been completely alien to Nicholas. The two compounds the doctors esteemed 'most precious' were Theriac of Mithridates and Alkermes. These were electuaries, syrups, their ingredients crushed into a fine powder and sieved through a 'tiffany searce' into a sweet solution, usually clarified honey. It was the adulteration of these powerful antidotes by 'criminal murders' that the College claimed as the chief reason for producing the *Pharmacopoeia*.

The recipe for *Confectio Alkermes* traced back to the Arabic physician Mesue the Younger (Yuhanna ibn Masawayh, AD 161–243), whose own dispensatory was one of the main sources used by the College. The name of the medicine came from one of its constituents: bright red dried kermes (*quirmis* in Arabic, from which the word crimson is derived). Kermes were then believed to be berries or galls, but were subsequently discovered to be scale insects (*kermes ilicis* – the red dye comes from the spawn of the flightless female, which dangles from the branches of oaks in Mediterranean climes). They gave the electuary a hot flavour, designed to enhance the effect of the other, supposedly therapeutic, ingredients, which included aloe wood, amber, musk, pearls, lapis lazuli, and gold leaf.

Theriac of Mithridates had been the sovereign remedy of the physician's pharmacopoeia since the Middle Ages, its very name coming from that of a king, Mithridates VI of Pontus in Asia Minor (132–63). His Greek physician Cratevas was said to have invented the recipe, which was developed by Damocrates and Andromachus and preserved by Dioscorides, a Greek army doctor who lived in the first century AD and whose *De materia medica* was another of the *Pharmacopoeia*'s principal sources. This Theriac or 'Treacle' opened up a new world to Nicholas, with its fifty ingredients coming from the four corners of the known earth, from the shores of the Levant to the grasslands of the Scottish mountains, and from the vineyards of Malaga to the groves of Cambodia. It contained myrrh, saffron, agrick (fungus, possibly *Polyporus officinalis*), ginger, cinnamon, spikenard (now better known as spignel or baldmoney, a root eaten in Scotland as a vegetable), frankincense, oil of nutmeg, turpentine, juice of *hypocistis styrax calamitis* (the balsamic resin of styrax, a deciduous tree), *cassia lignea* (a tree bark, similar to cinnamon and often used as a substitute), Macedonian parsley seed, the seeds of Cretan carrots, valerian, the bellies of skinks (lizards), the tops of St John's wort, and Malaga wine.

Containing such rare ingredients, authentic Alkermes and Mithridate (there were many cheap alternatives sold under the names) were only prescribed to richer patients, such as the Earl of Huntingdon, whose monthly bill from the apothecary Mr Cowper listed a 'pot' and a 'box' of Mithridate, priced at 2*s*. 3*d*. and 3*s*. 6*d*. respectively, substantial sums for doses that would probably last only a few days.[6] A more common remedy, a staple of most apothecary shops and one apprentices such as Nicholas would be expected to mix up in bulk, was another treacle, Theriac Londinensis, or London Treacle, the antidote so widely used during the 1625 plague.

The origins of the recipe are obscure, though one contemporary source ascribes it to an apothecary in Holborn called Walsh who was still practising when Nicholas became an apprentice.[7] Its ingredients were familiar and readily available: English herbs such as sorrel, peony, basil, angelica, rosemary, and marigold; spices such as nutmeg, mace, and cloves; and powdered deer antler (the only animal-derived ingredient). These were all mixed together and soaked in one part Malaga wine to three parts honey. The main therapeutic ingredient was a dram of opium. Opium was one of the apothecaries' stock items in the mid-seventeenth century, and relatively inexpensive, costing around twelve shillings a pound, the same price as aloes (or Aloe Vera, as the herb is now known), and considerably cheaper than rhubarb.[8]

Despite the popularity of medicines such as London Treacle, the *Pharmacopoeia* gave no hint as to their medicinal qualities. This was to confine the apothecaries to preparing medicines and to prevent them from prescribing them. As a measure, it largely failed. Just as they had overcome the difficulty of reading recipes in Latin by learning the English names parrot-fashion for the ingredients listed, the apothecaries shared enough collective medical lore to know which medicine treated which disease. In the case of London Treacle, it was well known that it helped resist 'pestilence', strengthened the digestion, and acted as an antidote to poisoning – three of the most common perils faced by Londoners, who not only had to contend with the constant threat of plague, but of contaminated water and food.

With his knowledge of Latin, Nicholas was able to study the recipes in the *Pharmacopoeia* closely, and he noticed discrepancies in some of them. For example, the book called for distilled waters to be prepared with fresh ingredients which, in England, could only be obtained dried. There were mixtures of herbs and inorganic materials such as mercury that were impossible to combine, and several herbs were confusingly listed under different names as though they were different ingredients.[9] The *Pharmacopoeia* itself acknowledged that there were deficiencies. In the section on plasters, the formula for *Emplastrum Ceroma seu Ceroneum Nicolai Alexandrini* includes among its ingredients opopanax and galbanum, which 'have been omitted from the list of simples'. 'If this seems inaccurate and defective as to precautions (it is not our intention to blame the antique authors),' the entry continues in Latin, 'it is quite permissible for the ardent seeker for information to consult another and no less scientifically compiled treatise, namely, that of the Parisian pharmacopolist Jean DuBois. Even the most experienced apothecary need not regret to have consulted his illuminating annotations on the compounding of medicaments, published some time ago.' But even the most experienced apothecary was unlikely to be able to consult an unspecified and antiquated volume published in Latin by a French author.[10]

By 1636, two years into his apprenticeship, Nicholas would have learned the basic skills of his craft: the preparation and storing of ingredients, the use of equipment such as the still and bain-marie, the mixing of compounds. He would also have served in the shop, dispensing prescriptions, selling tobacco, even demonstrating or performing simple medical procedures, such as using a quill to blow powdered liquorice into the eye to clear 'pin and web', the general term for a range of eye conditions. He would have fetched physicians' scripts and delivered treacles and troches, and accompanied White on visits, too, attending quietly while the physician made his diagnosis and drew up his prescription.

He may also have followed his master down to East India House in Leadenhall Street or the Royal Exchange at the junction of Threadneedle Street and Cornhill to buy produce from merchants, or to the Thames quayside to barter with spice traders from Aleppo and Constantinople or take tobacco samples from bales freshly shipped in from Virginia. He might also have accompanied his master on one of the Society's regular 'herbarizing' expeditions, when groups of apothecaries would set off to the countryside in the summer months to gather herbs. The veteran apothecary Thomas Johnson describes such a journey departing in two boats from a quay near St Paul's on the morning of 13 July 1629, a merry party bound for Rochester, from where they set off on a tour to sample the botanical treasures, as well as the taverns, of Kent.[11]

Perhaps these were happy years for Nicholas. He was in one of Europe's most exciting cities, learning new skills, meeting new people, with access to as much tobacco as he desired. But there are hints that life bound to Simon White may not have been all that easy. His master may have been abusive – Nicholas later wrote of the 'fear' of being an apprentice. In March of 1635, one of his fellow apprentices, a Thomas Hutchins, son of William of Salisbury 'gent', was 'turned over' – reallocated – to another master, Benedict Medeley. There are a number of reasons why this may have happened, but the most likely is that the master and apprentice had fallen out.

The confirming evidence that White was no good came in late 1636. His business went bust, and he absconded to Ireland with the money Nicholas had paid for his apprenticeship. Nicholas was now homeless, penniless, and, institutionally at least, fatherless once more.

The Society of Apothecaries stepped in to help. On 25 February 1637, Nicholas was turned over to a new master, Francis Drake, so that he could continue his apprenticeship. For a while, it looked as though he had fallen on his feet. Drake was in his early to mid-thirties and in charge of a well-established business in Threadneedle Street he had inherited from his father. He already had an apprentice, Samuel Leadbetter, the son of a Nottingham yeoman, who had been there since 1631.[12] Now in the final years of his apprenticeship, Leadbetter took the newcomer under his wing, inviting Nicholas to move into his lodgings.

Any pretence of paternalism was dropped. Nicholas's relationship with Drake was more as an equal than an apprentice. Drake asked Nicholas to teach him Latin, presumably agreeing to defray the cost of the lessons against the apprenticeship fees that Nicholas could no longer easily afford. However, two years later, Drake died.[13] On 19 February 1639 Nicholas and Leadbetter were turned over yet again, this time to Stephen Higgins. Higgins was a veteran of the Society of Apothecaries, a founder member and former Warden. He was now approaching the end of his career, and may simply have taken on the two apprentices as a formality so that they could serve out their terms. Whatever Higgins did for the two young men, it confirmed Nicholas's dim view of the apprenticeship system and of authority. He later described being an apprentice as 'seven years' care and fear', which 'makes a man never the wiser, nor a farthing the richer'. Following a master did not lead to the promised 'freedom' of enlightenment and security. You had to find your own way.[14]

Nicholas was by no means the only apprentice to feel that he had been failed by his masters. The streets of London thronged with disaffected and disgruntled youth. At the Middlesex Sessions and the Mayor's Court, young men clamoured to have their complaints of abandonment or abuse heard. One complained he had been so severely beaten up by his master, 'he could not go upright, and [spat] blood for a fortnight after'. Another had been taken by his master to a tavern to get drunk, and was then turned over to the sheriff to be imprisoned at Poultry Counter, the ancient, stinking prison next to Grocers' Hall.[15]

The authorities were not sympathetic. They viewed such incidents as the result, not of adult failure, but of youthful degeneracy. Apprentices flaunted the latter in their dress and in the length of their hair. The Court of Aldermen became so concerned it ruled that no apprentices were to be 'freed' (i.e. allowed to complete their apprenticeship) unless their hair was cut in 'a decent and comely manner'.[16] The injunction made little difference. A trainee wood turner called Robert Audley, summoned before the court of the Turners' Company for 'stubbornness and long hair', insolently presented himself with luxurious locks cascading onto a lace collar. A barber was brought to the Hall to cut his hair there and then. His collar was torn from his shirt and replaced by a handkerchief, and he was made to humble himself before his master. An order was subsequently issued demanding the 'decent apparelling of apprentices' and for hair to be 'round cut', presumably using a nicely-turned wooden pudding bowl.[17]

Nicholas later sported cascading tresses of dark hair, complemented by a jaunty moustache, which framed his long face and 'quick and piercing' eyes. He may have adopted the style in his apprentice days, along with his irreverent 'Knack of Jesting', which friends later described as 'inseparable to him', as were his outbursts of 'choler' – irascibility – which would 'macerate him very strangely'.[18]

He was also entering a profession that was linked with some of the murkier aspects of youthful exuberance. A telling incident occurred in September 1631, when the College Censors turned up to search the apothecary shop of one John Buggs. They found quantities of an unauthorized drug identified as 'hypomanes' – a medicine not listed in any known pharmacopoeia, but with a name suggestive of some mood-altering effect.[19] Asked why he had such a medicine in his house, Buggs 'smilingly answered divers young people asked for it divers times', indicating that drug abuse is a problem not confined to modern times.[20]

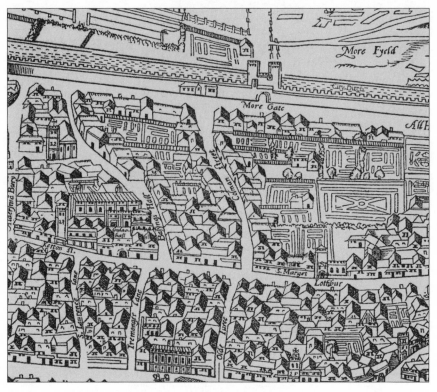

Coleman Street running north/south from Old Jewry ('Old Iuree') to the city wall. St Stephen's church is not shown.

Nicholas may have dabbled in drugs other than tobacco, but it was another dangerous activity that now became the main focus of his youthful exuberance: religious radicalism.

It was probably in the later years of his apprenticeship that Nicholas took, as a critic subsequently put it, 'the several degrees of Independency, Brownism, Anabaptism' by admitting himself to 'John Goodwin's School (of all ungodlinesse) in Coleman-street'.[21]

Coleman Street was a 'fair and large street' in the north of the City, 'on both sides built with divers fair houses' occupied by rich merchants. But, as in so many areas of London, poverty seeped into the opulent cladding of the main street through the alleys and 'small tenements in great number' that led off it. It was also known for its lawlessness, a shortage of constables arousing complaints from the neighbouring parishes of St Olave Jewry and St Margaret Lothbury.[22] At its southern end, it led into Old Jewry, named after the Jews who made the area their home before they were banished from England by Edward I in 1290. St Stephen's, the parish church, had once been a synagogue, before being converted into the chapel of St Olave's Church in Old Jewry and, in 1467–8, made into a parish church. All its monuments were defaced during the Reformation, and its parishioners remained staunchly Protestant, resisting all attempts by the bishops to reintroduce Catholic-style rites and sacraments. In 1590, the parishioners severed ties with the ecclesiastical authorities altogether by buying out the 'advowson', the right to the parish living, which gave them control over the appointment of the minister. In 1623 they asserted that right by ejecting the incumbent, Samuel German, for his 'many abuses in life and doctrine', despite strong opposition from the Bishop of London and the Crown.[23]

The man elected as German's replacement was John Davenport. He had been a curate at the nearby church of St Lawrence and lived in Milk Street, near Cheapside. Around the time of his appointment, an informant in the King's household accused him of being a Puritan, and the Bishop of London was commanded to investigate him for being 'factious and popular'. Davenport protested that, 'if by a puritan is meant one opposite to the present government, I profess ... the contrary'. He had always followed the prescribed liturgy, he claimed, and, far from agitating against the government, sought to 'persuade men to give unto Caesar the things that are Caesar's, and unto God the things that are God's'. Thanks to the support of the wife of a secretary of state, the charges were dropped and Davenport was allowed to take up his post.[24]

He proved to be a popular minister, attracting such crowds that a new gallery had to be built in the church nave to accommodate them. Meanwhile, in the streets, the parish's radicalism was being expressed in more sinister ways. John Lambe was the protégé of the hated royal favourite, the Duke of Buckingham, and had been implicated in the poisoning of James I. Just before the murder of his master in 1628, Lambe had tried to set up in medical practice, and soon came to the attention of the College of Physicians. William Harvey sat on a special Comitia convened on 18 December 1627 to interview the man whose name had been 'on the lips of everyone for some time, due to his knowledge of magic, astrology and other mystic sciences'. In fact Lambe revealed himself as ignorant of astrology as medicine, being forced finally to admit that 'all he did was trifles, fooleries, and babbles to get a little money'.[25] Six months later, while walking along Coleman Street, he was chased by a group of apprentices calling him the 'duke's devil'. He ran down the street into Lothbury, the thoroughfare leading east–west across the City, but was intercepted. The crowd stoned him and dragged his broken body off to the Poultry Counter, where he died. Soon after, a placard appeared in Coleman Street that read: 'Who rules the kingdom? The King. Who rules the King? The Duke. Who rules the Duke? The Devil.'[26]

This sinister graffiti expressed a widespread fear that Charles's court was full of papists bent on returning England to Rome. The man principally identified with this was Buckingham's former chaplain and confidant, William Laud, whom Charles had made Bishop of London in 1628, and Archbishop of Canterbury in 1633. Laud was a theological conservative who firmly believed that the bishops, not worshippers, should rule the Church, just as kings, not subjects, should rule the country. 'They, whoever they be, that would overthrow the *sedes ecclesiae*, the seats of ecclesiastical government,' he told Parliament, 'will not spare (if they ever get power) to have a pluck at the same throne of David. And there is not a man that is for parity, all fellows in the church, [who is] for monarchy in the state.'

Likening those set in authority to 'honest and good' surgeons, Laud called for the 'sinews' of government to be tightened up before they were 'broken or over-strained', resulting in a 'lame Church and a weak state'.[27] It was his job to perform this surgery, conducted in the name of the King – not the 'King in Parliament', the preferred formulation of MPs hoping to show they had a constitutional role in such affairs, but the King as head of the convocation of bishops. For this reason, he did not consider himself accountable to Parliament or any other representative body.[28]

Wielding a terrifying array of episcopal instruments, Laud set about the body of the Church with alacrity, insisting that communion tables set like kitchen furniture in the middle of the nave be replaced by proper altars surrounded by rails at the east end of the nave; that clerics should wear copes and surplices; that congregations should bow to the altar and receive the holy sacrament on their knees – reforms that invoked dark associations of Catholicism in the minds of Puritans.

Laud also instigated a series of high-profile cases against prominent Puritans at the High Commission and the Star Chamber, the two main extrajudicial 'prerogative courts', responsible for enforcing, not laws passed by Parliament, but the powers and privileges that the King exercised under the royal prerogative. These became the setting for a series of notorious show trials, in particular of the lawyer William Prynne, the author of *Histriomastix*, the cleric Henry Burton, and John Bastwick, a physician. In 1634, Bastwick was sentenced by the High Commission to a fine of £1,000, excommunication, and imprisonment for publishing two Latin tracts attacking the English bishops. At Laud's request, Simeon Foxe, the Censor so disrespectfully treated at the Apothecaries' Hall when Nicholas had been inducted, now President of the College of Physicians, backed up the judgment by calling for Bastwick's licence to practise medicine to be revoked, 'taking due notice of his misdemeanours and evil Carriage'.[29] Such eager cooperation showed where the College's sympathies lay on the matter, and put it at odds, not only with the Puritans, with but popular opinion throughout the City.

In 1637, Prynne, Burton, and Bastwick were all brought before the Star Chamber for continuing to produce seditious works and were sentenced to life imprisonment. They were also publicly branded in Westminster Palace Yard before a vast crowd of apprentices and shopkeepers, including Nehemiah Wallington, who watched as the letters 'S.L.' were cut into Prynne's cheeks, standing not for 'seditious libeller', as intended, but, in Wallington's view, for the scars of Laud.[30]

As well as the courts, Laud used spies and informants to monitor religious behaviour, and it was one of these who reported John Davenport in 1631 for administering the sacrament to worshippers while they sat. It marked the beginning of a concerted effort to unseat Davenport, and on 4 August 1633, the day after Laud was made Archbishop, he went into hiding. At a secret meeting of the parishioners, Davenport tendered his resignation and disappeared to Amsterdam.

The parishioners of St Stephen's were not intimidated and replaced Davenport with another radical, John Goodwin. Goodwin was dubbed by his critics the 'great Red Dragon' for his inflammatory views, which were blasted across London twice a week in lectures and twice on Sunday during sermons.[31] His message was visionary. Just as God had revealed the New World of America, there was a new spiritual world to be discovered, he told congregations packed into the pews. He quoted from the Book of Daniel: 'Knowledge shall abound, as the waters cover the face of the Sea.'[32]

Laud soon got to hear of Goodwin's unorthodox views and practices. An ecclesiastical spy called Hicks reported to the Archbishop that, during the 1637 Easter service conducted at St Stephen's, John Goodwin had, like his predecessor Davenport, given 'communion to divers strangers sitting'. Threatened with suspension, Goodwin professed obedience, but within months he was accused of continuing to flout the rules.[33]

The authorities, and some Puritans, became even more alarmed when 'independents', leaders of private religious groups unattached to the Church of England, began to appear in the back-alleys of Coleman Street. Anabaptists (who, believing infant baptism to be a meaningless formality, performed illegal adult baptisms) sprang up in White's Alley, and Millenarians (who believed that the Second Coming was imminent) appeared in Swan Alley. The home of a soap boiler called Thomas Lamb in Bell Alley became known as 'Lamb's Church', 'strange Doctrines being vented there continually'. The house and yard were regularly packed with apprentices and women who were encouraged to vote on who should 'exercise' or preach, those selected being expected to have no particular religious education, simply a fervent desire to spread the word.[34]

As well as 'strange Doctrines', these independents were full of excited talk of escape to a New World, which provides the first, rather convoluted link between Coleman Street and the fledgling religious and medical rebel Nicholas Culpeper. A number of rich merchants in the parish had backed the Massachusetts Bay Company, which received a royal charter to colonize New England in 1629. Several saw this as an opportunity to set up independent churches far beyond the reach of Laud's spies and strictures. In 1637, John Davenport returned from exile in Holland to organize an expedition of Coleman Street parishioners to Boston; they departed early in May and went on to found the colony of New Haven. Two years later Davenport was joined by another exiled nonconformist minister, the Revd Henry Whitfield. Rich, glamorous, with a preaching style possessing a 'marvellous majesty and sanctity', Whitfield had succeeded Nicholas Culpeper's father as rector of the parish of Ockley. Like Culpeper senior, Whitfield's patron was Sir Edward Culpeper of Wakehurst, whose daughter, Elizabeth, was married to Whitfield's brother, the prosperous merchant John. Nicholas Culpeper junior later identified John as both friend and 'kindred', dedicating one of his works to him. Henry Whitfield had been a popular parish minister, but in 1634 he joined the queue of clergymen brought before Laud's High Commission for nonconformity and, by 1638, had been ejected from Ockley.

Catalogue of the severall Sects and
With a briefe Rehear[

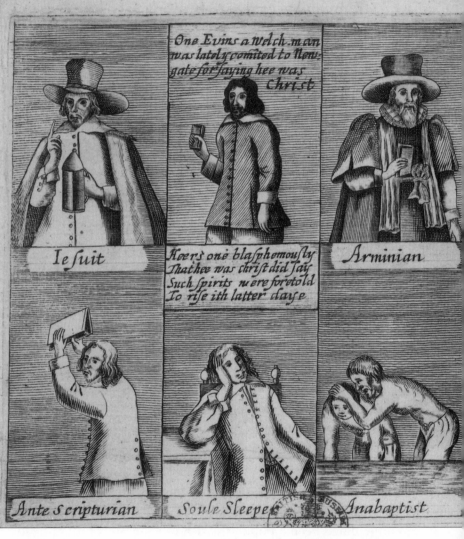

One Evins a welch man
was lately comited to Newgate for saying hee was
                    christ

Ie ſuit

Here's one blasphemouſly
That hee was chriſt did ſay
Such ſpirits n'ere foretold
To riſe ith latter claſe

Arminian

Ante Scripturian

Soule Sleeper

Anabaptist

Catalogue of London's religious sects,

Opinions in England and other Na
ll of their false and dangerous Tenents.

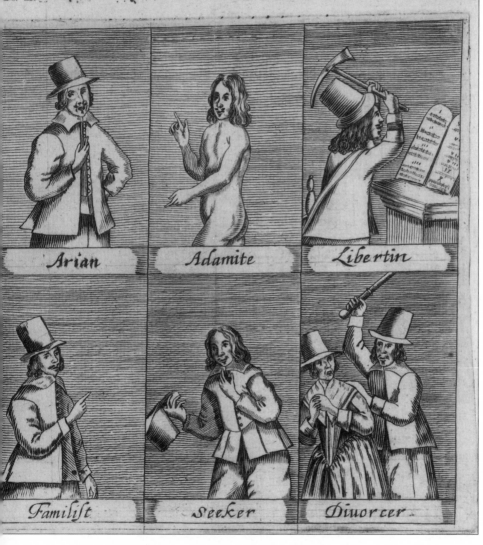

Arian   Adamite   Libertin

Familist   Seeker   Divorcer

s depicted in a pamplet of 1647.

After that he probably came to London and made contact with the Coleman Street Puritans – including, perhaps, Nicholas – and formulated a plan for another expedition to New England. In May 1639, he and around fifty others, including parishioners from Ockley and Coleman Street, together with John Davenport's young son, set off across the Atlantic. They were welcomed by Davenport himself at New Haven, who proclaimed their ship to have been 'guided by God's hand to our town'. Whitfield went on to found Guilford, Connecticut, named after Guildford, the prosperous county town near Ockley.[35]

If he had known about it, Attersoll would have been appalled that Nicholas was keeping the company of such sectaries, adventurers, radicals, and renegades. Worse still was the influence of John Goodwin. Though both could be described as Puritans, Goodwin disagreed with Attersoll on nearly every issue of politics and doctrine. Goodwin argued that no authority was beyond question, not even the champions of religious reform, Luther and Calvin. He was against the idea of strict predestination, that God had already decided who was to be saved, believing instead in the possibility that, through their own actions, even sinners might be redeemed – ironically, a position not dissimilar to his arch-enemy William Laud.

But Goodwin did not just pronounce on matters of theology. He voiced strong – and, to many, shocking – opinions on politics as well. He believed in the separation of Church and State, arguing that no government, whether royal, episcopal, or even Presbyterian, could set a magistrate between a Christian and his God. He challenged people to stand up against the authorities that repressed them: 'You shall break their cord asunder and cast their bands from you for ever,' he promised. Nicholas heard the call. He was to be bound no more.[36]

In 1639, Nicholas's fifty-five-year-old mother Mary discovered a
lump in her breast. Her health had been fragile since her son's
attempted elopement. She was now living in London to be near
him, leaving her father, William Attersoll, in Isfield to dwell on the
failings of his flock and his wayward grandson.

Cancer was then regarded as a matter of surgery rather than
physic, to be treated externally by applying plasters and ointments
or performing operations, rather than internally. Treatments could
be crude. The astrologer William Lilly, uninhibited by his complete
lack of experience or qualifications, once performed a mastectomy
using a pair of household scissors.[37] Mary was to receive less drastic
treatment, administered by the surgeon Dr Alexander Read.

Read was an unusual figure on London's medical scene. He was
one of the group of Scottish doctors who came to England with
James I and had been accepted into the College as a courtesy to the
new king. His views were conventional, his instincts conservative. In
his *Manuall of the Anatomy or Dissection of the Body of Man*, which
first appeared in 1634, more than a decade after Harvey published
his theory concerning the circulation of the blood, he described the
parts of the heart in conventional Galenic terms: the function of
the right ventricle was to 'minister nourishment to the lungs', that
of the left 'to be a store-house of vital blood'. He also dismissed
the novel theories of the 'chemists', in particular Paracelsus. It was
the 'safest course to insist on the foot-steps of the ancient' rather
than the modern, he argued.[38]

Such views were comfortably in line with those of the College;
but Read was never at home in Amen Corner. He was not clubbable,
and provoked grumbles at the Comitia by trying to avoid paying
for the annual College feast when it was his turn. More alarmingly,
he championed surgery – indeed he claimed it to be 'of all the arts
liberal ... the first which was invented' – whereas most of the
Fellows did not even consider it worth studying. In 1634, the Fellows
complained that he had joined the Company of Barber Surgeons
and threatened to throw him out.[39] But whatever the Fellows felt,

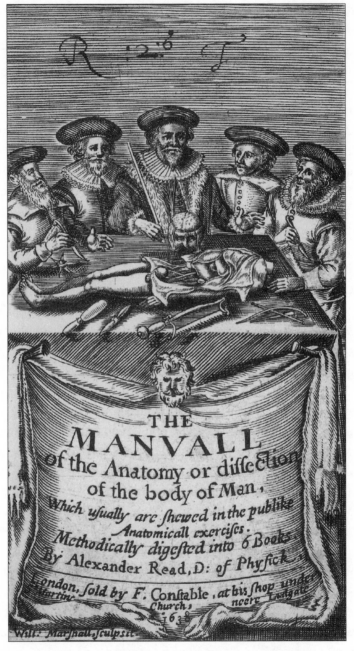

Title-page for Alexander Read's 1638 surgical manual.

Read was popular with his patients. He was also an expert on tumours and ulcers, having given a series of lectures on the subject, which made him well qualified to treat Nicholas's ailing mother.

Cancer was diagnosed when the tumour was hot and surrounded by veins 'full of black humour, which for the likeness, one may call the legs of the crab, as the round Tumour is the crab itself' (cancer being the Latin for crab).[40] It was recognized that the prognosis was poor, and that the range of effective treatments was limited. Queen Elizabeth's surgeon William Clowes, whose work Nicholas knew, wrote that breast cancer 'is hardly or never cured'.[41]

For Nicholas's mother, Read prescribed a powerful cooling, drying medicine: *Unguentum de miniosive rubrum Camphora*, or Ointment of Red Lead. This contained a great deal of lead: red lead (lead oxide), litharge (yellow lead oxide), and ceruss (lead carbonate), together with tutty (flakes of zinc oxide deposited in the flues of furnaces in which brass was melted), all pounded up in a lead mortar. These ingredients were mixed with camphor, wax, and oil of roses into a paste. Nicholas may have prepared the prescription himself at Stephen Higgins's shop, using the recipe in the *Pharmacopoeia Londinensis*. Read applied it to Mary by first rubbing the ointment into a cloth, and then placing it on the tumour. The aim was to reduce the inflammation. But, according to Nicholas, the medicine had no more effect on her breast than if he had rubbed on a 'rotten apple'. The sore broke, and she soon after succumbed.[42]

Perhaps Read's failure to keep Nicholas's mother alive contributed to his dislike of physicians, though elsewhere in his writings Nicholas treated Read with respect. He attended several of his anatomy demonstrations, when 'the doctors and chirurgeons [surgeons] were not high base [i.e. haughty] and denied you admittance'. These lectures, unconnected with the Lumleian lectures conducted by Harvey at the College, were held at the new Barber-Surgeons' Hall near Cripplegate, designed by Inigo Jones and modelled on the anatomy theatre at Padua where Harvey had learned his craft. Read performed public dissections there on Tuesdays and Nicholas saw

a post-mortem of a woman who had died in childbirth and a
dissection of a 'yard' or penis, which prompted him to marvel at
blood vessels 'woven together like a Net'. These lectures provided
the basis of his assessment that Read was a 'good Anatomist'.[43] Read
also endorsed attempts to spread medical knowledge by translating
Latin medical texts into English. His own English-language works
on surgery were advertised in Nicholas's books.[44]

Within a year of Mary's death, William Attersoll died in Isfield,
leaving £400 to his son William junior, who had dutifully fulfilled
his father's expectations and become a member of the clergy, and
forty shillings to Nicholas, who was instructed to collect his inheritance from a bookshop. He put on a brave face. 'This small sum he
received with a smile,' a friend recalled.[45] 'I had once an estate in
this world,' Nicholas wrote in 1650, 'yet can I never say the loss . . .
made me live a sad hour.' Attersoll had written that children should
expect to inherit 'not so much of their Father's Lands and livings,
of their wealth and worship, as of their virtues, goodness, and
godliness'. He had apparently decided that Nicholas's wayward
behaviour had deprived him of both.[46]

Forty shillings would not be enough to pay the fees and living
expenses of two more years of apprenticeship, on top of the £2
(including a silver spoon to the value of 13s. 4d.) required to redeem
his 'freedom' – his right to practise as an apothecary.[47] Nicholas's
decision to abandon his apprenticeship, therefore, was probably
provoked by economic necessity. But it was a move he was ready
to make. Inspired by the example of his friends in Coleman Street,
he had decided to break away from the established institutions and
become an 'independent'.

Having broken his bond, he could no longer live with his friend
Leadbetter, and so he began to look for alternative accommodation.
He also took a wife – Alice Field, the daughter of a wealthy London
merchant, 'a gentlewoman of good extraction', who, 'besides her
richer qualities, her admirable discretion, and excellent breeding
. . . brought him a considerable fortune'. She was also a woman

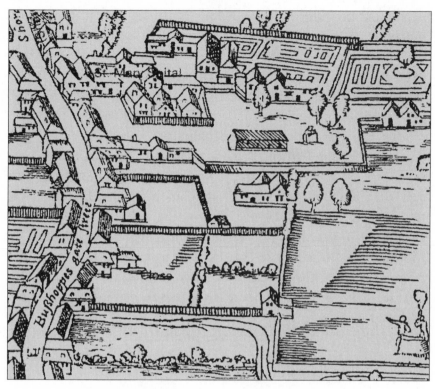

*Nicholas's neighbourhood showing St Mary Spital to the left,
and the Artillery Yard to the right.*

'at her own disposing', as a friend diplomatically put it. In their
subsequent, sometimes troubled marriage, she certainly showed herself to be strong-willed as well as an astute businesswoman, arousing
respect among some of Nicholas's associates for loyally backing her
husband in the face of often violent abuse, as well as criticism from
others for exploiting his name.[48]

Nicholas and Alice set up home outside the city, in the precincts
of St Mary Spital, a former hospital to the north of the city ('Spital'
being the medieval contraction of 'hospital', a place of Christian
charity and hospitality). St Mary's, attached to the Augustinian
priory of St Mary without Bishopsgate, had been one of London's

largest and best known. Founded in 1197 by London merchants, its
ninety or so beds tended to the poor and destitute wandering on
the still wild frontier of the city's suburbs. It also catered for pilgrims
from the north on their way to the shrine of St Thomas à Becket
at Canterbury, and the occasional emergency case, such as a man
pole-axed after he urinated in someone else's shoes.[49]

After the Dissolution of the Monasteries in 1538, St Mary's was
taken over by the Crown. The prior, canons, and sisters were pen-
sioned off, twenty-seven 'fothers' (tons) of roofing lead were
stripped from the dilapidated priory church, and the buildings sold
to a court favourite. In the intervening century, the precincts
became crowded with houses and tenements built out of stone
robbed from the church and bricks made from brick earth excavated
from a field over the eastern wall. It was one of the tenements that
probably became the setting for Nicholas's new home and business,
and it proved to be perfect.

Though no longer operating as a hospital, the area's associations
with healing and charity were still well known to London's citizens.
A play published a few years before Nicholas moved there recalled
how at St Mary Spital:

> . . . all distressed Christians,
> Whose travails this way bends the Hospital,
> Shall free succour be, for three days, and three nights'
> Sojourn, for diet, and lodging, both sweet, and satisfying;
> And if their need be such, as much in Coin,
> As shall for three days more defray their further travail.[50]

St Mary Spital had also been associated with radicalism. From its
famous open pulpit in the old hospital churchyard many an
inflammatory sermon had been preached. One had sparked off the
most violent apprentice riots of the sixteenth century. Nicholas
himself would have been able to overhear one delivered by the
preacher Calybute Downing in 1640, which proclaimed that 'for

defence of religion, and reformation of the church, it was lawful to take up arms against the king'.[51]

Being beyond the city walls, and within the 'liberty' of a former ecclesiastical property, the site was remote, if not immune from the reach of the royal and city authorities, including the College of Physicians and Society of Apothecaries. It was the perfect setting, in other words, for an unlicensed medical practice.

It also offered a few practical benefits for the budding physician, such as a ready supply of herbs. Recent archaeological excavations of St Mary Spital's drains and cesspits recovered seeds for a variety of medicinal plants, such as common mallow (*Malva sylvestris*, infused with fennel and parsley to treat fevers), henbane (*Hyoscyamus nigra*, the leaves of which soothe inflamed eyes and sore joints), hemlock (*Conium maculatum*, used to treat external ailments, including priapism), and vervain (*Verbena officinalis*).[52] Many of these were probably still to be found growing wild around the old hospital, and Nicholas would have had no trouble in identifying them.

Other herbs were within easy reach. At nearby Finsbury Fields, he found a spot 'beyond the windmills' where Star Thistles (*Centaurea colcitrapa*) grew, which he prescribed for fistulas (a kind of ulcer). A little further west, at St Pancras and Paddington, he discovered Burnet (*Sanguisorba officinalis*), one of his favourites, 'the continual use of [which] preserves the body in health, and the spirits in vigour'. Yet further west, at Longford (now subsumed into Heathrow Airport), and to the east at Bow, the heart of modern London's East End, grew wild honeysuckle, which country people called 'meadow trefoil' and used to treat snake bites. A little further north, in Hampstead wood, there were clumps of Tutsan (*Hypericum androsaemum*), a variety of St John's wort used for treating cuts and other wounds. To the south, in Peckham fields, there was Mithridate Mustard (*Thlaspi arvense*, also known as Penny Cress), one of the ingredients for the plague remedy Mithridate. One of the most fertile places was just outside the city walls, at the Inns of Court, where a small pasture was irrigated by leaks from Lamb's Conduit, which brought water from the Fleet River. There, Nicholas picked such choice herbs as Winter Rocket and Saxifrage (*Saxifraga granulata*).[53]

St Mary Spital was also conveniently located for the city. A short walk past the statues of Madness and Melancholy marking the entrance of Bethlehem or 'Bedlam' took him to Bishopsgate and Threadneedle Street. There stood the shop of his old master, Francis Drake, now run by his friend and former fellow apprentice Samuel Leadbetter. In 1640, Leadbetter had completed his apprenticeship and been freed to practise as an apothecary. He had taken over Drake's business and offered to let Nicholas use the premises to prepare medicines and treat patients. Nicholas and Leadbetter drew up an 'indenture' formalizing the arrangement. They both signed it, then tore it in two, each retaining a half. In the event of a dispute, the halves could be reunited, the join proving to any third party that the two pieces came from the same document. Thus their bond, and Nicholas's future in medicine, appeared to be sealed.[54]

SELF-HEAL

Prunella vulgaris

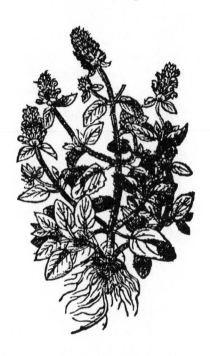

The common Self-heal is a small low creeping Herb, having many small roundish pointed Leaves somwhat like the Leaves of Wild Mints, of a dark green colour without any dents on the edges, from among which rise diverse square hairy Stalks scarce a foot high, which spread somtimes into Branches with diverse such smal Leaves set thereon, up to the tops, where stand brown spiked Heads, of many smal brownish Leaves like scales and Flowers set together, almost like the Head of Cassidony [Lavandula stoechas, *French*

lavender], which Flowers are gaping, and of a blewish purple, or more pale blew, in some places sweet, but not so in others: The Root consists of many strings or fibres downward, and spreadeth strings also, whereby it encreaseth: The smal stalks with the Leaves creeping upon the ground, shoot forth fibres taking hold of the ground, wherby it is made a great tuft in short time.

It is found in Woods and Fields every where . . .

It is an especial Remedy for all green Wounds to solder the lips of them, and to keep the place from any further inconveniences: The Juyce hereof used with Oyl of Roses to anoint the Temples and Forehead, is very effectual to remove the Headach: and the same mixed with Honey of Roses, clenseth and healeth all Ulcers in the Mouth and Throat, and those also in the secret parts.

And the Proverb of the Germans, French, and others is verified in this, That he needeth neither Physitian nor Chyrurgion, that hath Self-heal and Sanicle to help himself.

The Germans called it Brunellen, because it cured an inflammation of the mouth they called 'die Breuen'. The corruption of this name gave the plant its Latin name 'Prunella'. Gerard was as keen on self-heal's medicinal properties as Culpeper, writing that a 'decoction of Prunell made with wine and water doth join together and make whole and sound all wounds, both inward and outward'.[1]

rom his house in St Mary Spital, and at Leadbetter's shop in Threadneedle Street, Nicholas quickly established a popular practice, drawing as many as forty patients a morning from across the capital. With his apothecary training, his university education, his botanical knowledge, and a touch of pastoral concern picked up from his church background, he was well placed to provide basic care. He also drew the attention of the College of Physicians, though he somehow managed to evade the summonses of the Censors, perhaps by exploiting demarcation disputes with the Society of Apothecaries over responsibility for renegade apothecaries.[2]

The main principle of his practice was to offer medical help to anyone who needed it, no matter how poor – 'Jupiter delights in equality, and so do I', as he put it, using an astrological image. 'I wish from my heart our present State would . . . take a little care for the lives of the poor Commonalty, that a poor man that wants money to buy his wife and children bread, may not perish for want of an angel to see a proud insulting domineering Physician, to give him a Visit,' he wrote – Robert Burton's idealism here enlivened by his instinctive pugilism.[3]

His policy kept him very busy. London's streets were full of sick paupers. A continuous stream of royal orders and proclamations complained about the gathering ranks of 'impotent poor people, not able by their labours to get their livings' who 'wander up and down the City and country begging, or which is worse, maintain themselves by filching and stealing'.[4] The problem was particularly acute in London, where greedy landlords divided up the already high density of properties into ever smaller units to increase their rental income. In 1636, the King's Privy Council issued a decree pointing out that the number of 'new buildings and dividing of tenements have daily more and more increased, and such numbers of poor dissolute and lewd persons are therein harboured, that in many parishes ... there are far more households and families that live by begging, and other unlawful ways, and by relief and alms of the parish, than are in the same parish to live by their own means and vocation'. The numbers had grown so high, 'the wealthy are not able to relieve the poor in time of health, much less in time of sickness or infection'. The result, the Privy Councillors observed, was that the 'sick and infected have gone among the whole'.[5]

They had nowhere else to go. By the late 1630s and early 1640s, medical facilities in the capital were stretched to breaking point. As early as 1633, the hospital governors at St Bart's were concerned that 'the poor of this house are increased to a greater number than form'ly have been, to the great charge of this hospital & to the greater labour & more necessary attendance of a physician', a situation not helped by Harvey's regular absences on royal duties.[6]

Nicholas's tiny practice in St Mary Spital could by no means hope to fill such a gaping hole in medical provision, but he did believe that he could make a difference. He emphasized the need for education, to encourage hygiene and healthy living. 'A little medical knowledge about cleanliness and care can do more good than many costly potions from the apothecary,' he argued. Patients often presented themselves with conditions that did not need medicating. 'Many a times I find my patients disturbed by trouble of conscience and sorrow and I have to act the divine before I can be a physician. In fact our greatest skill lies in the infusion of hopes, to induce confidence and peace of mind.'[7] Where old Attersoll had considered visitations of the sick as being superstitious and spiritually distracting, Nicholas saw healing as having a pastoral as well as a medical dimension: it was about salving the soul as well as the body, the health of the one being intimately tied to that of the other. He prescribed treatments for nightmares just as he did for nits, considering the former to arise from 'gross cold Phlegm, as also from melancholic blood settled about the Heart and Veins of the Breast, from whence cold vapours are belched'.[8]

When medicines were needed, Nicholas insisted that they should be based on local ingredients simply prepared. Exotic, expensive medicines, such as opium, were prescribed by doctors 'for lucre of Money[;] they cheat you, and tell you 'tis a kind of Tear, or some such like thing that drops from Poppies when they weep, and that is some where beyond the Sea, I know not where, beyond the Moon'. 'Lay by your Learned Receipts,' he insisted. His patients could 'take so much Senna, so much Scammony, so much Colocynthis, so much Infusion of Crocus Metallorum, &c' – the exotic, sometimes toxic medicines preferred by the College – or they could take a simple, an herb such as Common Groundsel (*Senecio vulgaris*): 'This herb alone preserved in a Syrup, in a distilled Water, in an Oyntment shall do the deed for you in all hot Diseases [such as fevers], and it shall do it, 1. Safely, 2. Speedily.' And best of all, 3. Cheaply.[9]

Though Nicholas supported Paracelsus' ideas about chemical medicines, they were of little help to the sorts of patients he treated. He was more interested in discovering traditional remedies than novel ones, and would search through manuscripts looking for recipes. There is a report, for example, of him discovering an ointment 'in an old Manuscript written anno dom 1513' which seemed to be effective in treating wounds.[10] He approved of many foreign methods and mixtures, and of foreign uses of ingredients that were available in England; but he strongly disapproved of using herbs that could not be grown locally.[11] Warmer climes may yield sweeter, fatter, more colourful and more pungent plants, but they might not suit the constitution of English people, which he believed to be closely linked, like the plants, to the soil and climate in which they had been raised. 'I do not intend to send you to the Canaries for a Medicine,' he wrote.[12] The prominent exception to this rule was tobacco. The addiction he had picked up at Cambridge to the Virginian weed was as strong as ever.

His method of treatment was, first, to 'strengthen . . . the part grieved', then attend to the disease caused 'so Nature may be able to help on in the Cure'.[13] One of his main criticisms of physicians was that they concentrated on the disease rather than the patient. He also condemned those who diagnosed through the inspection of urine samples. To illustrate why, he told the story of a woman 'whose Husband had bruised himself'. She 'took his Water, and away to the Doctor trots she':

The Doctor takes the Piss and shakes it about. How long hath this party been ill (saith he)?

Sir, saith the Woman, He hath been ill these two days.

This is a man's water, quoth the Doctor presently (this he learned by the word HE). Then looking on the water he spied blood in it.

The man hath had a bruise, saith he.

Indeed, saith the woman. My Husband fell down a pair of stairs backwards.

Then the Doctor, [knowing] well enough that what came first to danger must needs be his back and shoulders, said the Bruise lay there. The woman, she admired at the Doctor's skill, and told him, that if he could tell her one thing more she would account him the ablest Physitian in Europe.

Well, what was that?

How many Stairs her Husband fell down.

This was a hard Question indeed, able to puzzle a stronger Brain than Mr Doctor had. To pumping goes he, and having taken the Urinal and given it a shake or two, enquires whereabout she lived, and knowing well the place, and that the Houses thereabouts were but low built Houses, made answer (after another view of the urine, for fashion['s] sake) that probably he might fall down some seven or eight stairs; ah, quoth the woman, now I see you know nothing, my Husband fell down thirty; thirty! quoth the Doctor, and snatching up the Urinal, is here all the water saith he? No saith the woman, I spilt some in putting of it in. Look you there quoth Mr Doctor. There were all the other stairs spilt.[14]

Nicholas's mischievous portrayal of the doctor as a quack would have appealed to many of his poorer patients and readers, but it was not altogether fair. Clauses in the College of Physicians' statutes specifically condemned the practice of receiving 'ignorant persons and females who carry around chamberpots'. Nevertheless, some physicians persisted with the practice. As late as 1664, one doctor was happy to inspect a sample from a young man 'newly married' whose urine 'resembled Distilled Simple water only with some filaments flying in it'. He diagnosed an 'abundance of Aphroditical Salacitie', i.e. lechery – a harsh judgment for a newlywed.[15]

Nicholas's diagnostic method was more sophisticated and relied on an assessment of the patient's entire physical and spiritual disposition. He would inspect the face, the eyes, the lips, the deportment or the manner in which he or she lay in the sickbed. As well as looking, he would sniff. Breath odour provided the 'best judgement' on the state of the 'spirits, heart and lungs'. He may have been suspicious of urine's diagnostic value – 'there is no digestion found in the urine' – but he was interested in the state of other bodily 'excrements', such as spittle and faeces. Spittle that was clear and 'well digested, not viscous' was a good sign; if it was 'tough and knotty' it was a bad one; spittle containing blood (or, even worse, that was black) indicated a fatal condition. Faeces had to be examined with reference to the patient's diet, he insisted, 'for take this for a certain rule, and you shall find it never vary without a miracle: how much the excrements are different from [the patient's diet], so much worse is the sign'. His conclusion was: 'He is fitter to make a Hangman then a Physician that takes no care of his Patient go[ing] orderly to stool.'[16]

One of the first patients to visit Nicholas's practice was the sixty-year-old former physician to the Emperor of Russia, Dr Arthur Dee, suffering from a liver condition. He was hardly typical of the other patients Nicholas saw, except in one important respect: he was a medical outcast. He had regularly attracted the attention of the College Censors, and during the Star Chamber trial against the apothecaries had spoken on behalf of the renegade Edward Cooke.

There were other factors that may have brought Dee to the door of this twenty-four-year-old upstart. They were distantly connected via Nicholas's friend John Whitfield, brother of the Revd Henry Whitfield of Ockley. Whitfield lived at Mortlake, where Arthur's father, Dr John Dee, had built his world-famous library. Another link was astrology. Dr John Dee had been Queen Elizabeth's unofficial astrologer, advising her on a number of occasions on the significance of astronomical phenomena, such as the appearance of a new star in the constellation Cassiopeia in 1572 and the passing of a 'blazing star' or comet over Windsor in 1577. Arthur had been directly involved in his father's occult interests and activities, and had pursued them himself in adult life, producing a book on alchemy published in Paris in 1631.[17]

Nicholas, too, had become an astrologer. It is not clear who taught him the art, but it was to become the most prominent and controversial feature of his medical practice. Time and again, from the seventeenth century through to the twentieth, this was used to belittle his contribution to medicine, allowing critics to dismiss him as a 'figure-flinger', a 'quack salver', and even 'inconsequent'.[18]

It certainly put him in bad company. London swarmed with astrologers, offering services ranging from medical consultations to identifying lovers. One of the most prominent was William Lilly, who provided a rogues' gallery of astrological practitioners in his memoirs. There was John Evans, for instance, a lapsed cleric who became Lilly's astrological tutor. Evans was a striking figure, 'the most perfect Saturnine person my eyes ever beheld', according to Lilly, 'very abusive and quarrelsome, seldom without a black eye or one bruise or another'. He had set up shop at the sign of the Magpie in Gunpowder Alley, a narrow passage of 'mean' lodgings near Fleet Street with a cockpit at one end and a Puritan sect at the other.[19] There he started giving astrological consultations dressed in his old surplice. He also began to sell antimonial cups and had published a pamphlet entitled *Universall Medicine* extolling their medicinal virtues. Antimony, a flaky, silvery metal, was used to fashion goblets, out of which patients were advised to drink claret, muscatel, or malmsey wine. The contaminated drink provoked vomiting to clear the gut of toxins and infestations; but used in excess, the treatment was dangerous and there were several reports of patients being killed. In 1635, the College Censors tried to stop Evans practising, but officially he was still in holy orders and therefore under the authority of the Archbishop of Canterbury. William Harvey led a deputation to the Archbishop, who happily ordered Evans to cease practising and further ordered that copies of his *Universall Medicine* be destroyed.[20]

Another colourful character was Captain Bubb of Lambeth Marsh, a handsome, well-spoken man 'but withal covetous and of no honesty'. According to Lilly, Bubb was once approached by a butcher who wanted to know who had robbed him of £40 when he was on his way to a fair. Bubb promised to help the butcher catch the thief 'for £10 in hand paid'. He told the butcher on 'such a night precisely to watch at such a place, and the thief should come thither'. When this happened, Bubb told the butcher to apprehend the man 'by any means'. 'The butcher attends according to direction. About 12 in the night there comes one riding very fiercely upon a full gallop, whom the butcher knocks down and seized both upon man and horse.' The man turned out to be Bubb's own servant, who, despite being warned by his master, had obviously underestimated the butcher's ability to stop him, 'for which the Captain was indicted and suffered upon the pillory, and afterwards ended his days in great disgrace'.

Lilly also knew a certain Alexander Hart of Houndsditch,

formerly a soldier, 'a comely old man of good aspect' who 'professed Questionary Astrology, and a little of Physic'. His greatest skill was apparently guessing the outcome of games of dice. He, too, was a cheat, and was pilloried for accepting money from a 'rustical fellow of the City, desirous of knowledge' to raise a spirit that failed to appear.

Then there was William Poole, best man at Lilly's first wedding. Though professing astrological expertise, Poole would turn his hand to anything, including the theft of a silver cup from a tavern, for which a magistrate issued an arrest warrant. 'Poole, hearing of this warrant, packs up his little trunk of books (being all his library) and runs to Westminster; but hearing some months after that the Justice was dead and buried, he came and enquired where the grave was; and after the discharge of his belly upon the grave, left these two verses upon it, which he swore he made himself: *Here lieth buried Sir Thomas Jay, Knight, Who being dead, I upon his grave did shite.*'

There was also William Bredon, 'a profound Divine, but absolutely the most polite person for Nativities in that age, strictly adhering to Ptolemy, which he well understood'. In other words, he was something of an academic, with a scholarly understanding of astrological principles; but 'he was so given over to tobacco and drink that when he had no tobacco, he would cut the bell ropes and smoke them'.[21]

Lilly himself had a thriving practice in the Strand, where he combined astrological readings with his own brand of medicine. In the autumn of 1641, for example, a woman turned up at his doorstep with chamberpot containing a urine sample. It had been produced by Bulstrode Whitelocke. Whitelocke was now an MP and since organizing the masque commemorating Charles I's return from his Scottish coronation had undergone a significant change of heart, leading the protests against the King's continuing efforts to rule without Parliament. Whitelocke was suffering from a serious illness that his physician, Francis Prujean, a friend of Harvey's and future President of the College, had failed to cure.

Lilly cast a 'figure', or horoscope, using the 'questionary' or 'horary' method practised by Alexander Hart, which required drawing up the horoscope for the time the consultation was made. His prognosis was that Bulstrode would recover, he announced, 'but by means of a surfeit would dangerously relapse within one month'. While convalescing at the house of the MP Thomas Sandys near Leatherhead in Surrey, Whitelocke ate too much trout with the predicted result. 'Then I went daily to visit him, Doctor [Prujean] despairing of his life, but I said there was no danger thereof and that he would be sufficiently well in five or six weeks, and so he was.' Whitelocke's own diary makes no mention of urine samples or surfeits of trout, but it does confirm that Lilly's intervention helped him pull through.[22]

Nicholas, however, condemned such methods. Those who cast horoscopes over chamberpots he dismissed as 'piss prophets'.[23] He rejected the 'horary' astrology practised by the likes of Bubb and Bredon, refusing to see scores of clients who turned up hoping for the magical identification of a burglar or a lover. His attitude to fortunetelling (as well as drinking) was illustrated by a story. An unidentified country doctor came to St Mary Spital to 'try' Nicholas's astrological abilities. The visitor 'had no sooner after he had knocked entered the Parlour, but Mr Culpeper was got half way on the stairs, and asked him bluntly (as his manner was) what he would have:

> The Doctor told him that he had come some miles to be resolved of an Astrological question and that he would be very grateful to him. Before he could almost speak these words, Mr Culpeper turning himself round to go up stairs told him that he would have nothing to do with this question. Yes, but you would, replied the Doctor, and laughed, if you knew what it were. What it were, says Mr Culpeper! Why what is it? Says the Doctor, Whether you will go to the Tavern and drink a glass of Sack. I'll resolve you that question presently, says Mr Culpeper, takes his Cloak, and immediately goes with him, in such an humour his friend might demand of him what he pleased, and never fail of an ingenuous and civil satisfaction.[24]

Nicholas's astrological method was 'decumbiture'. With horary consultations, the astrologer simply drew up a chart based on the moment the client approached them with a question (or a chamberpot), plotting the position of the sun, moon, and planets against the zodiac for that time and place. This meant that there was no need to inquire about the patient or the disease, or the circumstances in which the latter had arisen. Decumbiture, in contrast, required that a chart be drawn up for the moment the illness manifested itself, usually when the patient had taken to their bed (the term 'decumbiture' comes from the Latin for 'lying down'). This was considered to be the moment the cosmological forces revealed by the zodiac were most forcefully expressed through the patient's body – the time the illness was 'born'.

To demonstrate how decumbiture worked, Nicholas recorded the case study of a patient of the distinguished physician Dr John Fage, a French exile, possibly a Huguenot.[25] Dr Fage's patient was a young woman who had come to London following the break-up of her marriage and gone into service. One December midnight, she awoke with 'a furious disease', and Fage was summoned, the household fearing she may have contracted plague. Fage confirmed the diagnosis, noting the patient had many 'tokens' or symptoms of the disease. Nicholas, who 'came accidentally to the house' the following morning, found 'all the household weeping' and a joiner 'busy pulling down the bedsteads' as the family prepared to evacuate their home. Nicholas examined the girl privately; he found her 'in a strong Fever, that's true: but I could see no tokens, unless 'twere tokens of the Doctor's ignorance'.

Over the following days, the patient's condition deteriorated, and she became 'increasingly bound in body, not going to stool in a week'. Fage, who had taken up residence, responded by prescribing a regular course of 'strong purges', including scammony, one of the College's listed poisons. The treatment seemed to make her condition worse, so Nicholas persuaded the nurse to administer secretly a medicine that would counteract its effect. He also drew up an astrological chart based on the time the patient had contracted the fever. From this he concluded that the true cause of the disease was, as he put it, 'hid, or at least very obscure, [as] plainly signified by so many planets being under the earth' – in other words, beneath the horizon at the time the sickness broke. He noted such positions as Jupiter in Virgo, indicating a blockage in the bowels, and Venus afflicted by the 'Scorpion's Heart', the star Antares, suggesting a violent fever.

A few days later, the 'very obscure' cause of the disease was disclosed: smallpox. The patient suffered two further 'crises' in her condition, but gradually recovered, and within a month was better. 'And thus whoever lost,' Nicholas concluded, 'the joiner he got money by the bargain on both hands: First, pulling the bedsteads and tables to pieces, and for setting them together again: And thus you see 'tis an ill wind that blows no body no profit.'

The case study is a revealing one, but not for the reasons that Nicholas provides. It suggests that astrology did not have the central role in his medical practice and philosophy that he makes out. He used it to provide a prognosis, and to post-rationalize the outcome; but when it came to diagnosis and treatment, he relied upon more obviously medical principles, such as examining the patient and studying the 'signs' of the disease. This is borne out by his other works. For example, in treating the sort of liver complaint presented by Dr Arthur Dee, Nicholas's Herbal recommends a number of plants, such as agrimony (*Agrimonia eupatoria*), hart's tongue (*Phyllitis scolopendrium*), or the lichen liverwort (*Peltigera canina* – one of a number of 'worts' prefixed with the condition or organ they treated, such as woundwort and pilewort). The latter was a 'singular good Herb for all the diseases of the Liver', not because of its astrological properties, but because it was 'an excellent remedy for such whose Livers are corrupted by surfeits which causeth their bodies to break out, for it fortifies the Liver exceedingly and makes it impregnable'.[26] All of these plants were ruled by the planet Jupiter, which also ruled the liver. This, Nicholas argued, explained why they worked so well on that particular organ. However, what in the end recommended them was not their Joviality, but the fact that they had the right balance of qualities to treat the condition presented and had worked in the past.

Given this, why did Nicholas allow himself to become so closely associated with astrology, with Lilly's disreputable crew of frauds and the bell-rope smokers? It was not a love for the occult. Nicholas treated Dr Dee's liver condition successfully, and in gratitude Dee gave him the magic crystal used by his father in a series of séances with his notorious medium or 'skryer', Edward Kelley. The jewel was little larger than a button, but via it Kelley had supposedly disclosed to Dee a series of angelic messages that would lead them both, together with young Arthur, across Europe. Nicholas experimented with the crystal, even tried to use it to cure illness, but became terrified by the 'lewd' images he saw glinting in the glass. He put it away and never looked at it again.[27]

What attracted Nicholas to astrology was the very feature that made it so controversial: it was unauthorized. Its practice was not regulated by a college or livery company, it was not controlled by royal charter, it was not prescribed by scripture or canon. The political, medical, and religious establishment despised it because they could not control it. It was the knowledge system of outcasts.

ROSA SOLIS, OR SUN-DEW

Drosera rotundifolia

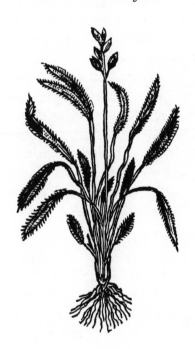

It is likewise called Red-rot, and Youth-wort.

It hath diverse small round hollow Leaves, somewhat greenish, but full of certain red hairs, which makes them seem red, every one standing upon its own Footstalk, reddish hairy likewise. The Leaves are continually moist in the hottest day, yea the hotter the Sun shines on them the moister they are, with a certain sliminess that will ripe (as we say) the small hairs always holding this moisture: Among these Leavs rise up small slender stalks, reddish also, three or four

*fingers high, bearing diverse smal white Knobs one above
another which are the Flowers, after which in the Heads
are certain smal Seeds: the Root is a few small hairs.*

*It groweth usually on Bogs, and in wet places, and
sometimes in moist Woods.*

*Rosa Solis is accounted good to help those that have
salt Rhewm distilling on their Lungs which breedeth a
Consumption, and therfore the Distilled water thereof in
Wine is held fit and profitable for such to drink, which
Water will be of a gold yellow colour: The same Water is
held to be good for all other Diseases of the Lungs, as
Phtisicks, Wheesing, shortness of Breath, or the Cough; as
also to heal the Ulcers that happen in the Lungs, and it
comforteth the Heart and fainting Spirits . . . There is an
usual Drink made hereof with Aqua vitae and Spices frequently, and without any offence or danger, but to good
purpose used in qualms and passions of the Heart.*

Sun-dew is exotic by the standards of Britain's restrained flora. It is a
carnivore. Droplets of sticky 'dew' form on the red hairs, trapping small
insects that are slowly digested by enzymes secreted by the leaves. It can
still be found in large colonies in acid peat-bogs and damp moorland. A
'sundew "meadow" against the setting sun is a dramatic spectacle, the rufous
leaves and beads of dew catching and sparkling in the light', according to
Richard Mabey. Its method of entrapment gave it a reputation, which was
still current in the 1960s, as a love-charm, suitors slipping the leaves into
the pockets of those they desired.

A nineteenth-century American herbal noted that it was particularly effective for treating the 'expulsive or explosive, spasmodic' coughs associated
with measles and whooping-cough.[1]

iscount Hugh Montgomery, a young Irish noble 'with a good complexion, and habit of body', stood before Charles I and opened his shirt. A metal plate was attached to the lower side of his left breast. He removed the plate to show the King a hole in his chest. The King inserted his fingers, the royal touch probing the orifice until it reached a 'fleshy part sticking out, which was driven in and out by a reciprocal motion'. Others who had beheld this medical marvel had assumed the motion to be that of the breathing lung, beneath a membrane of scar tissue. William Harvey, who had brought Montgomery to show the King, said it was the pulsing of the young man's heart.

News of Montgomery's punctured chest had circulated through the court in 1640, and the King had commanded Harvey to investigate the matter. Harvey had gone to Montgomery's lodgings and beheld a sprightly eighteen-year-old in such good health he could not believe the young man had suffered so serious an injury. 'But having saluted him, as the manner is, and declared unto him the Cause of my Visit, by the King's Command, he discovered all to me, and opened the void part of his left side, taking off that small plate, which he wore to defend it against any blow or outward injury.'

Montgomery explained that, as a boy, he had fallen and fractured his ribs on the left side. The injury had suppurated and subsequently produced 'a great quantity of putrified matter', which continued to flow for some time. It eventually healed, leaving the hole Harvey now inspected.[2] Montgomery had adapted well to the injury. Each morning, his valet would cleanse it with an injection of warm fluid, and cover it with the specially-made protective plate. This prepared him 'for any journey or exercise' and allowed him to live 'a pleasant and secure life'. In his late teens, he felt healthy enough to leave Ireland and tour Europe, eventually ending up in London.

Harvey soon established that the movement he felt when he probed the hole did not synchronize with Montgomery's breathing but with his pulse, leading him to realize that what lay beneath could not be the left lung but the 'cone or substance' of the pericardial sac. The hole was an aperture on the living human heart.

This was too good an opportunity to miss. Instead of providing an 'Account of the Business' as requested, Harvey decided Montgomery must be presented to the King in person 'that he might see, and handle this strange and singular Accident with his own Senses; namely, the Heart and its Ventricles in their pulsation'. And here he was, the King probing the orifice, Harvey explaining how the movements he felt with the tips of his fingers illustrated Harvey's hypothesis that each beat injected blood into the arteries.

Harvey felt he owed Charles such a demonstration of the circulation of the blood because he had published his theory in the King's name. After years of gestation, it had first appeared in 1628, in his *Exercitatio anatomica de motu cordis*, 'Anatomical Exercises on the Motions of the Heart'. *De motu cordis*, as it came to be known, was a distinctly foreign production. It was written in Latin – another quarter century would pass before it appeared in English, the unofficial translation being produced by a physician based in Rotterdam. The publisher of *De motu cordis* was William Fitzer of Frankfurt, the English son-in-law of the famous German printer Johann Theodore de Bry. Harvey had apparently chosen Fitzer because his friend and fellow College member Robert Fludd had discovered that German publishers offered authors better terms. Nevertheless, the treatise was aimed at the home market, bearing fulsome dedications to Dr John Argent, President of the College of Physicians, and to Harvey's master, King Charles.

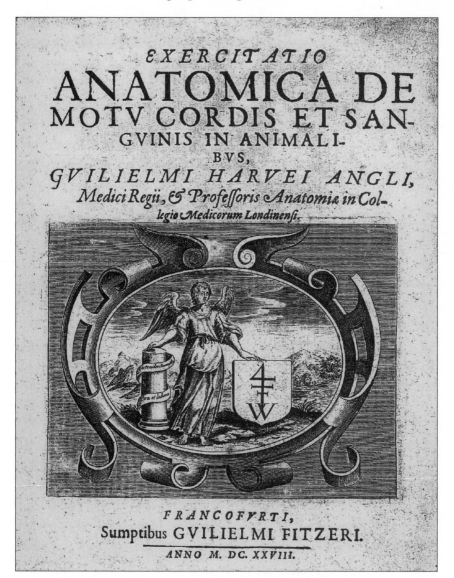

To Dr Argent he wrote of how he was 'greatly afraid to suffer this little Book, otherways perfect for some years ago, either to come abroad, or go beyond the Sea, lest it might seem an action too full of arrogancy', but he was reassured by the fact that he had been allowed to 'maintain what I proposed in the presence of you & our College'. Furthermore, 'I do not endeavour, nor think fit, to defraud any of the ancients', in particular Galen, 'of the honour due to them, nor provoke any moderns', such as Paracelsus.

This unthreatening tone provoked nods and murmurs of approval among the Fellows. The book may contain revolutionary ideas, Harvey was saying, but there was no need for them to challenge medical orthodoxy or upset medical practice. The College could simply carry on as before, which is what it did. There were some critics. Dr Edward May, the occultist and physician to Queen Henrietta Maria, claimed in a pamphlet published in 1639 that his discovery of a serpent in the heart of a young man showed that the theory could not be true (Harvey assumed the 'serpent' must be a blood clot). May inspired a more considered, but not much more effective, critique from the Regius Professor of Medicine at the University of Paris, Jean Riolan, who was also physician to Queen Henrietta Maria's mother, Marie de Medici. Riolan's arguments rested on such Galenic issues as the effect of blood rushing through the vessels on the balance of humours through the body. In reply, Harvey wrote a respectful letter dealing with Riolan's objections one by one, and demolishing them all.[3]

Harvey aimed to win over Charles with a bolder strategy. In the royal dedication that introduced *De motu cordis*, he wrote: 'The heart of animals is the foundation of their life, the Prince of all, the Sun of their Microcosm, on which all growth depends, from whence all vigour and strength does flow. Likewise the King is the foundation of his Kingdoms, the Sun of his Microcosm, the Heart of his Commonwealth, from whence all power, all grace proceeds. I was so bold to offer to your Majesty things which are written concerning the Heart, so much the rather, because ... all things human are according to the pattern of man, and most things in a King according to that of the Heart; Therefore the knowledge of his own Heart cannot be unprofitable to a King, as being a divine resemblance of his actions.'[4] With the young Viscount Montgomery now before him, the King could discover this divine resemblance for himself, feel the same pulsating power that radiated from the sun across the universe, and from the throne across the nation.

Harvey was by now one of the King's closest courtiers. In December 1639, he was formally promoted to the position of the King's personal doctor, provided with a 'diet of three dishes of meat a meal', lodgings at Whitehall, and an annual pension of £400.[5] A year later, they were exchanging Christmas gifts. Charles gave Harvey 24 ounces of silver plate, and Harvey reciprocated with 'a box of marmalade', a preserve, possibly boasting medicinal qualities prepared with the help of the royal apothecary, Adrian Metcalf.

As well as presents, the King gave Harvey more practical resources. Like his father, Charles was a keen hunter, with herds of deer 'wandering at liberty in the Woods or Forests, or inclosed and kept up in Parks and Chases'. He allowed Harvey to pick out specimens, and during 'rutting time . . . when the Females are lusty and admit the Males', he had 'a daily opportunity of dissecting them, and of making inspection and observation of all their parts, which liberty I chiefly made use of in order to [dissect] the Genital parts'. In a landmark series of anatomical exercises, he explored the way embryos form and develop, at one point laying before Charles and Queen Henrietta Maria a 'foetus of the magnitude of a Pease-cod, cut out of the uterus of a Doe, which was complete in all its members (so that it was apparently a Male by the parts) . . . It did swim, trim and perfect, in such a kind of White, most transparent, and crystalline moisture (as if it had been treasured up in some most clear glass receptacle) about the bigness of a Pigeon's egg.'[6]

Equally remarkable to the King was Harvey's discovery that, in the early stages of pregnancy, the wombs of impregnated does contained no trace of the stags' semen. It was widely believed that the male seed was the source of fertility, the female egg merely providing the raw material for its development. If there was no semen in the womb, how could the does possibly become pregnant? When the King told his keepers and huntsmen of this curiosity, they assumed the does Harvey had dissected had not been impregnated. There had been a drought that year, and it may have depressed the fertility of the stags. Members of the King's medical staff were equally sceptical. In an effort to settle the matter, Charles commanded a group of does to be locked away after the start of the rutting season. Those that were dissected were found to have no semen in their wombs, yet some of those that survived became pregnant and produced healthy young.

Harvey himself was unable to explain this discovery, and would remain undecided on the issue of the respective roles of the male seed and the female egg for the rest of his life. In the fly leaf of his own copy of *De Generatione Animalium* (1651), the book in which he eventually published the results of his work on the King's deer, he speculated on whether fertilization might be like a venereal disease or rabies or smallpox, laying dormant in its host for a period of time before producing its symptoms. Or perhaps it worked in the same manner as the fermentation of alcohol.

Whatever the solution, such questions could only be properly considered in stable, orderly, controllable conditions. The chaos of city life, the politicking of Amen Corner, the bustle of St Bartholomew's Hospital – these were no places for proper science. It demanded the quiet of a university college – or a king's palace. At Hampton Court, Greenwich, Whitehall, or Richmond Harvey could continue his investigations free of financial constraints and domestic distractions, generously supplied with equipment and experimental samples. The sorts of advances in medical science that he was producing might challenge the *status quo*; but they also depended upon it.

The presentation of Viscount Montgomery to the King was a chance to demonstrate to Charles how much Harvey had managed to achieve as a result of royal benefaction. But the episode did raise one puzzling issue. As the royal fingers had pressed upon the pulsating membrane at the base of the hole, Harvey noted that Montgomery reported feeling nothing other than the 'sensation of the outward skin'. It appeared that the heart, the sovereign of the body, lacked feeling.

On 10 August 1641, Harvey once again accompanied the King on a progress to Scotland. Since the coronation, Scotland had moved towards outright rebellion against Charles's religious policies, and Charles in turn had mobilized his forces in an attempt to assert his authority, marching an army up to the Scottish borders. But he was forced to back down due to lack of funds. In a desperate attempt to raise money to renew his campaign, he called a parliament in England on 13 April 1640, thereby ending the eleven years of 'Personal Rule'. An unusually large number of the seats for the elections to this parliament were contested (in the past, by far the majority of MPs were elected by default), producing an influx of politicians eager to make their mark. The leading Puritan radical John Pym, adapting the medical metaphor used by Harvey, set the tone by proclaiming that 'parliament is as the soul of the commonwealth, that only is able to apprehend and understand the symptoms of all such diseases which threaten the body politic'. It was, he added for good measure, the 'intellectual part which governs all the rest' – the brain, not the heart.[7]

The heart of the commonwealth missed a beat to hear such words, and Charles dismissed what became known as the Short Parliament after just three weeks. But he was forced to recall it again in November, after the rebelling Scots invaded the north of England, a skirmish at Hexham, near Newcastle, finally settling the matter in favour of the Scots. This time, Parliament was to stay put, passing an act in May 1641 prohibiting the King from dissolving it without its consent. For good measure, it abolished the courts of the Star Chamber and High Commission and ordered the release of the persecuted Puritans Prynne, Burton, and Bastwick.

It was in these desperate circumstances that the King left for Scotland. The situation demanded haste. It had taken weeks for him to travel north for his coronation. He and his cumbersome cortège managed the journey this time in just four days, arriving in Edinburgh on 14 August. He spent the next few weeks trying to negotiate a settlement with the 'Covenanters', the leaders of the Scottish rebellion. As at his coronation, he turned to ceremonials to reassert his royal authority. In an attempt to show that his powers remained intact, he offered to touch acts passed by the Scottish Parliament with his sceptre, the traditional way of conferring royal assent. But a pretext was found to prevent him from doing so. The magic had gone out of the monarchy.

Harvey, meanwhile, went with the King's apothecary, Adrian Metcalf, to Aberdeen, the city having remained loyal to the King during the recent hostilities. There they were made honorary burgesses, receiving 'five shillings in a white purse, as is the custom'. The purpose of the visit may have been to merge Aberdeen's two colleges into a new Caroline University. If so, it failed, and Harvey's presence aroused protests from local Covenanters, who stirred up anti-royal feeling against 'spending the common good upon wine and other things, superfluously' to curry favour with the King's officials. Apparently the wife of one Alex Roland had been paid eighteen shillings to provide the visitors with duck, bread, and a quart of wine.[8]

The royal party arrived back in London on 14 November and was 'entertained of the citizens joyfully and sumptuously' on four courses of meat, brawn, and fish. 'And the Lord Mayor and Aldermen, with some of the chief of the city, went to meet the King on horseback, and the city streets had rails all along for all the company to sit in when the King came through, and brave coverlids hung over the penthouses all the way he went.'[9] For a moment, it looked as though England had escaped the convulsive disease that had seized Scotland, and that the regal heart of the nation could return to a gentler, more restful beat.

But the mood was misleading. In Parliament, a 'Grand Remonstrance' was introduced in the House of Commons. It listed a multitude of grievances that had built up over the years of Personal Rule and interrupted parliaments: the 'enlargement' of royal forests into private property, the abuse of the monopolies of 'Soap, Salt, Wine, Leather, Sea-Cole and, in a manner, of all things common and necessary', the 'restraint of the Liberties of the subjects in their habitation, Trades, and other Interests', the 'fines, imprisonments, stigmatizings, mutilations, whippings, pillories, gags, confinements, banishments' imposed by the Star Chamber, the 'suspensions, excommunications, deprivations and degradations' inflicted by the bishops, and, most particularly, the papist 'Faction' in the King's court 'grown to that height and entireness of power'.[10]

As this catalogue of complaints was being read out, the mood of anger deepened with news of a Catholic rebellion in Ireland. Many Puritans had friends and relatives directly involved. Nehemiah Wallington's brother-in-law Zachariah Rampaigne, for example, was a wealthy Ulster planter with estates near Enniskillen. Nehemiah heard that when the rebellion broke out, Zachariah had tried to leave the country with his family but was waylaid on the road to the coast by a group of rebels who stabbed him, 'which his wife beholding did on her knees beg for his life, as also his children, crying pitifully, "O do not kill my Father".'[11]

Reports of this sort arrived by the day, each more lurid than the last, many exaggerated, many fabricated. They had their effect, steeling opinion against Catholics, and encouraging suspicions that the 'Faction' in the King's government was somehow complicit. The Grand Remonstrance was passed, though with a thin majority of 159 votes to 148.

Among the 148 dissenters was Sir John Culpeper, a distant relation of Nicholas's. He was MP for Kent, and had backed many of the parliamentary measures that had challenged the King's authority.

The Grand Remonstrance was a step too far for him and he joined a clique of MPs who switched their loyalties to the King. As a reward, Charles made him Chancellor of the Exchequer, in charge of managing the royal finances.

In the city, crowds started to gather to deliver remonstrances of their own. It has been estimated that, in the coming month, the petitions delivered in support of Parliament bore the signatures of thirty thousand apprentices, accounting for almost all working in London.[12] William Lilly watched from his house a daily tide of protesters flowing up and down the Strand, 'men of mean or a middle quality themselves, having no aldermen, merchants or Common-Council men among them . . . modest in their apparel but not in their language'. The wood turner Nehemiah Wallington wandered the streets, electrified by 'the charge of the strength of our city'.[13]

The mood of militancy intensified with the return of the three Puritan martyrs, Prynne, Burton, and Bastwick, all bearing the livid branding scars meted out by the Star Chamber. On 7 December at Blackheath, a windswept heath to the south-east of the capital long associated with rebellious gatherings, Wallington joined a procession of 'many coaches and horse and thousands on foot' to welcome Bastwick home. The doctor, who had spent the last four years locked up in the Star Castle on St Mary's, one of the Scilly Isles, was greeted with garlands of rosemary and bay, the herbs of remembrance and victory, which the welcomers waved over their heads.[14]

These developments provoked political jostling at Amen Corner. Harvey and the other royal physicians could no longer attend its meetings, and the College found its royal associations were becoming a liability. Earlier in the year, it had petitioned the Commons as part of its ongoing dispute with the apothecaries, seeking parliamentary support on the grounds that, in 1627, the Society had been 'condemned by Parliament' for splitting from the Grocers. This required a deft reversal of its own position, as it had originally been in support of the split, and had opposed Parliament's intervention.

Having now put its grievances in the hands of the MPs, it had to decide what to do about the returning hero it had so peremptorily dismissed for his 'misdemeanours and evil Carriage' in 1634. At a special session of the Comitia held on 18 December, the Fellows voted to reinstate Bastwick with immediate effect.[15]

Few took any notice of the College's decision. Events outside were spiralling into chaos. On Sunday 26 December, 1641, Lord Mayor Sir Richard Gurney, one of the few among the City élite still openly supporting the King, warned the royal court that the apprentices were ready to riot. On Monday, a crowd 'flocked' around the House of Commons, calling for the ejection of the bishops and lords from Parliament. The apprentices' shaven heads, once enforced by city regulations, now adopted as a mark of collective pride, led them and parliamentary supporters thereafter to be called 'roundheads'.[16] Whether shaven or tousle-haired, Nicholas Culpeper was somewhere among them. People power, press freedom, religious toleration – these were the causes for which he would fight, and here on the streets battle was joined.

The next day, the roundheads, joined by shopkeepers and merchants, were back at Westminster, forcing one of the doors of the Abbey, demanding the destruction of its 'popish relics'. On Wednesday evening, a crowd of two thousand apprentices armed with clubs, swords, and spears gathered in Cheapside, London's main market, following the outbreak of a fight at Whitehall between protesters and palace servants. On Friday and Saturday, according to Wallington, the King ordered that powder and ammunition for five hundred men be fetched from the armoury at the Tower of London and carried to Whitehall. In response, the Commons abandoned Westminster and reconvened at the Guildhall and Grocers' Hall, where they were 'pompously seated, and fawningly courted', as one of the King's supporters observed.[17]

On Sunday, 3 January 1642 the King wrote to the exiled House saying he would guarantee the safety of members who returned to Westminster. At noon, a group proceeded together back up the

Strand towards Whitehall 'with much fear'. That night, provoked by rumours that the House planned to impeach the Queen herself, the King announced charges of treason against five radical MPs: John Pym, Denzil Holles, Sir Arthur Haselrig, John Hampden, and William Strode. Tipped off that Holles was meeting his accomplices in his study, a detachment of the King's men was sent to seize them, but they erupted into an empty room. They sealed it up, together with the rooms of the other four members. Pym meanwhile found himself 'dogged' by two men on the streets. He confronted them, giving a 'push to the adversary', and they slipped off into the dark.

The fraught atmosphere intensified when a detachment of cannoneers was sent to the Tower, 'which put the city to much trouble and great fear' and instigated a struggle between the King and Parliament for control of London's commanding citadel. In response, some of the city's aldermen and sheriffs set guards at the gates and drew chains across the streets. Householders were knocked up and told to fetch their weapons and stand by their doors. As the sun rose over the wary city, shops remained shut in anticipation of a bloody confrontation.

That lunchtime of 4 January, William Lilly was dining at Whitehall with a group of politicians. He noticed that the room was filled with chests packed with the arms recently brought from the Tower. Mid-meal, one of the King's knights burst into the room and started to break open the chests, 'which frighted us all that were there', Lilly recalled. However, one of his companions had the presence of mind to slip from the room and run down to the House of Commons, where the members were alerted 'that the King was preparing to come into the House'.[18]

At 3 p.m., Charles I proceeded from Whitehall Palace to Westminster, escorted by a detachment of four hundred armed supporters. Parliament was packed. Eighty of the King's men brandishing swords and pistols pushed into the lobby, jostling members, and pulling the doorkeepers from the entrance to the chamber. The King passed through, and was received with a deferential reflex, the members standing up and doffing their hats. The King responded by raising his and bowing to the assembly. He made his way towards the Speaker's throne. 'Mr Speaker,' he said, 'I must for a time make bold with your chair.' The Speaker gave up his place. 'Gentlemen,' said the King, 'I am sorry for this occasion of coming unto you. Yesterday I sent a Sergeant-at-Arms upon a very important occasion, to apprehend some that by my command were accused of high Treason, whereunto I did expect Obedience, and not a Message.'[19]

The mood of gallantry evaporated. The King asked for the whereabouts of John Pym. The House was hushed. The King asked for the whereabouts of Denzil Holles. No reply. The King then asked the Speaker if he knew whether the offending MPs were present. Upon bended knee, the Speaker 'did very wisely desire his majesty to pardon him saying that he could neither see nor speak but by command of the House'. 'Well, well, 'tis no matter,' replied the King. 'I think my eyes are as good as another's.' He then peered along the ranks of faces looking at him 'a pretty whiles to see if he could espy any of them'.[20]

The five MPs had in fact already slipped away to avoid 'Combustion in the House'.[21] They had made straight for the City, to the one place where they knew they would find sympathy and support: the Star tavern in Coleman Street.

Charles left the Commons chamber 'in a more discontented and angry passion than he came in', his supporters clearing a way for him through the crowd with cries of 'a lane, a lane'.[22] For the rest of the day, the City was tense. Shops remained shut, shopkeepers like Wallington on their guard. The following morning, the King and members of the Privy Council marched to the City, to demand of the Commons now reassembled at the Guildhall that the five MPs be surrendered. His wish denied, Charles set off back to Whitehall, escorted by Lord Mayor Gurney and the City Aldermen. As they approached Temple Bar, where, before Simon White's old shop, the Mayor would take his formal leave of the King, a gang of 'rude persons' started to jostle the parade. One group were 'in a most undutiful manner, pressing upon, looking into, and laying hold' of the King's coach, trying to throw seditious pamphlets through the window. Another pulled the Mayor and some of the aldermen from their horses. The humiliated City leaders were forced to complete the journey at the head of the royal escort on foot.[23] The previous year, a waterman had warned 'it was Parliament time now' and that 'the Lord Mayor was but [our] slave', and so it now seemed.[24]

Within hours of these events, news-sheets rolled off presses in the print works around the Royal Exchange and the secret garrets of Coleman Street. With the abolition of the Star Chamber and Court of High Commission, both the Crown and the Church had been deprived of their main instruments for controlling the press. With nothing as yet put in their place, printing was effectively unregulated, creating a surge in demand for news and opinion which new, faster presses efficiently met. Parliamentary speeches, petitions, 'faithful remonstrances', sermons, and incendiary reports poured out like flames from a burning building. A visiting Bohemian intellectual was astonished by the number of bookshops in the capital. George Thomason, who made a point of buying up every pamphlet and tract published in the capital, collected 24 items in 1640, 721 in 1641, and 2,134 in 1642.[25]

The streets became littered with new ideas and conflicting reports: the five MPs had been captured, reported one pamphlet; they are still at liberty, claimed another. Stories scurried through the streets of murder, conspiracy, invasion. An army of fierce men was marching from the north, a secret weapon that stuck in the body and could not be pulled out was being prepared for deployment, hit-lists of radical MPs and citizens were being drawn up.

Our main protagonists are lost among the confusion of protesters, petitioners, patrols, and search parties. Harvey was in London, probably at his grace-and-favour apartment in Whitehall when not at the King's side. He did not attend any of the College Comitias during this period – he would not be seen again at Amen Corner for eight years. Nicholas would have been at his house in St Mary

Spital, Leadbetter's shop in Bishopsgate, or at Coleman Street. That he was actively involved among the protest groups at some level is shown by his participation in the coming hostilities.

On Thursday 6 January 1642, just two days after the crisis had begun with Charles's uninvited entry to Parliament, anticipation became panic. It was an evening 'I desire might never be forgotten,' wrote Wallington. At around 9 p.m. there was a sudden sound of shooting and fights. It later emerged that they were produced by the accidental discharge of a carbine and the riotous noises of duelling courtiers in a Covent Garden tavern.[26] However, at the time, the disturbances were taken as the sound of invasion. A watchman at Ludgate heard that the King's forces were on their way. At Culpeper's tenement in St Mary Spital, at Lilly's house on the Strand, at Wallington's shop in Eastcheap, there was 'a great bouncing at every man's door to be up in their arms'. 'Both in the City and Suburbs,' Wallington recorded, 'we heard (as we lay in our beds) a great cry in the streets that there was horse and foot coming.' Women and children 'did then arise, and fear and trembling entered on all'. Some, Wallington claimed, died of shock, including the wife of a neighbour, Alderman Adams.

But nothing happened. 'Although some might slight, jest, and scoff at this and think and say there was no cause, and that we were more fright than hurt,' wrote Wallington, 'yet it is certain enough, that had not the Lord of His mercy stirred us up to bestir ourselves, it would have gone hard enough with us.'[27]

A moment of quiet, and then suddenly hordes of petitioners from across the kingdom descended upon the capital, from Kent to Cumberland, Gloucestershire to Suffolk, of every occupation and class, seamen and silk-throwers, landlords and labourers. They had come to protest to Parliament, not about the King, but about the 'papists' they supposed to have infected his court and policies. From Chester in the north, the citizens presented their most 'humble and heart thanks to the Parliament', and asked that it 'remove from His Majesty's most Sacred Person, all pestilent troublers of this Church,

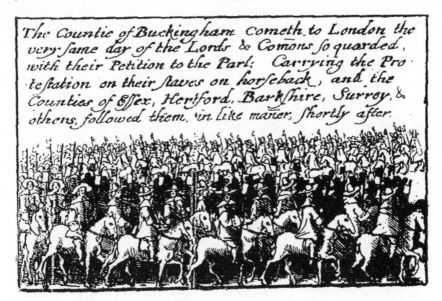

*Contemporary cartoon of petitioners from Buckinghamshire descending on
Parliament, 11 January, 1642.*

and State'. From Devon in the south, the knights, gentlemen and
yeomanry pledged their support to Parliament in apprehending the
'Priests and Jesuits lurking here and there' who 'stir up sedition,
Rebellion and insurrection'.[28]

It was not just burgesses and knights who crowded around Parliament. Hundreds of 'gentlewomen, tradesmen's wives and many
others of the female sex' presented themselves. Likened to the
'woman of Tekoah', a biblical reference to a wise woman who made
an appeal to King David, they complained of the 'great decay of
their trading, occasioned by the present distempers and distractions'. When they approached the Duke of Lennox outside the
House of Lords with their petition he waved them off with his
cane. 'Away with these women', he said, and they, 'interrupting his
passage, catched hold of his staff'.[29] Eventually Lord Savage was
persuaded to present their case to the House.

Just beyond the back wall of Nicholas's home in St Mary Spital, the sound of muskets became ever more insistent. It was London's citizen militia or 'Trained Bands', practising in the neighbouring Artillery Ground. The Ground was a walled-off yard between St Mary Spital's precincts and Spitalfields (the fields formerly belonging to the hospital) to the east. It had turf embankments at each end for target practice by musketeers and heavier artillery, and a stone and brick armoury used to store five hundred sets of arms.[30]

The Trained Bands drilled twice a week. The capital had as many as six thousand militiamen, 'very good troops', a Spanish spy reported, 'and . . . well armed', even though they were 'commanded by merchants'.[31] They were volunteer reservists, their service being seen as a form of taxation. They were also required to purchase their own weapons, which provided an opportunity to show off their social status. Many were seen strutting around with 'arms of . . . such extraordinary beauty, fashion and goodness for service, as are hard to be matched elsewhere'.

But by the spring of 1642, the drills were being performed in earnest. In December 1641, the balance of power of London's government had shifted decisively from the Lord Mayor and the Aldermen to the Common Council. Under the old arrangements, the Lord Mayor had the power of calling the Council whenever he chose, and he rarely chose. However, the Common Council elections of 28 December 1641 had returned an overwhelming number of Puritans and Parliamentarians. 'Fears and jealousies had distracted the City,' a supporter of the King noted. In place of the 'grave, discreet, well-affected Citizens' of the past were voted a motley crew of craftsmen and itinerants, 'Fowke the Traitor, Riley the squeaking Bodice-maker, Perkins the Tailor, Norminton the Cutler, young beardless Coulson the Dyer, Gill the wine-cooper, and Jupe the Laten-man [tinker] in Crooked-Lane'.[32]

On the very day the King attempted to arrest the five MPs, these tinkers and tailors called for the setting up of a 'Committee of Safety' to oversee the defence of the City. The Committee was also given powers to compel the Mayor to summon the Common Council, and would later take direct control of the Trained Bands.

This development had a neat symmetry with Parliament's own efforts to assert its position: the Common Council had challenged the authority of the Lord Mayor and the Aldermen; the House of Commons had done likewise with the King and the Privy Council; both had given themselves the power to determine when they assembled and to raise an army. A royalist news-sheet noted that they had become 'as two strings set to the same tune . . . on two several viols . . . if you touch one, the other by consent renders the same sound'.[33]

The Committee of Safety quickly set about preparing London for the coming military confrontation. On 4 April 1642, Parliament gave the Committee powers to raise and train forces and deploy troops, not just within the bounds of the City, but beyond. On 15 April, the Aldermen and Common Council members of each City ward were instructed to identify 'able' men for enlistment. On 10 May, the full complement mustered under the command of Major General Philip Skippon at Finsbury Fields, just to the west of Spitalfields, under the turning sails of its three giant windmills. Eight thousand men assembled, divided into six regiments, named after, not kings or counties, but the colours of the rainbow.

MPs were invited from Westminster to survey this magnificent new militia, and were opulently entertained in a large tent at a cost of nearly £400. It was an impressive spectacle, the display of military might and preparedness only momentarily marred by the sight of Alderman Thomas Atkins, Colonel of Red Trained Band, being toppled from his horse when it was startled by a discharge of musketry (the incident was gleefully reported in the royalist news-paper *Mercurius Aulicus*, which recorded that Atkins 'was troubled with a yearning in his bowels').[34]

The following month, news reached the capital that the King was forming a bodyguard at York and calls went out for money and plate to finance the raising of a parliamentary cavalry force. A huge consignment of arms was delivered from Hull, originally stored there by the King in readiness for the war on Scotland, which a local MP had managed to keep from royalist hands on Parliament's behalf. The bounty was distributed throughout the capital, one load being delivered to the Apothecaries' Hall.[35]

In July, Parliament formally voted for the setting up of a national army under the command of the Earl of Essex, a veteran of the wars in Holland and Germany and the son of Elizabeth I's impetuous favourite Robert Devereux, who had been executed when the Earl was ten.

Further thousands enlisted at the Artillery Ground in late July, their numbers swelled by three thousand apprentices who had been promised their freedoms on discharge from the army at the end of the conflict.[36] As the army performed manoeuvres at Tothill Fields, an area of low-lying ground to the west of Westminster, many anxiously contemplated what lay ahead for both city and nation. In the speech of a lifetime, Bulstrode Whitelocke warned the Commons that they stood 'at the pit's brink, ready to plunge ourselves into an ocean of troubles and miseries . . . It is strange to note how we have insensibly slid into this beginning of a civil war by one unexpected accident after another, as waves of sea.' 'I am not for a tame resignation of our religion, lives and liberties into the hands of our adversaries who seek to devour us,' Whitelocke told his fellow MPs, 'nor do I think it inconsistent with your great wisdom to prepare for a just and necessary defence of them.' Negotiation, though, might yet deliver the country from war. 'Accommodation' was the word; everyone prayed for an 'accommodation'.[37]

But to be on the safe side, security was stepped up across the capital. Cripplegate, Bishopsgate, and Moorgate to the north, Aldgate and the Postern Gate to the east, Aldersgate, Newgate, and Ludgate to the west were all locked and their cullises lowered. Streets were barricaded with posts and chains, some even bricked up. The homes of royal sympathizers were searched and ransacked. In the house of one Mr Molleins in Baldwin's Gardens near Gray's Inn

Lane, ammunition was discovered for twenty men, together with '2 great pieces of ordnance, one culverin, one great murdering-piece, and four small brass murdering-pieces'. Suspicious groups of people were seen entering the house of the Queen's painter. It was sealed off by Trained Bands, but no one emerged, and a search of the property revealed 'a private way down into a vault under the ground, in which they might go a quarter of a mile, leading them to the Thames-side where they might privately take a boat and escape'.[38]

Harvey's apartment in Whitehall Palace was targeted. He had obviously left in haste, or in the expectation of imminent return, as all his possessions and papers lay unprotected in his rooms. The soldiers who broke in 'not only spoiled me of all my Goods', Harvey later recalled with 'a sigh or two', 'but also (which I most lament) have bereft me of my Notes, which cost me many years industry'.[39] Among the losses were papers on the generation of insects, respiration, the movement and structure of muscles, sex in animals, nutrition – a collection of incalculable value to 'the Commonwealth of Learning', as Harvey immodestly but accurately put it. Perhaps the most significant work he claimed to have lost was entitled 'A Practice of Physic conformable to . . . the Circulation of the Blood'. Harvey's theory had raised important questions about standard treatments, such as blood-letting, cupping, and purgation, all of which rested to some extent on the assumption that blood seeped rather than circulated through the body. Harvey never made fully known his views on the implications of his theory for medical practice. If he had committed any to paper, they expired in the ransacking of his apartment.[40]

The King had slipped out of the capital on the night of 10 January, 'driven away by shame more than fear, to see the barbarous rudeness of those Tumults'.[41] Harvey followed him. On the advice of Sir John Culpeper, the royal party had headed for York, to start rallying support among the northern gentry, who were assumed to be more dependable. Just as Londoners conceived of forces massing beyond the city walls, so the royal party imagined the capital disgorging rebels armed to the teeth. Rumours were spread of 'continual, not small distillations, but floods of men, money, ammunition, and arms descending from the head city, and metropolis of the kingdom'.[42]

The struggle was now on for Charles to raise a force of his own. Reviving yet another feudal instrument, he issued 'Commissions of Array', instructing local supporters to rally troops. Now was the time for sides to be taken, when men had to choose between friendships and loyalties, families and political principles, rebellion and the *status quo*. Several Culpepers joined Sir John on the royalist side, probably including Sir Thomas, another MP and author of a famous tract on usury. On the parliamentary side would stand Nicholas and, somewhat less prominently, one other notable member of the family: Sir William Culpeper, son of Sir Edward of Wakehurst, to whom Nicholas would later dedicate a book on the 'fall of monarchy'.

Those that chose to be with the King were instructed to come to Nottingham, where, on 22 August 1642, Charles 'floated' the royal standard, announcing his readiness to fight. It was a largely symbolic event, and the expected numbers did not materialize.

William Harvey stood steadfast beneath the flag, though he temporarily removed himself to visit a medical friend, Percival Willughby, who lived in Derby, fifteen miles away. It provided a brief respite from politics, which Harvey clearly detested, the two choosing to talk about uterine rather than national disorders.[43]

A few days later, Charles dispatched Sir John Culpeper to Westminster to initiate peace negotiations. Sir John received a hostile reception. Though still an MP, he was refused permission to take his seat in the Commons and was forced to stand at the bar of the House, 'looking more like a culprit than a Privy Councillor', as one member observed from the benches. He was not even allowed to speak, and handed over the King's message in silence, which was answered with a refusal to treat until the charges of treason against the five MPs were dropped and the royal standard was lowered.[44]

The latter condition was fulfilled by the weather, a strong wind blowing the standard down two or three nights after it had been raised. After such a desultory and humiliating showing, the King had no choice but to move on.

In September, Charles and his retinue settled at Shrewsbury, where they had more luck. The King had abandoned his Commissions of Array in favour of granting commissions to noblemen and gentlemen, allowing them to raise regiments in his name. This strategy attracted a significant force, numbering some twelve thousand by mid-October. He had also been joined by his nephews, Princes Rupert and Maurice. Rupert, only twenty-three, was the model of the cavalier: exquisitely dressed, nobly born (son of Frederick V, Elector Palatine, and Charles's sister Elizabeth, Queen of Bohemia), loyal, ruthless, and ready to gallop into any fray with his pet poodle Boy on his lap. A veteran of the Thirty Years War, he was given command of the King's cavalry. The royalist forces were now ready to engage, and set off for London.

News of the King's movements reached London in days, and, thanks to the quickening heartbeat of the presses, circulated through the capital within hours. On 9 September, the Earl of Essex mounted his horse at Temple Bar and, 'guarded with most of the Trained Bands of the City of London', processed through the city, up Ludgate, through St Paul's churchyard, into Cheapside, and past the Royal Exchange. Leaving London through Moorgate, he marched via St Albans and Northampton to Worcester, where, approaching the city, his cavalry unexpectedly ran into Rupert's. The young prince sent the parliamentary horse galloping, before wheeling round and returning to the King in Shrewsbury, brimming with confidence.[45] Now just fifteen miles apart, the two armies groped towards each other until they finally collided on 23 October at Edgehill in Warwickshire, between Banbury and Warwick, where the first substantial engagement of the Civil War took place.

The King himself was on the scene of the battle from the start, taking part in the first advance of the royal infantry, marching to its rear, his position advertised by a scarlet standard. He had decided to bring his two children, the Prince of Wales, aged twelve and armed with his own pistol, and the Duke of York, aged just nine. After parliamentary ordnance started to explode around them, it was quickly decided that the children should be withdrawn. The Prince of Wales refused to go, reportedly cocking his pistol and crying 'I fear them not.' His princely petulance was ignored, however, and he and his brother were carried off. They were deposited at a small barn surrounded by a hedge that was being used as a dressing station for wounded men. It was there that they were put in the care of William Harvey.

Harvey was no warrior. War destroyed the settled order, stirred emotions, wasted resources, interrupted his studies. He had already witnessed the terrible consequences of the Thirty Years War during a tour of the Continent in 1630. In a letter home, he was moved to uncharacteristic intensities of emotion, noting 'the relics of the war & the plague, where famine had made anatomies [of the people]. It is scarce credible in so rich, populous & plentiful countries as these [once] were that so much misery, desolation & poverty & famine should in so short a time be as we have seen.'[46] Now war threatened to make the same alteration to his homeland.

The accounts are confused, but he was presumably at the barn helping to treat the wounded. He was withdrawn from these duties and put in charge of the children. All he could think of doing was taking cover with them in the nearby hedge and reading from a book he happened to have in his pocket, most likely a medical tome. As his lecture notes show, he could hold an audience's attention, and no doubt managed to distract the boys with accounts of gruesome surgery or grisly wounds, while beyond the bushes such horrors were being turned into reality. But he was interrupted by the 'Bullet of a great Gun', which 'grazed on the ground near them' and was forced to 'remove his station', perhaps taking the children to safer refuge at the rear of the royalist positions.[47]

That night, as the frost gathered on the ground, Harvey was relieved of the King's children and returned to treating the

wounded. One was Sir Gervase Scrope. He had been left for dead
in the field, awaking from a coma at midnight and drawing a dead
body to his barely living one for warmth. Found by his son, he was
taken back to the royal encampment and treated by Harvey, who
was credited with saving his life.

In return for his help at Edgehill, the King later gave Harvey a portrait of the Prince of Wales being presented with a helmet by his
younger brother. Not yet a teenager, Prince Charles is depicted as
already aged by the responsibilities of his rank, holding a staff over the
decapitated head of Medusa while the battle rages in the background.
Harvey would have no further part in the terrors portrayed.[48]

Two days after Edgehill, news reached London that Essex had
achieved a 'little victory', but was on his way back hotly pursued
by the King. Under the direction of the Committee of Safety, the
capital once again went into a spasm of defensive activity. 'It were
endless,' a royalist in London observed caustically, 'to relate all the
means used to heighten the fears of this miserable City.' The women,
he noted, who had 'hugged their Husbands into this Rebellion',
provided 'hot water (besides what they sprinkled for fear) to throw
on the Cavaliers; joint-stools, forms, and empty tubs are thrown
into the Streets to intercept the Horse'.[49]

Sheds clustered around the city walls were pulled down to prevent
them being used to breach the defences, arms were taken from the
Tower (now under parliamentary control) and dispersed, a census
was made of the capital's horses, guard posts were further reinforced
with wooden barricades and 'great chains of iron', volunteers and
members of the Trained Bands were put on 24-hour alert with
orders to 'seize and arrest all suspicious persons, Ammunition or
Arms passing through their Parishes', and fourteen troops of horse
were dispatched to patrol the highways at night, reporting anyone
seen travelling towards the city.[50]

Dwarfing all these initiatives was the construction of the 'Lines
of Communication'. On 10 August 1642, Parliament had issued a
set of 'Directions for the Defence of London', which called for the

mobilization of tens of thousands of citizens to build a vast defensive barricade surrounding the entire conurbation.[51] To aid the effort, all shops were ordered to shut while citizens gathered according to their livery company or trade, with whatever tools they possessed, and then set off for the city's perimeter. Eight thousand tailors assembled, together with seven thousand watermen, five thousand cobblers, and a thousand 'oyster women' from the fish market at Billingsgate. A Scots visitor witnessed the immense mobilization: 'The daily musters and shows of all sorts of Londoners here were wondrous commendable, in marching to the fields (as merchants, silk-men, macers, shop-keepers &c,) with great alacrity, carrying on their shoulders iron mattocks and wooden shovels; with roaring drums, flying colours, and girded swords.' The companies were 'interlarded' with women and girls, walking two by two, carrying baskets of provisions to sustain the workers, many of whom 'fell sick of their pains'. It was early winter, and the conditions were freezing. Nevertheless, they did not 'even cease to work on Sunday', noted the Venetian ambassador, 'which is so strictly observed by the Puritans'. Royalists thereafter greeted advancing parliamentary troops with choruses of 'Round headed cuckolds come dig'.

The digging unearthed some interesting material, notably at Mile End in the east Sir Kenelm Digby, who was trying to reach the royalist forces in disguise. Digby was a member of Queen Henrietta Maria's household and had been exiled to France by Parliament. He had just returned to England after killing a French nobleman, who had insulted Charles I, in a duel. He was a flamboyant figure, a Catholic with an interest in magic and medicine. He had tried to conjure up a spirit with William Lilly's tutor John Evans, the pedlar of antimonial cups. Digby was also famous for his unorthodox remedies, such as the 'Powder of Sympathy', which he claimed could heal a wound by being applied to the weapon that caused it, and a cure for bad breath which involved sufferers holding their mouths open over a privy.[52]

By December 1642, just four months after work had begun, a

An
EXPLANATION
of the
several FORTS, *on the*
Line of
COMMUNICATION.

1 *A Bulwark & half on the Hill*
at the North-end of Gravel Lane.

2 *A Hornwork near the Wind-*
mill in White-chapel Road .

3 *A Redoubt with 2 Flanks ,*
near Brick Lane .

4 *A Redoubt with 4 Flanks ,*
in Hackney Road, Shoreditch.

5 *A Redoubt with 4 Flanks , in*
Kingsland Road, Shoreditch.

6 *A Battery & Breastwork ,*
at Mountmill .

7 *A Battery & Breastwork ,*
at St. John's Street End .

8 *A small Redoubt , near*
Islington Pound .

9 *A large Fort with four*
half Bulwarks , at the
new River upper Pond .

10 *A Battery & Breastwork on*
the Hill E. of Blackmary's hole.

11 *Two Batteries & a Breast-*
work , at Southampton , now
Bedford House .

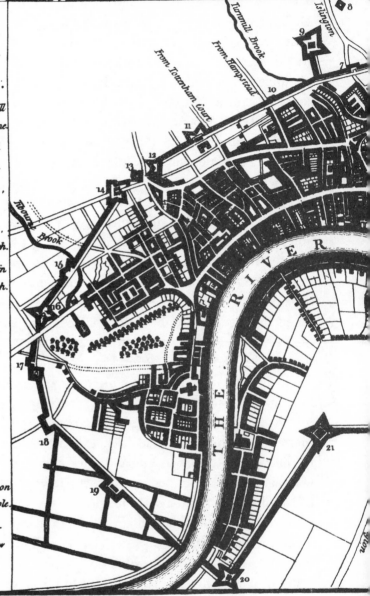

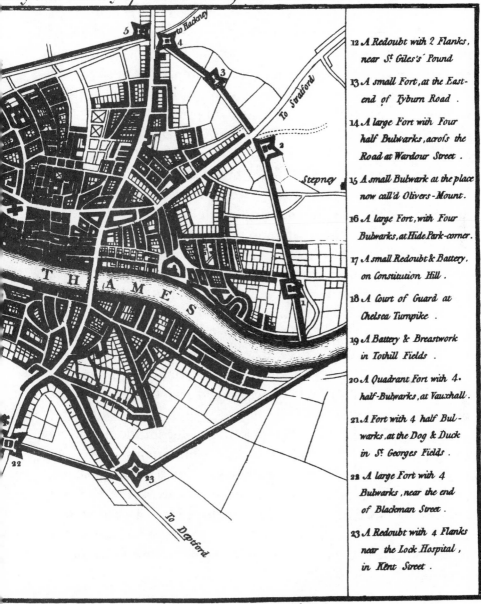

12 *A Redoubt with 2 Flanks,*
   near S.ᵗ Giles's Pound

13 *A small Fort, at the East-*
   end of Tyburn Road.

14 *A large Fort with Four*
   half Bulwarks, across the
   Road at Wardour Street.

15 *A small Bulwark at the place*
   now call'd Olivers-Mount.

16 *A large Fort, with Four*
   Bulwarks, at Hide Park-corner.

17 *A small Redoubt & Battery,*
   on Constitution Hill.

18 *A Court of Guard at*
   Chelsea Turnpike.

19 *A Battery & Breastwork*
   in Tothill Fields.

20 *A Quadrant Fort with 4.*
   half-Bulwarks, at Vauxhall.

21 *A Fort with 4 half Bul-*
   warks, at the Dog & Duck
   in S.ᵗ Georges Fields.

22 *A large Fort with 4*
   Bulwarks, near the end
   of Blackman Street.

23 *A Redoubt with 4 Flanks*
   near the Lock Hospital,
   in Kent Street.

ed *by* Order *of* PARLIAMENT, *in the* Years *1642* & *1643.*

99, at the Kings Arms, N.ᵒ 16, Paternoster Row.

continuous fortification stretched from Wapping to the east to
Chelsea in the west, from Islington in the north to Nine Elms in
the south: 'eighteen Kentish miles' of trenches, ditches, and dykes,
with twenty-four forts, some very substantial. They were ungainly
angular structures, with several jutting ramparts 'contrived and
reared after the modern model of an impregnable citadel', bristling
with twenty or more cannon mounted on platforms of sturdy oak,
protected by roofs tiled with stone. One of the largest fortifications,
a pair of four-sided 'redoubts' straddling the Great North Road
at Shoreditch, stood less than two hundred yards from Nicholas
Culpeper's front door. He would have seen it rising up in the latter
months of 1642, if he did not actually help build it.[53]

The Lines of Communication were an astonishing achievement,
arousing awe among visitors and pride in Londoners. To many of
those who had toiled over its walls and embankments, it was a
monument to Protestant resolution. Many had heard through
foreign bulletins of the fate of Magdeburg, a prosperous German
city on the front line of the Protestant Reformation. In 1631, after
withstanding a two-year siege, it was sacked by Catholic imperial
forces, who butchered twenty to thirty thousand citizens and laid
waste the buildings. These defences would save the godly citizens
of London from a similar fate.

But not everyone saw it that way. Even as the fortifications were
being constructed, there were sporadic demonstrations in favour of
peace, and protests about the enormous tax burden the capital was
having to bear to pay for the parliamentary forces. The Venetian
ambassador noted of the forts that 'the shape they take betrays that
they are not only for defence against the royal armies, but also against
tumults of the citizens and, to ensure a prompt obedience on all
occasions'.[54]

As the winter of 1642 set in, and the fortifications reached completion, Parliament and its supporters published ever more lurid reports of royalist atrocities. The Earl of Cumberland, whose troops of northerners were particularly feared by Londoners, was said to be cutting off the hands of any who refused to lend money to the royalist cause; at Henley, Prince Rupert hanged a man from a tree near a bowling alley for alerting townsfolk to the army's approach; at Brentford, just ten miles west of the city, twenty local parliamentary sympathizers were tied up and thrown into the Thames.

Intermingled with this news, the wood turner Nehemiah Wallington noted other, ominous portents, such as a tempest in Norwich, 'the thunder sounding distinctly as if great pieces of ordnance had been shot off', and which in a nearby village raged so violently that an 'abundance of rooks and [jack]daws sitting upon the trees were stricken dead, insomuch that one hundred and eleven of their carcasses were found the next morning ... [with] their bones and bodies terribly rent and shattered, and not one drop of blood was to be seen, either upon the ground, the trees, or their carcasses'. He heard of 'divers great flashes of fire' seen in the north-west, like flashes of cannon fire, and of a mysterious glow in Suffolk on a moonless night, bright enough to read by. It was as if heaven was rehearsing the terrible conflict about to erupt on earth. 'Suddenly every man was to let his servant be tested to go forth in his arms with all expedition.' Among them was William Grant, Wallington's apprentice since 1637. During the night, Nehemiah lay awake, listening to the rumble of wagons carrying shot and powder through the city.[55]

On 12 November 1642 a deputation went to the Common Council to plead for London's Trained Bands to be called up. Until now they had played no part in the hostilities, as they were supposed to have a non-partisan, defensive role. However, the Council agreed that the time had come for them to be deployed. Under the leadership of Major General Skippon, they marched along the Strand, through St James's, and on to Hammersmith, beyond which lay 'the great guns ready to be drawn up as there should be occasion'. 'Come on my brave boys,' Skippon called as he rode between the companies. 'Let us pray heartily and fight heartily.'

BRYONY, OR WILD VINE

Bryonia dioica

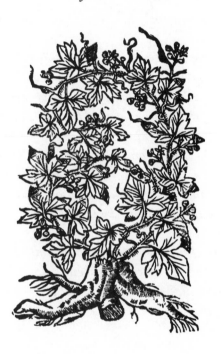

The Common white Briony groweth ramping upon the Hedges, sending forth many long rough very tender branches at the beginning with many very rough broad Leavs theron, cut (for the most part) into five partitions, in form very like a Vine Leaf, but smaller, rougher, and of a whitish or hoary green colour . . .

The Berries [are] separated one from another more than a Cluster of Grapes, green at the first, and very red when they are through ripe, of no good scent, but of a most loathsom tast provoking Vomit: The Root groweth to be exceeding great with many long Twines or Branches grow- ing from it of a pale whitish colour on the outside, and more white within, and of a sharp, bitter loathsom tast.

It groweth on Banks, or under Hedges, through this Land the Roots lie very deep.

It Flowereth in July and August, some earlier and some later than others.

The Roots of the Briony purge the Belly with great Viol- ence, troubling the Stomach, and hurting the Liver, and therfore not rashly to be taken, but being corrected is very profitable for the Diseases of the Head, as Falling-sickness, Giddiness, and Swimmings . . .

The Leavs, Fruit, and Root, do clens old and filthy Sores, are good against al fretting and running Cankers, Gangrenes, and Tetters [skin eruptions such as eczema], and therfore the Berries are by some Country People called Tetter-Berries.

The Root clenseth the Skin wonderfully from al black and blew Spots, Freckles, Morphew, Leprosie, foul Scars, or other deformity whatsoever: as also al running Scabs, and Manginess are healed by the Pouder of the dried Root, or the Juyce therof.

In France white bryony is called *Navet du Diable*, or Devil's Turnip, because of the violent and dangerous action of the milky juice that oozes from its fleshy root. Gerard recalled being shown by Queen Elizabeth's surgeon, William Godorous, a bryony root as big as a one-year-old child, weighing half a hundredweight (56 lb).[1]

According to a nineteenth-century herbal, the roots were used to make counterfeit mandrakes. The mandrake (*Mandragora autumnalis*, a member of the nightshade family) was a plant attributed with extraordinary magical and aphrodisiac powers. When it was pulled from the ground it was said to emit a scream, and the shape of the root that emerged often resembled a human body. But mandrake, which grew commonly in southern Europe, was hard to cultivate in colder English climes, so impostors would use bryony to manufacture fakes:

> The method which these knaves practised was to open the earth round a young, thriving Bryony plant, being careful not to disturb the lower fibres of the root; to fix a mould, such as is used by those who make plaster figures, close to the root, and then to fill in the earth about the root, leaving it to grow to the shape of the mould, which is effected in one summer.[2]

he astrologer John Gadbury studied Nicholas Culpeper's birth-chart or 'nativity' soon after his death. Under a section entitled 'The Accidents by which this Nativity was verified' he noted that for the year 1643 the stars signified that Culpeper was subject to 'directions of so evil Tendency and Import, that might very well have ruined a king'. And so it proved to be.

He had already run into serious trouble. Some time after his marriage he had fought a duel. When, over what and with whom is unclear, but as a result he had to pay for his opponent's treatment and flee to France for three months, presumably to escape a warrant for his arrest. Then, in December 1642, as the Trained Bands were mobilized for war, he faced an even more serious charge: an accusation of witchcraft. A widow named Sarah Lynge visited Nicholas at St Mary Spital seeking medical help. After consulting him, she started to 'waste away', and continued to do so for a month. On the basis of this, she accused Nicholas of using witchcraft upon her. The charge was taken seriously, and led to Nicholas being arrested in January 1643. He was gaoled, probably in Newgate Prison, one of London's toughest gaols.[3]

Accusations of witchcraft were not rare at this time. For the accused to be a man was unusual, but not unknown; and in the fraught atmosphere produced by the threat of London's imminent invasion, denunciations of all sorts filled the air.[4] Widow Lynge may have been seeking redress for Nicholas's failure to cure her, or for making her condition worse. The most obvious recourse for such a complaint was to the College of Physicians, but since the

King had left the capital the Censors had become timid. The House of Commons, meanwhile, had decided to launch a review of medical practice and was proving itself dangerously attentive to the complaints of the College's critics.

The College had pragmatically adapted to the changing situation by becoming more parliamentarian, at least in appearance. In 1640, the President, Simeon Foxe, had been calling for volunteers 'to serve his Majesty in the war intended', and helping to appoint Fellows to act as physicians to the royalist army. But by 1643 both he and John Argent were dead, removing two of the leading conservative figures. Foxe's replacement as president was Othowell Meverall. He adopted a policy of acceptance towards the parliamentary regime, in return for the maintenance of the College's privileges, such as exemption of Fellows from military service. Under his presidency, the College agreed to raise money for and administer oaths of loyalty to the parliamentary cause. It also patched up its relationship with the City, and in return the 'quill' or water supply, which had been cut off for a decade, was reconnected. The Comitia had even allowed Humfrey Brooke, a physician well known for his radical sympathies, to become a Fellow, whilst discouraging the fully-qualified Walter Charleton for no detectable reason other than his obstinate royalism.[5] By 1642 they were proving so eager to appear submissive that Ralph Bishop, Vice-Chancellor of Cambridge University, was complaining that the university's medical students were no longer bothering to graduate because they could so easily practise in London without degrees.[6]

It was in this context that Nicholas Culpeper found himself under arrest. Perhaps Sarah Lynge thought, or was encouraged to believe, that the courts would provide a more punitive response than the subdued College of Physicians. If so, she was wrong. Nicholas was tried before a jury in mid-January 1643 and acquitted.

However, within days, he was under attack again, this time through his association with his former fellow apprentice Samuel Leadbetter. On 31 January 1643, the court of the Society of Apothecaries, possibly at the behest of the College, passed a motion ordering that 'Mr Leadbetter's plaster shall be destroyed'.[7] A subsequent entry, dated 3 June, 'ordered and warned' Leadbetter 'to put away Nicholas Culpeper who so now employed in his shop'.

It is odd that the Society of Apothecaries should have spent so much effort prosecuting Nicholas in the midst of a national emergency. The apothecaries' court at this time was overwhelmed by much weightier concerns: demands for contributions to city funds and Parliament's war chest; the invasion of its hall by members of the Trained Bands trying to find secure storage for their arms; and the Society's own armaments programme, which had resulted in the purchase of muskets, helmets, swords, pikes, and armour and two barrels of gunpowder. The court was also concerned about the lack, rather than excess, of apothecaries in the capital. At the time, a substantial number of apprentices had broken their bonds or had won their freedom and chosen not to practise. The reasons for this are unclear, but presumably many had signed up to fight, and many more could not see themselves making a living in London at a time of such economic and political chaos.[8] All this leaves the distinct impression that Nicholas was under attack for more than medical misdemeanours.

At the outbreak of the Civil War, one of the charges levelled against radicals was the biblical nostrum that 'Rebellion is as the sin of witchcraft'. The royalist newspaper *Mercurius Aulicus* claimed that witchcraft was a 'usual attendant on former rebellions', and others noted that, since the outbreak of hostilities, the number of witches had proliferated, 'more ... ever this Island bred since the Creation'. The *Parliamentary Journal* observed that 'it is the ordinary mirth of the malignants of this city to discourse of the association of witches'.[9]

Perhaps, then, Nicholas was under attack for his links to political radicalism. At around this time, opinion within the city was polarizing between those wanting to fight for political liberties and those anxious to reach a settlement – the so-called 'war' and 'peace' parties. John Goodwin led the rallying cry for the war party. In 1642 he published *Anti-cavalierisme* with a subtitle clearly indicating its tenor: *Truth pleading, as well the necessity as the lawfulnesse of this present warre, for the suppressing of that butcherly brood of cavaliering incendiaries, who are now hammering England, to make an Ireland of it.* It was an extraordinary production, drawing great dark clouds of political fury from the cauldron of Coleman Street. The royal prerogative had expanded to a 'monstrous & most unnatural proportion', and Londoners must fight to contain it, else their liberties would be lost. 'Give me leave in that which remains, to excite and stir you up, from the greatest to the least, both young and old, rich and poor, men and women.' For Goodwin, war was being joined not just with the King, but with the anti-Christ, in an apocalyptic struggle being conducted by Protestants across the world, 'amongst which likewise I comprehend those plantations of our Brethren of this Land, in America, and other Western parts, at least between all that are truly faithful'.[10] People who backed Goodwin's view attacked Parliament's conduct of the war as pusillanimous, held back by aristocratic sensitivities and special interests. Graffiti appeared showing the Earl of Essex, the leader of the parliamentary forces, lounging in an easy chair, holding a glass of wine in one hand and a pipe in the other.

On the opposite side, a 'peace' party, made up of peers and wealthy citizens, was active. It was not an homogenous group, ranging from parliamentary appeasers to outright royalists, but its members wielded considerable influence. They included Sir George Binyon, a leading merchant, Sir Paul Pindar, a financier, and Sir Nicholas Crispe, a slaver, Master of the East India Company, and, while secretly financing the King's army, until 1642 a member of the Society of the Artillery Garden.[11]

There was also the Westminster Assembly of Divines, made up of 121 ordained ministers and a selection of lay members drawn from Parliament. It was set up in July 1643 to run the Church, replacing the bishops. As it gained strength, cracks emerged between the 'Presbyterians', followers of the Scottish model who emphasized centralized discipline, and 'Independents' who wanted congregations to have more power over their own religious affairs. Several of the Independent members of the Assembly, the so-called Dissenting Brethren, who had been exiles in Holland during the Laud era, protested at the Presbyterians' increasing authoritarianism, and a clear split opened up between the two factions. One manifestation of this was the Presbyterians' increasing hostility to the unorthodox ideas and practices associated with independency, in particular astrology.[12]

It was in the midst of these fractures and arguments that Nicholas, medical astrologer and alumni of Goodwin's 'school of all ungodliness', found his own fortunes coming under attack.

'Novelty beyond novelties', one bewildered observer described it in the summer of 1643: the palace of Whitehall, the hub of royal government, lay empty. Holbein Gate, once portal to Henry VIII's seat of power, was patrolled, not by plumed bodyguards but by motley citizens. 'And which was more rarer', in the courtyard around the King's house, the grass grew deep.[13] London had ceased to be part of the kingdom. It was an independent republic, with its own army and government.[14] 'The proud, unthankful, schismatical, rebellious, bloody city of London', one royalist pamphlet called the capital. John Berkenhead, the Oxford academic and protégé of Laud, reached for a medical metaphor: London would 'dissolve the nerves, and luxate [dislocate] the sinews of this admirable composed government'. The only remedy was 'reducing this stubborn city either to obedience or ashes'.[15]

But Charles was not yet ready to administer such drastic treatment, and the expected confrontation over control of the capital failed to materialize. The best that could be managed was a face-off at Turnham Green, to the west of the city, between Prince Rupert's troops and the combined forces of the Trained Bands and Essex's army, which, following the indecisive battle of Edgehill, had marched swiftly back to London via the Roman road of Watling Street. Rupert, outnumbered two to one, withdrew without a bullet being fired, leaving the London militiamen to celebrate by feasting on 'many Cartloads of provisions and wine' sent by their wives. For many who were there, the apprentice wood turners, lawyers, and watermen, this was their first experience of deployment, and it was exhilarating. The MP Bulstrode Whitelocke, who had volunteered to 'trail a pike' among the foot soldiers of John Hampden's regiment of Buckinghamshire greencoats, was so overcome with excitement that he nearly ended up on a charge for questioning the Earl of Essex's orders.[16]

The King withdrew to Oxford, where he set up a court and later a parliament in exile. The royal party found the university atmosphere convivial. William Harvey was especially at home among the colleges. While his loyalties to the King remained as firm as ever, he was in his sixties and wanted nothing more to do with the war. His only desire was to continue his scientific work, and Oxford, though garrisoned and hectic with military and diplomatic traffic, provided something of a refuge. On 7 December 1642, shortly after his arrival, he was awarded an MD (doctorate in medicine) by the university on the basis of his previous medical education (over which the university records are confused, describing him as 'incorporated' at Cambridge, though there is no evidence of him ever having studied there).[17] He soon started to take an active interest in the university's affairs and to avail himself of its unparalleled academic facilities. However, the impositions of war could not be completely ignored. When asked by a colleague if his affairs were satisfactory, Harvey replied: 'How can they [be] . . . when the Commonwealth is surrounded by intestine troubles? . . . If the comfort of my studies, and the remembrance of many things, long since fallen under my observation, were not some refreshment to my mind, I know not what could prevail upon me to survive the present.'[18]

In the winter of 1642, Harvey's twin brothers Matthew and Michael, who were in London, both fell gravely ill. He could not visit them, and they came under the care of Dr Baldwin Hamey – an enthusiastic uroscopist who diagnosed illness from urine samples even when the patient was not present.[19] Though he used such discredited methods, Harvey trusted him.

Matthew died on 21 December 1642. Three weeks later a letter got through to Harvey at Oxford about Michael, 'who also frequently threatens departures'. Addressing Harvey as 'Excellency', Hamey's report is written in ornate Latin (Hamey was a classicist, eager to promote the medical use of Greek and Latin as well as urine), filled with references to Hippocrates and Galen, and describing in detail Michael's symptoms, which he was 'safe in agreeing with your opinion and with ancient opinion' indicated scurvy. Hamey had prescribed a clyster, a 'julep of specifics for liver and spleen', a 'light vomitory', which yielded a great quantity of phlegm. This produced temporary relief, which was confirmed by Hamey's examination of Michael's urine, which 'became free from all sediment, deposits or reddish clouding'. He was 'fortified by an electuary of antiscorbutics', but soon relapsed. His humours becoming 'tartaric and malignant', Hamey treated him with a course of emetics and purgatives. His efforts were in vain. By the time Harvey received Hamey's letter, Michael too was dead.[20]

Soon after, Harvey received more bad news. His post as physician at St Bartholomew's Hospital had been confiscated and given to Dr John Micklethwaite, one of a new generation of Fellows. Micklethwaite was friendly to parliamentary supporters, and was an angling companion of the astrologer William Lilly.

With his personal, professional, and political links with London now severed, Harvey devoted himself to life at Oxford. The memoirist and gossip John Aubrey, then a young student, remembered seeing him at the university, though 'too young to be acquainted with so great a doctor'. He recalled Harvey making regular visits to Trinity College to see George Bathurst, a theological scholar, 'who had a hen to hatch eggs in his chamber, which they daily opened to discern the progress and way of generation'. Harvey's work with Bathurst was to inspire some of the most accomplished scientific writings of his career.

Harvey also continued as best he could to foster the fraternal values of the College of Physicians for those, like him, exiled from Amen Corner. He secured a doctorate in medicine for his friend Charles Scarbrugh, who had been assisting him on some of his embryological experiments. Scarbrugh (1614–93) was a more belli-cose royalist, and eager to fight for the King. When he left to join the royalist army, Harvey wrote to him protectively, 'Prithee leave off thy gunning and stay here. I will bring thee into practice.'[21]

Harvey went on to become Warden of Merton College, in the face of objections from rivals who claimed he was ineligible because he was a 'stranger' – not a member of the college. The protests were quashed by the intervention of the King himself, who, in a letter to the college, announced that it was 'Our Will and Command . . . that according to your accustomed manner you forthwith receive and admit the said Dr William Harvey . . . to have and enjoy the Warden-ship of the said house or College, with all the rights, Emoluments and profits thereunto belonging'. Furthermore, these rights, emoluments, and profits were to be enjoyed in 'as ample and beneficial manner' as those of the previous Warden, who had been forced from his position due to his sympathies with the parliamentary cause.[22]

Harvey continued to practise medicine at Oxford and was also called upon to make occasional emergency excursions. In October 1643, he went to Milton Abbot in the south-west of the country to attend Prince Rupert's brother Maurice, who had come down with a fever, assumed to be the 'ordinary raging disease of the Army', which Harvey decided, being 'very dangerous and fraudulent', should be treated with 'very little physic, only a regular diet and cordial antidotes'.[23]

Harvey may also have been tangentially involved when a parliamentary commission arrived from London in the spring of 1643 to negotiate with the King. Among them was the conciliatory MP Bulstrode Whitelocke, who, while negotiating with the King's counsellors over a possible peace treaty, 'fell extreme sick of a violent fever'. A Dr Turner, a royal physician, offered to help. Whitelocke had met Dr Turner before the outbreak of the war and liked him, knowing him to be 'much addicted to drollery or raillery & plain speaking'. Having 'asked many questions' about Whitelocke's 'distemper, & considered of it above an hour together over several pipes of Tobacco, at length he told Whitelocke that he was very ill indeed, & in much danger'. Turner then announced that, although Whitelocke 'was a Traitor & a Rebel against his King, yet as to his own person he knew him to be an honest man, & would prescribe him that which would recover him'. Such tokens of gallantry were a peculiarity of these troubled times, at least in the participants' recollections, and stood in relief to the gruesome treatment combatants meted out to each other on the battlefield. Turner wrote a prescription and advised Whitelocke to 'send for it to his own Apothecary' so there was no suspicion of poisoning, which Whitelocke did, against the advice of the other commissioners. After taking the medicine, he 'slept reasonably well that night, & within a few days after was abroad again'.

During his illness, Whitelocke was lodged at Merton College. Harvey was not yet the Warden, but, given his prominent role in the royal medical team and his links to the college, he was likely to have known about, and perhaps even advised on, Whitelocke's treatment.

Despite the intervention, and Whitelocke's recovery, the commission failed, in a manner that became characteristic of the endless, fruitless negotiations to follow. As Whitelocke put it:

> The King in this Treaty shewed great abilities, in his apprehension, reason & judgement, but his unhappiness was to trust

others judgement more then his own, to his prejudice, for having agreed with the Com[missione]rs upon a point of the Treaty, they prayed his answer accordingly, but the King told them it was then too late to write it, being midnight, but bid them come to him the next morning & they should have it in writing as he had agreed it. They attended him the next morning & then he gave them his answer in writing to that point, quite contrary to what he had agreed the night before.[24]

What Whitelocke did not know was that before they had even arrived in Oxford, the King had already made arrangements for an armed rising in London. A group of seventeen prominent citizens, including the Recorder of London, Sir Thomas Gardener, were instructed to 'consult, advise, and resolve of all such things, and of such ways and means as . . . you shall think fittest, for the raising of Forces both of Horse and Foot' to take the city. The King's plot was discovered and two of the leaders were hanged outside their own houses, hefty bribes saving most of the others.[25]

The episode did not ease tensions in the capital. At the end of July 1643, days after 'very great Storms, or Rain' had soaked the city, news arrived that the King had taken Bristol; a 'great loss', recorded Wallington, which 'discontented me that I could not settle about anything, nay, I could neither write, read, nor pray'.[26] August offered no consolations. There were shortages of food and fuel across the capital. 'Our rich Men are gone, because the City is the Place of Taxes and Burdens; Trade is decayed, and Shops shut up in a great measure; Our Poor do much increase,' the House of Commons was told.[27] Parliament wobbled. An MP who dared voice the thought that the country would be better off without the royal family was expelled from the House and given a fortnight in the Tower. A set of propositions amounting to surrender was passed by the House of Lords, and only just rejected by the Commons, the slenderest of majorities sustained by the sound of an angry mob of five thousand in Palace Yard accusing the pacifiers of treason.

Meanwhile, on the tenth of the month, Sir John Culpeper stood at the head of his regiment of cavaliers on the outskirts of Gloucester as a message was sent in to the city ordering its parliamentary governor, Colonel Edward Massey, to surrender. Massey refused, and the inhabitants living in the suburbs set fire to their properties and withdrew behind the city walls, where they became besieged.

In London, news of the siege once again tipped the volatile mood into panic. Within days of one mob calling for war, another, made up mainly of women, battered at the doors of the Commons demanding peace. The House of Lords emptied, as peers withdrew to their country seats, or to the King at Oxford. Though the economy was close to collapse, shops were ordered to shut to allow members of the Trained Bands to rejoin their regiments. The relief of Gloucester was urged from every pulpit. This was retribution for the city's failure to follow the Lord, 'God's axe to hew his people', warned a preacher at St Mary's Abchurch.[28]

Writing as these events unfolded, a royalist pamphleteer living anonymously in London (probably John Berkenhead, the Oxford academic and protégé of Laud), recalled: 'You may well remember when the Puritans here did abominate the Military-yard or Artillery-Garden, as Paris-Garden itself. But at last when it was instill'd into them, that the blessed Reformation intended could not be effected but by the sword, these places were instantly filled with few or none but men of that Faction.'[29] Nicholas Culpeper, now out of gaol, hopped over his back wall and was among them. He had formally joined the 'war' party, enlisting in the Trained Bands, or one of its auxiliary regiments.

'London was now about to throw its sword into the scale', as the historian S. R. Gardiner put it. No more peace, no more procrastination. In Oxford, William Harvey gazed at the 'great Metamorphosis, and wonderful alteration' of a chick forming in its egg, the war a distant distraction through the leaded glass of a college window. In London, Nicholas Culpeper took up arms for the great Metamorphosis and wonderful alteration of the State. He was preparing to fight, not merely for an adjustment of constitutional niceties, a parliamentary privilege acquired here, a royal prerogative surrendered there, but, urged on by Goodwin, for education and liberty, freedom of expression, religious toleration, and equality before the law. For, as another radical cleric put it, none could now arbitrate 'our supreme disputes' as they had become 'so full of new Revolutions, and Interpositions, especially now, when an Almighty power seems to mingle, and incorporate his own Interests with ours, and engage us upon new Fundamentals'.[30]

William Attersoll had warned against this. Quoting Livy's *History of Rome*, he wrote of Capua, 'a city flowing with wealth and super- fluity of all ... infected most with the licentious looseness of the Commons, who exceeded beyond all measure and abused their liberty'. During the second Punic War, when Hannibal's army descended from the Alps to attack the might of the Roman Empire, the people of this corrupt state, manipulated by an unscrupulous senate, lost their independence and became enslaved by Rome. This was what happened when the 'beast of many heads', the populace, prevailed.[31]

Nicholas ignored the warning. On 25 August, he was among the massed ranks of the Trained Bands who marched out of London in a great cavalcade, urged on by their wives and leaders, to relieve their brethren besieged at Gloucester.

They arrived at nearby Brentford at one in the morning and, after their first night of military life, many 'who seemed very forward and willing at the first to march with us' lost their nerve, made their 'fair excuses', and returned home, hiring others to go in their place.[32] Those who remained, Nicholas among them, joined a vast army of 14,000 that marched off on 25 August, brushing past Oxford on 31 August, and reaching Prestbury Hills, overlooking Gloucester, by 5 September 1643. Following an artillery attack on the royalist encampment, they quickly raised the siege. Having succeeded in their mission, many officers of the Trained Bands urged Essex to let them go back to London. According to the royalist newspaper *Mercurius Aulicus*, letters were being intercepted regularly from the wives of the London militiamen pleading for their husbands' return. 'Why could you not come home with Master Murphy on Saturday?' Susan, wife of one John Owen of the Blue regiment, wrote on 5 September. Master Murphy must have been among those who had made their 'fair excuses' at Brentford and turned back. 'Could you not venture as well as he? But you did it on purpose to show your hatred to me . . . Everybody can come but you.'[33]

Commanding so many soldiers untested on the field of battle, forced from the warmth of a chimney corner or the bustle of a workshop to a cold, sodden field half way across the country, Essex was loath to engage in open confrontation with the King's battle-hardened regiments. He decided to make his way back to London circuitously, feigning a movement north to split the royalist forces. Interrupted by skirmishes along the way, he managed to get as far as Hungerford, near the strategic Reading road back to London, in just over a week. There his forces rested, 'much distressed for want of sleep as also for other sustenance', one soldier recalled. 'It was a night of much rain and we were wet to the skin.'

The following day, as the troops made their way towards the town of Newbury, a curious incident occurred that later became notorious. According to a contemporary pamphlet, a group of soldiers had become separated from the main body of the army 'by reason of their loitering by the way in gathering nuts, apples, plums, blackberries and the like'. One of their number climbed a tree, 'being pursued by his fellows . . . in waggish merriment', and, looking over towards the river Kennet, which passes through Newbury, saw a tall, slender woman who, to his 'amazement and great terror', was 'treading of the water with her feet with as much ease and firmness as if one should walk or trample on the earth'. Fearing her to be a witch, the soldiers seized the woman and attempted to shoot her, one aiming his 'carbine close to her breast, where discharging, the bullet back rebounded like a ball and narrowly . . . missed his face'. Infuriated by her cackles at their futile efforts, a member of the company recalled hearing that a witch's power could be neutralized by 'piercing the temples of the head'. 'The woman hearing this knew that the Devil had left her and her power was gone, whereupon she began aloud to cry and roar, tearing her hair and making piteous moans, which in these words expressed were: "And is it come to pass that I must die indeed, why then his Excellency the Earl of Essex shall be fortunate and win the field", after which no more words could be got from her, wherewith they immediately discharged a pistol underneath her ear at which she strait sunk down and died.'[34]

The story of the witch of Newbury surfaced later, partly to counteract royalist propaganda. The witch showed that Satan was working for the cavaliers. On a more practical level, some said she was a royalist agent, sent to destroy Essex's ammunition store. However, it is more likely that the story of her gruesome killing was circulated less for political reasons than to express the traumatic experience of the engagement to come, one of the earliest in England in which the injuries and outcome were primarily the result not of hand-to-hand combat and cavalry charges, but of gunpowder and artillery.

Essex approached Newbury on 19 September, to learn from his scouts that an advance guard of the King's troops had got there first, and was blocking the way. The town was already occupied by Prince Rupert's cavalry, which was swiftly reinforced by the Life Guards, 'composed of the noblest and wealthiest cavaliers . . . with casque and plume and glittering cuirass'.[35] As Newbury was now occupied, Essex's exhausted troops were forced to spend the night in the open fields to the west of the town. They had to contend with several skirmishes before dawn disclosed the full ranks of the King's army in battle formation before them, blocking the way to London. Beyond lay Newbury, providing a safe haven to which the royalists could retreat – a formidable advantage for Essex's forces to overcome.

Nicholas Culpeper was likely to have been among the foot soldiers on the right flank, where the Trained Bands were positioned under the command of their Major General, Philip Skippon. The troops drew up to their positions at about 5 a.m. and made an immediate advance towards the main battery of the King's heavy guns, ranged along a rough earth platform in the centre of the battlefield. They pushed forward for half an hour under heavy fire without cover from their own ordnance, during which time 'the enemy's cannon did play . . . against [us]' and 'men's bowels and brains flew in our faces'.

After three hours of fighting, advancing one moment, sheltering behind hedges and banks the next, assailed by artillery throughout, they managed to reach a 'little hill', the western slope of the plateau where the heart of the King's army stood. For half an hour they repulsed an attack by two regiments of royalist infantry in their efforts to hold the ground before finding themselves surrounded by two regiments of cavalry, forcing them to charge the line of horses, 'which was performed by us with a great deal of courage and undauntedness of spirit, insomuch that we made a great slaughter among them and forced them to retreat'.[36]

The manoeuvre was crucial, securing the right flank while Essex advanced with his troops on the left. But the royalist retreat did not bring an end to the battle. A Frenchman noted that 'nothing but night could separate these furious Englishmen, who seem'd delighted to shed the blood of each other'. As darkness fell, the exhausted militiamen bivouacked on the positions they had just secured. They had no food and, despite the sodden conditions, little fresh water. One officer was reported to have offered ten shillings for a quart of refreshment. Skirmishes continued, the combatants finding each other by 'the glimmer of the matches and flashing of the fire-arms'.

The next day, the work of tending to the wounded and gathering the dead began. Estimates of the number of casualties varied from five to eight thousand. Reports circulated of sixty cartloads of dead and wounded royalist troops being transported back to Newbury. Among those found on the battleground were the thirty-three-year-old Lord Falkland and his horse, both riddled with bullets. Once a supporter of the Long Parliament who had joined the King with Sir John Culpeper, Falkland had found 'that the very agony of the war, and the view of the calamities and desolation which the kingdom did and must endure took his sleep from him and would shortly break his heart'. On the day of the Battle of Newbury he had dressed in clean linen, and announced he would 'be out of it ere night'. And so he was.[37]

But it was the clusters of more anonymous casualties that shocked onlookers. One parliamentary soldier saw a hundred bodies stripped naked strewn across the site of one clash. A royalist cavalryman came across six men decapitated by a single cannon shot, the burst skulls lying on the ground like a row of scythed poppy heads.

The dead were buried in mounds and covered over with earth to create great tumuli. Dotted across the centre of the battlefield, they would be landmarks for centuries to come. The antiquarian John Fuller, writing twenty years later, could not resist the melancholy pun that it was as if 'Newbury were so named by a sad Prolepsis' or prophecy, 'sore-signifying that that Town should afford a new burying place to many slain'.[38]

Even more striking was the state of the survivors. The combination of cannon, musket, and cavalry flying into formations of foot soldiers had left hundreds horribly maimed. A parliamentary trooper reported 'such crying . . . for the Surgeons as never was the like heard'. They were on the field, working behind the lines, administering to the wounded where they lay, but many lost or had to abandon their surgical equipment in the heat of the battle, and when the action died down they became overwhelmed by the number of casualties. They also had to struggle with new types of wounds, the most perplexing being the burns and internal trauma caused by artillery fire. Alexander Read, the surgeon who had unsuccessfully treated Nicholas Culpeper's mother, wrote: 'Man in every age doth devise new instruments of death . . . we have in our age, *Gun-shot*, the imitation of God's thunder.'[39] Nicholas would have been in no position to help the wounded. He lay among them. He had been struck by God's thunder, a bullet or shrapnel wound to the chest producing an injury from which he would never fully recover.

Few in England had experience of treating artillery wounds on this scale. The *Pharmacopoeia Londinensis* did not list any remedies specific to the terrible burns and ruptures such weapons inflicted. It listed some compounds used for treating wounds, such as *Syrupus de Pilofella* (Syrup of Mousear) and *Emplastrum de Betonica* (Plaster of Betony, 'to unite the skull when it is cracked, to draw out pieces of broken bones and cover the bones with flesh'), but none of these treatments were practical in battlefield conditions, even when the ingredients (which included frankincense, wine, and mastic tree gum) were available.

However, two important surgical textbooks had recently appeared in English which at least provided some guidance for hard-pressed field surgeons. One was an updated edition of *A profitable and necessarie booke of observations, for all those that are burned with the flame of gun powder* by William Clowes (1544–1604), Queen Elizabeth's surgeon. First published in 1596, it was reissued in 1637 by Peter Cole, who would later become Nicholas's publisher. Clowes had little experience of war wounds and most of the case studies he mentioned were the result of accidents (such as two 'gentlemen' who were blown up by a sample of gunpowder they were mixing in a heated brass pan). He advised that the burns be left alone and that ointments made with soap, honey, and lard be applied.[40]

The other book drew on experience of the Thirty Years War on the Continent, where brutal artillery battles of the sort fought at Newbury had become a sorry familiarity. It was a translation of a treatise by the German surgeon Wilhelm Fabry von Hilden (known by his Latin name Gulielm Fabricius Hildanus), rushed out in 1642. Wounds such as Nicholas's were, according to Hildanus, 'very dangerous' because they were liable to gangrene and 'sphacelus' (necrosis). The signs that this might happen were 'the skin, muscles, flesh, veins, arteries &c [being] dried and drawn together, so that the blood cannot flow to the offended part', and the intense pain causing an accumulation of humours, in the form of blood and mucus, which 'increase the burning heat'.

Hildanus' proposed treatment was that, as soon as possible, the 'blisters are to be cut and the water that floweth by reason of the Combustion, to be dried with a cloth or sponge' (Clowes had advised against such drastic measures, on the grounds that they 'will cause your patient to be in intolerable pain'). Within a day or two of the injury being sustained, the wound was to be 'separated, or at least to be cut away almost as close to the flesh, whereby the humour which is retained under the hard crust may flow forth, the Medicines may enter, and whatsoever is . . . hardened by reason of the heat may soften'.[41]

As for the medicines, there were several options. Hildanus suggested an ointment made using basil followed by a wrap soaked in a hot, soapy emulsion. Nicholas's own suggestions, had he been in a fit state to offer any, would have been simples. One remedy that he knew had been used by the Germans was saracen's confound (probably *Senecio fluviatilis*, a variety of ragwort), which grew in the sort of moist woodlands and groves surrounding the battlefield. *En route* for Gloucester, he may have anticipated the suffering he and his fellow troopers faced by picking leaves of clown's wound-wort (*Stachys germanica*), which grew in ditches 'frequently by Path sides in the Fields near about London, and within three or four miles distance about it'. It provided the basis for an effective wound dressing. The botanist Gerard heard of a man cut across the shin by a scythe who 'crept unto this herb, which he bruised with his hands, and tied a great quantity of it unto the wound with a piece of his shirt, which presently staunched the bleeding, and ceased the pain'.[42] Whatever treatment Nicholas received – probably no more than a dirty dressing – he faced an uncomfortable ride home on the back of a wagon.

The outcome of the previous day's action meant the main road to the capital was now open, and Essex was anxious to press on. London's Trained Bands had proved themselves formidable fighters, suffering 'too cheap an estimation' by their military peers, as even the royalists now accepted. One of the King's supporters, who had managed to remain in London during the war, wrote that, when he had first seen the apprentices and shopkeepers, merchants and servants drilling at the Artillery Ground in Spitalfields in 1641, 'we were wont you know to make very merry at their Training, some of them in two years' practice could not be brought to discharge a Musket without winking'. Now he was forced to concede that 'we did little imagine then, that they were ever likely to grow formidable to the State, or advance to that strength, as to be able to give the King Battle'.[43] But these men had no stomach for a drawn-out campaign. They belonged back home, at the side of their neglected workbenches and anxious wives.

On the morning of 21 September, Essex drew up his forces on the battlefield and resumed the march east for the capital. They got as far as the village of Aldermaston, near Reading. While passing through a narrow passage, their rear guard came under attack from Prince Rupert's indefatigable cavalry. Wagons tumbled, troops scattered, and horses bolted before the soldiers managed to rally and fire back. Their attackers, lacking infantry support, were eventually forced to retreat, but not before both sides suffered yet more casualties. After a stop at Reading to rest and celebrate their victory, the parliamentary army proceeded to London.

The troops arrived on 28 September to find the streets lined with thousands welcoming them home. At Temple Bar, the Lord Mayor and Aldermen in scarlet robes officially greeted them. Among the reception committee stood the MP Bulstrode Whitelocke, who presumably only now heard the news of the death of his friend Lord Falkland. Musing on the accolades ringing through the streets, he told Essex that, in the event of defeat, it would have been jeers rather than cheers that welcomed the general home. They 'honoured no man for his own worth', Essex ruefully concurred, 'but for the good they received by him'. But honour was due to these men now parading before him, who were prepared to 'leave a soft bed, close curtains and a warm chamber to lodge . . . upon the hard and cold earth'. They had left 'the choicest . . . meats and wine for a little coarse bread and dirty water, with a foul pipe of tobacco', 'the pleasing discourse and conversation of friends, wives and children for the dreadful whistling of bullets, and bodies dropping dead at one's feet'. And then, another thought passed into Whitelocke's mind, provoked by the image of the tumuli of mangled corpses on the fields of Newbury: why did so many have to die? Now it mattered to none of them whether they were royalists or rebels, Catholic or Puritan: 'All were Englishmen, and pity it was that such courage should be spent in the blood of each other.' Later, he discovered that Falkland had left a ring to his old friend Bulstrode in his will.[44]

Whitelocke's colleagues in the House of Commons did not share his qualms. Though the outcome of Newbury had not been decisive, they sensed that the tide had turned and called for a public thanksgiving 'to be given in all churches for the great success it pleased God to give the army under the command of the Earl of Essex', a collection for the wounded, and motions of thanks for the commanders.

But no such welcome or thanks awaited Nicholas Culpeper. Despite gallant participation and grievous wounds, he returned to find that, while he had been away fighting the royalists, he had been under attack at home. On 22 September, two days after the Battle of Newbury, as he lay wounded in a wagon, jostled along rutted roads back to London, his old partner Samuel Leadbetter had been formally warned by the court of the Society of Apothecaries 'not to employ Culpeper in the making or administering of any medicine, who promised to obey the same'. Leadbetter had evidently been roughly interrogated by the court. To show that Nicholas had been legitimately employed, Leadbetter produced his half of the indenture formalizing their arrangement. The court responded by demanding that he produce Culpeper's half.

By the following spring, Leadbetter had somehow managed to retrieve the other half of the indenture from Nicholas, even as his friend recovered from his wounds. On 13 May, Leadbetter pledged to the Society that he had 'discharged' Nicholas, handing over the missing section to the Society as evidence. As the pieces of paper were reunited, the partnership and friendship between Nicholas and Leadbetter was dissolved. An associate of Nicholas's later noted that he had 'divers pretended Friends, but was rather prejudiced then bettered by them; and when he most stood in need of their Friendship and Assistance, then they most of all deceived him'.[45]

The medical authorities could now claim to be free of Nicholas, but equally Nicholas could claim to be free of them. The world had changed since he had last been in Leadbetter's shop – 'turned upside down', in a favourite biblical phrase of the time – and those pushed to the bottom now felt themselves rising to the top.[46]

HEMLOCK

Conium maculatum

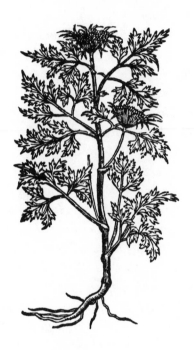

The Common great Hemlock groweth up with a green stalk four or five foot high or more, ful of red spots somtimes, and at the Joynts very large winged leavs set at them which are divided into many other winged leaves, one set against another dented about the edges, of a sad green colour branched towards the top where it is full of Umbles of white Flowers, and afterwards with whitish flat Seed: The Root is long, white, and somtimes crooked and hollow within, the whol Plant and every part hath a

strong, heady, and ill favor'd scent, much offending the Senses.

It groweth in all Countries of this Land by Wals and Hedges sides, in wast Grounds and untilled places.

It Flowreth and Seedeth in July, or there abouts.

Hemlock is exceeding cold and very dangerous, especially to be taken inwardly:

It may safely be applied to Inflamations, Tumors, and Swelling in any part of the Body (save the Privy parts) as also to St Anthonies fire Wheals, Pushes, and creeping Ulcers that rise of hot sharp Humors, by cooling and repelling the heat. The Leavs bruised and laid to the Brow or Forehead, is good for their Eyes that are red and swollen, as also to take away a Pin and Web growing in the Eye, this is a tried Medicine; Take a smal Handful of the Herb and half so much Bay Salt beaten together, and applied to the contrary Wrest of the Hand for twenty four Hours, doth remove it in thrice dressing. If the Root hereof be roasted under the Embers, wrapped in double wet Papers, until it be soft and tender, and then applied to the Gout in the Hands or Fingers it will quickly help this evil.

If any shall through mistake eat the Herb Hemlock instead of Parsly, or the Root instead of a Parsnip (both which it is very like) whereby hapneth a kind of Phrensie, or Perturbation of the senses, as if they were stupified or drunk, the Remedy is as Pliny saith, to drink of the best and strongest pure Wine, before it strike to the Heart, or Gentian put into Wine or a draught of good vinegar, wherewith Tragus doth affirm that he cured a Woman that had eaten the Root.

Saturn claims Dominion over the Herb, yet I wonder why it may not be applied to the privities in a Priapismus, or continual standing of the Yard, it being very beneficial for that Disease.

Though better known as the deadly poison that Socrates was condemned to drink, hemlock has been used as a medicine since antiquity. The active constituent is Coniine ($C_8H_{17}N$), a colourless, oily liquid universally described as having a 'mouse-like' odour. In modern times, medicines derived from this alkaloid have been used to treat insomnia, restlessness, and 'sexual excesses'. Toxic doses produce thirst, nausea, dizziness, staggering gait, paralysis, dilated pupils, and convulsions terminating in death. 'In rare instances coma ensues, but usually consciousness and the intellect remain unimpaired until death.'[1]

‘he Lion of righteousness being dead, there shall arise a White and Noble King in Britain: first of all flying, after that riding on horseback; some time after that departing or descending, and in that his decease or departure he shall be limed or ensnared. Moreover it shall be reported, and pointed as it were with the finger, yonder is the White and Noble King.’[2]

So began the ancient prophecy of an anonymous Welsh sage. The astrologer William Lilly claimed to have come across these words in Sir Robert Cotton's cramped library next to Westminster Palace, among bookcases, each topped by a bust of a Roman emperor, that contained over a thousand books and scrolls.

Lilly published the prophecy in a book, *A Prophecy of the White King, and Dreadfull Dead-man Explaned*, which appeared on 6 August 1644, sold by John Sherley and Thomas Underhill at the sign of the Golden Pelican in Little Britain, near Smithfield. It was the first English version of the text, though Lilly, whose Latin was not very advanced, does not mention who made the translation. It is possible the work was done by Nicholas, who was certainly in the right place at the right time, with connections that may have brought him into contact with Lilly during the period. He was later identified as Lilly's collaborator and protégé.

The Golden Pelican was inundated. Eighteen hundred copies were sold within three days of publication, making the work the bestseller of the time by a wide margin.[3]

Lilly had already made a name for himself as an astrological seer. In April 1644, he had published an almanac called *Merlinus Anglicus*

Junior, an early test case for the censorship regime set up following the outbreak of the Civil War.

Censorship was in chaos after the courts of the Star Chamber and High Commission were banned in 1642 as they had been the government's primary instruments of press control. Parliament had tried to regain control by passing an ordinance 'for the regulating of printing, and for suppressing the great late abuses and frequent disorders in printing many false, scandalous, seditious, libellous and unlicensed pamphlets, to the great defamation of religion and government'. It authorized 'the masters and wardens of the Company of Stationers to make diligent search, seize and carry away all such books as they shall find printed, or reprinted by any man having no lawful interest in them, being entered into the hall book to any other man as his proper copies'.[4] The ordinance did not have the desired effect, as by the time it was introduced, in June 1643, the capital was awash with so many printing houses, booksellers, and readers (between seventy and eighty per cent of London's male population could read) that it proved impossible to police.[5] Furthermore, many of Parliament's supporters were emphatically against press control. John Goodwin, for example, proclaimed from his pulpit in Coleman Street that 'the setting of Watchmen with authority at the door of the Press, to keep errors and heresies out of the world, is as weak a project . . . as it would be to set a company of armed men about a house to keep darkness out of it in the night'.[6]

Lilly's original manuscript of *Merlinus Anglicus Junior* had been full of the sorts of 'scandalous, seditious, libellous' claims Parliament was trying to stifle. Even though they were favourable to the parliamentary cause, they were too inflammatory to be allowed a public airing. The book was brought to the attention of John Booker, the 'mathematical licenser' responsible under the new regulations for authorizing the publication of astrological works at the Stationers' Company. He demanded several 'impertinent' changes, Lilly recalled, and they were duly incorporated in the first edition. However, within months Lilly had managed to get an unexpurgated version into circulation, and Booker was unable or unwilling to get it withdrawn.[7] It was in this context that *A Prophecy of the White King* appeared.

Lilly makes no mention of the identity of the White King of the title, but few who bought the book could have been in any doubt that it was Charles I, who had famously chosen to wear white robes for his coronation rather than the traditional royal scarlet. The reason for Lilly's reticence was not censorship so much as sales. In 1644, after two years of bloody war, most still assumed that elusive 'accommodation' would be found. Even radicals held back in their discussions of the alternatives. In *Anti-cavalierisme*, John Goodwin had pointed out that 'a King or Kingly Government is . . . an ordinance of man, or an human creation', an ordinance that the people could withdraw, if the government violated the Law of God. This was why the fight was 'just, and holy, and good: there is nothing in it that should make you ashamed either before God, or justly-judging men, nothing that needs make you tender, or holding off in point of conscience'. The citizens of London were right to stand up 'in the defence of your Lives, your Liberties, your Estates, your Houses, your Wives, your Children, your Brethren'. Yet even he accepted that the sovereign was 'to be obeyed and submitted unto', at least when he acted according to God's law. The nation's woes were caused by the 'vile persons that are gathered around' the King, 'as an ivy about an oak', not by the King himself.[8]

Thus Lilly insisted he was not interpreting the prophecy, merely 'paraphrasing' it. Yet, as each page was turned, so the parallels with the present became ever more obvious.

'Then shall a multitude of his people, and of his ships assembled together, and this company shall be taken from him; and then there will be chopping and changing, as if men were dealing for Horse and Ox,' the prophecy continued. 'Men shall labour for emendation of the times; but none will be; unless one head for an other; some

shall then go towards the Sun rising, and others towards the Sun
setting.' The sun rises in the east, sets in the west, and it would
not have escaped Lilly's readers, that the eastern side of the country
was by 1644 predominantly parliamentarian, the west, where the
King had his court-in-exile at Oxford, royalist.

'After these things, it will be noised all over Britain, there is a
King; nay there is no King' – a kind of 'interregnum', Lilly called
it – 'as if his Regal power should be executed by others for some
years in his so long absence', which again accurately described the
current position, with the King's rule, at least in London, arrogated
by Parliament.[9]

'After these things he shall lift up his head, and shall signify that
he is a King by his many Commissions or Actions &c, but yet no
reparation made ... See what pilling and polling, what shedding
of blood here is? Ovens are held in as much esteem as many
Churches. What man sows an other reaps, the prolonging of a
miserable life prevails, a few men are left in whom any found
charity abides.' This section seemed clear enough, and needed little
elaboration, but then came a strange – comic, Lilly admitted –
image: 'Afterwards the chicken of the Eagle will come with the Sun
upon wooden horses from the South, sailing into Britain upon a
rousing high spring tide. And then making speed to the high house
of the Eagle, thirsting, he presently thirsts after another.' The
wooden horses were obviously ships, a sort of cavalry, commanded
by this 'chicken of the Eagle'. 'Who this *Pullus Aquilae* may be; or
who the Eagle here intended, is, or was; I am silent as a man
that have no revelations; much mischief comes by such particular
interpretations,' wrote Lilly, but added: 'Eagles shew a royal regal
Family, and Chickens are harmless Creatures, during their youth,
but after they will shew of what house they are; this *Pullus Aquilae*
will prove himself a Cock of the game.' He pointedly specified that
the eagle 'does not represent the Austrian family', the Hapsburgs,
rulers of the German empire. He made this exclusion to signal that
it was linked to the Prince of Bavaria, whose armorial insignia bore

an eagle with one head, as distinct to the Imperial eagle, which had two. The Prince of Bavaria was Rupert, Charles's cousin and the commander of the royalist cavalry.

'Mercury shall then be in no esteem,' the prophecy continued, 'but every man takes care how to preserve his own, and get away goods from others.' This clearly referred to the pillaging by unpaid troops that had blighted the conduct of the war since it began. 'Afterwards the White and Noble King shall go towards the West, invironed or guarded with a great company to an antient seat near a running River' – 'near or in some ancient Town', Lilly speculated, 'perhaps Wallingford, Kingston or Reading' or perhaps further west at Oxford, Bristol, Bath, or Salisbury.

This all fitted well with events being reported in the news-sheets that daily circulated through the streets of London. Following the Battle of Newbury, the main engagements of the war had continued in the west, drawn out by the parliamentary army's lack of central command. The next part of the prophecy seemed to address this deficiency directly: '[The White King's] enemies shall then meet from all parts and shall order the battle against him . . . At that time he shall be assaulted before and behind, or on all sides, and then the white and noble King shall die.'

In October 1644 Lilly issued *England's Propheticall Merline*. Where the *Prophecy of the White King* was not overtly concerned with astrology, it did place the prophecy in the context of a number of planetary 'marvels', notably the 'eclipse of the Sun in May 1639 . . . and the three Conjunctions of Saturn and Mars'. *England's Propheticall Merline*, in which Lilly now explicitly identified himself as successor to the Arthurian wizard, developed this theme further. Astrology was, he claimed, the key to understanding what was going on. Merlin's prophecies could not be 'unlocked' without it. However, care must be taken. 'These times suffer not all truth to be unmasked,' he warned; nevertheless, 'some will find my key . . . Rex is not always a King, nor homo a man, words have severall explications &c.' What he was presenting to the reader was a way of breaking the cosmic code of prophecies and planetary movements, but in a way that was itself encoded.[10]

Many (including Lilly's modern biographer) have characterized Lilly's astrological predictions as deliberately vague, on the assumption that they were designed to cover eventualities he had not foreseen. As the historian Ann Geneva has shown, this is certainly not the case. The manner in which he expressed his interpretations was circumspect, but the interpretations themselves were not. 'Should I speak Verity in its proper Colours,' he wrote elsewhere, 'it might procure me a lodging in Newgate [Prison].'[11]

In *England's Propheticall Merline*, there was a lengthy disposition on the conjunction (when two planets appear next to each other in the zodiac) of Saturn and Jupiter, the two largest planets. This event occurred with remarkable regularity: once every 19 years, 318 days, and 12 hours, according to the calculations of the time. It was also noted that each conjunction occurred in a different sign, but within the same 'trigon', one of the four groups of zodiacal signs associated with each of the four elements, earth, fire, water, and air. This would happen for ten successive conjunctions, then they would start to occur in a different trigon. This 200-year interval was considered to be an astrological epoch, during which time earthly affairs would be shaped by the character of the ruling trigon. In 1603, Lilly noted, a new epoch had begun, when Saturn and Jupiter conjoined in Sagittarius, a fiery sign. Entry into a fiery trigon was, Lilly claimed, associated with the rise of great monarchies. That year, he also noted, James I ascended to the English throne, thus starting the era of the Stuart dynasty.

The next conjunction, in 1623, had occurred in Leo, another fiery sign. However, in 1643, the conjunction had occurred in Pisces. Pisces was a watery sign, and it was the watery trigon that the conjunction had just left. This, as far as Lilly was concerned, was an astrological event so contrary to the natural movements of the heavenly bodies as to denote a divine portent, one that suggested a reversal of the events connected to the conjunction of 1603.

Lilly did not spell out the significance of this perversion of the cosmic order, but many of his readers would have understood. Just as 1603 marked the rise of the Stuart dynasty, so 1643 must betoken its fall. The question was not if, but when, and on that matter he was prepared to make some suggestive speculations. '1643 and 1644 we shall have very great action, nor shall it determine, or much cease,' he wrote. This was daily confirmed by the news-sheets. One compared the conduct of the war to a football game 'where one side does give the other a kind of overthrow and strikes up another's heels, but presently they rise and give the other as great a blow again'.[12] The royalists had suffered a serious defeat at Marston Moor, then the parliamentarians had surrendered at Lostwithiel in Cornwall. Innumerable battles, skirmishes, and sieges were won and lost, but not the war.

Two weeks after *England's Propheticall Merline* appeared, both armies had come full circle, facing each other across the fields of Newbury as they had done a year before. In the ensuing clashes, the advantage once again swung from one side to the other. At one point, the King himself narrowly escaped capture and was forced to withdraw. At another, his army managed to recover control of Donnington Castle, where, according to one parliamentary report, he had stored not just his artillery but his crown, his papers, and the Great Seal of State. In the end, the parliamentary general, the Earl of Manchester, judged the time was not right for an all-out assault and allowed the King's army to march away. Oliver Cromwell, now emerging as a leading figure on the parliamentary side, protested. Manchester was 'afraid to conquer', he complained.[13] Parliament was prompted by this into a complete review of the conduct of the war, which resulted in the decision to take the running of military affairs out of political hands and entrust them to the generals, who were to set up a new, professional army properly financed by taxation. These developments made Lilly's other main prediction in *England's Propheticall Merline* appear particularly pertinent: 'And so it may be hoped by this order of direction, that in the year 1645 towards the latter end thereof, we shall have a great likelihood of being in a better condition that now we are in.'

Perhaps emboldened by this forecast, in 1645 he published another pamphlet, *The Starry Messenger*, which contained his most explicit prophecy yet of the King's demise, an outcome that for most people was still unthinkable. The clue came in the pamphlet's subheading: 'An Interpretation of that strange Apparition of three Suns seene in London 19 Novemb. 1644 being the Birth Day of King Charles'.[14] The sun, everyone knew, was the sovereign of the skies. 'The King [is] the sun of the world around him, the heart of the republic,' as Harvey had put it in the dedicatory epistle of *De motu cordis*. Lilly had received several reports that on the morning of Charles's forty-fourth birthday, two 'mock suns' had appeared on either side of the real one. In the countryside, the phenomenon was well known – in Nicholas Culpeper's Sussex they were known as the 'hounds of the sun'. The scientific term is 'parhelia'. They are concentrations of light, sometimes of dazzling intensity, that appear in the sun's halo, often, as depicted on the title-page of *The Starry Messenger*, in combination with rainbows above or below.

Even in Lilly's time, some considered the phenomenon to be natural. 'Many Philosophers are of the opinion, that these false Suns ... do especially appear, when many subtle moist Clouds are betwixt us and the Sun,' Lilly wrote. 'But if that collected Clouds, or multitude of vapours, or any Natural cause, produced such a rare and unusual Apparition, why have we not such Sights oft?'[15] In Lilly's opinion, they were divine portents, like the rainbow, sent by God as a reminder of the Deluge. What, Lilly then speculated, was the meaning of a mock sun?

He first considered the question by looking at previous occurrences, noting that each appearance coincided with misfortune to a sovereign: the overthrow of a king, the outbreak of rebellion, a dispute over succession. As recently as 1622, three suns had appeared at Heidelberg, at the time of 'woeful calamities' that befell the German Palatine.[16]

THE STARRY
MESSENGER;

OR,

An Interpretation of that strange Apparition of three Suns seene in *London*, 19. *Novemb.* 1644. being the Birth Day of King CHARLES.

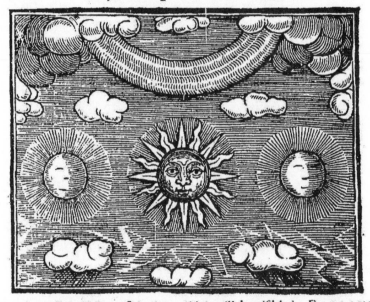

The effects of the Eclips of the Sun, which will be visible in ENGLAND, 11. *August*. 1645. whose influence continues in force, from *January*, 1646 to *Decemb.* 1647. almost two whole yeares; and cannot but be the fore-runner of some extraordinary mutation in most Common-wealths of Europe, but principally in ENGLAND. *With an Answer to an Astrologicall Judgement.* *Printed at Oxford, upon his Majesties present March.*

By WILLIAM LILLY Student in *Astrologie.*

LONDON,

Printed for *John Partridge* and *Humphry Blunden*, and are to be sold at the Signe of the *Cocke* in Ludgate Streete, and the Castle in Cornehill, 1645.

To consider the significance of the parhelia seen on Charles's birthday, Lilly turned from the examples of history to the more coded language of astrology. He reproduced a 'scheme' or astrological chart for the 'middle-time' of the apparition, 9.35 a.m., which revealed that the 'Lord of the tenth' was 'in the seventh House, Retrograde'.[17] The casual reader might think little of the observation, but it released a meteor shower of warnings and equivocations: 'Our prime men, of all Qualities, are intended to share in the Mischief hereby portended,' Lilly wrote. 'Kings, Princes, Nobility . . . I particular out no one . . . What man would run such a hazard of danger? . . . What an Ass were the Astrologian, saith Paracelsus, if upon the appearance of a Prodigious Sight in the Elements, he should say, to the face of a Prince, King or Emperor: Such a thing shall happen unto thee, Thou shalt be slain, knockt in the head with a Bullet; Thy subjects shall spoil thee, and cast thee out of thy Kingdom.' It was the identity of the 'Lord of the Tenth' that provoked this anxious outburst. The planet that rules the tenth house is Saturn. In his earlier almanac, *Merlinus Anglicus Junior*, Lilly had written that astrologers 'take the signification of the Kings or Princes from the sun, Saturn, and the planet casually posited in the tenth house'.[18] The collector George Thomason bought a copy of *Merlinus* on 12 June 1644 and annotated a 'key' provided by Lilly, writing 'Charles' in the tenth house, and 'Parlement' in the first, showing these identifications were well understood by at least some of Lilly's readers. Therefore, the king, prince, or noble Lilly refused to 'particular out' would have been relatively easy to identify as Charles, who, being 'retrograde', was to share the 'mischief hereby portended'.

'Mischief' was hardly the word. Other astrological patterns betokened a 'sudden and violent death', more explicitly still, 'that some very great man, what King, Prince or Duke, or the like, I really affirm I perfectly know not, shall, I say, come to some such untimely end'.[19] The disingenuous declaration of ignorance would have fooled few readers: Lilly was predicting the downfall of monarchy.

As *The Starry Messenger* was being prepared for printing, Lilly saw a copy of an 'Astrological Judgement' written by a rival, the royalist astrologer George Wharton, under the unfortunate pseudonym Naworth, which Lilly and other parliamentarian astrologers inevitably corrupted to 'No-worth'. Wharton launched an attack on Lilly and also on the censor John Booker, who by now had overcome his and Parliament's qualms and embraced the publication of increasingly explicit astrological attacks on the King. Their 'sole endeavour', Wharton claimed, 'hath hitherto been by most disloyal and ambiguous Phrases to animate and hasten on the Rebels and other Conspirators to plot and attempt Mischief against His Majesty'. Wharton's deciphering of the cosmic code produced a very different message from theirs. Analysing a chart drawn up for a march of the King's forces from Oxford on 7 May 1645, he concluded: 'the several Positions of the Heavens duly considered and compared among themselves ... do generally render His Majesty and his whole Army unexpectedly victorious and successful in all his Designs: Believe it (London) thy miseries approach, they are like to be many, great and grievous, and not to be diverted, unless thou seasonably crave pardon of God for being Nurse to this present Rebellion, and speedily submit to thy Princes Mercy.'[20]

Wharton's words struck a chord. A few weeks before, Parliament had dispatched its reformed 'New Model Army', now under the command of Sir Thomas Fairfax, to engage the full might of the King's forces. London jangled with anxiety. The costs of the war were eating away at the capital's economy. 'There is a general muttering that money is hard to come by,' noted a Scottish visitor, 'and that is, because all kind of trades and trading begin to decay ... Weekly taxes are great, levied to maintain the Parliament's army.'[21]

The lawyer and MP Bulstrode Whitelocke had been netting over £100 a year in fees at the beginning of the decade. Now he was forced to sell his plate and dig up some coins he had buried in case of invasion by the King's army 'to buy bread, having then nothing else to live upon'.[22] Standing at his stall, the wood turner Nehemiah Wallington faced even tougher times, taking just sixpence one market day, 'for I sold but a sack bottle, two pence, a pair of nipples, three pence, and a top, a half penny, and all in brass farthings, so that I took no silver all this day'.[23] An unexpected delivery of wood from his lumber merchant threw his finances into crisis. He was forced to accept one loan of five pounds from a widow leaving for New England, and another from his brother, whose terms included Nehemiah having to endure 'some tart words' about financial mismanagement.[24]

In his response to Wharton's warnings, Lilly added a hasty postscript to *The Starry Messenger* reassuring his readers. Ridiculing 'No-worth', he claimed: 'God is on our side; the Constellations of Heaven after a while will totally appear for the Parliament.' He also produced his own interpretation of the chart for the King's march: 'The figure doth at the beginning promise success, but the end of this march will be unlucky, and foreshow some wilful obstinate Commanders on his Majesty's side, will afford us an absolute victory over you.'[25]

On 9 June 1645, as copies of *The Starry Messenger* were coming off the presses in the Old Bailey, Bulstrode Whitelocke wrote of 'accidentally in the streets meeting with his kind friend Mr Lilly, who asked him of the news of the 2 Armies being near one another'. He was now living near to Lilly in Middle Temple, in chambers sequestered from a royalist supporter, and had intelligence that the armies were very likely to engage. 'Mr Lilly replied, if they do not engage before the eleventh day of this month, the Parliament will have the greatest victory that they ever yet had.'

Five days later, on 14 June, *The Starry Messenger* was published at the sign of the Cock in Ludgate Street, and of the Castle in Cornhill. On that day, the two armies met near Naseby, a small village in Northamptonshire. The outcome of the ensuing battle sealed the fate of the royalist cause, and the reputation of William Lilly as England's new Merlin. The battle was fought 'with great

Courage on both sides, & was exceeding bloody', wrote Whitelocke, who laid the blame for a royalist rout on an impetuous charge by Prince Rupert, the 'chicken of the Eagle', against the parliamentary left flank. 'Of their Army were slain & wounded about 1000 officers and soldiers. The King did perform his part very gallantly, the Parlemt here gained a Compleat victory.' Among the spoils was the personal cabinet of the King himself, stuffed with papers confirming the monarch's double-dealing with 'papists' and foreigners. Lilly had predicted that the Parliament could expect 'the greatest victory that they ever yet had', '& it proved accordingly', Whitelocke observed.[26]

On 14 February 1647, a group of astrologers gathered for a 'Feast of Mathematicians', the inaugural meeting of the Society of Astrologers. The venue was Gresham College, founded on a bequest from the merchant and Lord Mayor Sir Thomas Gresham (1518–79) to promote new, practical teaching methods and ideas aimed at London's merchant classes.

That first feast attracted a diverse range of figures. William Lilly was prominent, possibly as one of the organizers. Lilly's friend Bulstrode Whitelocke was a supporter, and may have looked in, though he appears to have been too busy with parliamentary business to stay. John Booker, the Stationers' Company censor, was there, as was George Wharton, the 'No-worth' ridiculed by Lilly in *The Starry Messenger*. Elias Ashmole, a thirty-year-old lawyer and a staunch supporter of the King, was there. He had slipped into London three months earlier, ignoring a post-war ban on royalists coming within twenty miles of the capital. He cut a cavalier dash amidst the Puritan austerity, wearing a cornelian ring in his ear, his hair slicked back with an ointment he applied daily to his scalp in the hope of reversing his premature baldness.[27]

Another figure who attended was the thirty-year-old Nicholas Culpeper. He had yet to publish any works of his own, but the astrological aspects of his medical practice would have been well known.

Friends and enemies, veterans and newcomers, this diverse group were all brought together in the common cause of astrological 'science', which, as they later wrote in a letter to Whitelocke thanking him for his support, 'was hardly known to this (herein unhappy) Segment of the Terrestrial Globe or (if at all) but lodged in the retired bosoms of some few', and which the Society now saw its function to make 'publique to the Benefit of this Nation'.[28]

The astrologers discussed their common interests and ideas over a lavish lunch, afterwards removing to the convivial surroundings of the White Hart Inn in the Old Bailey. Ashmole records attending the event in his diary. He was suffering with constipation at the time, concerned at his 'late stool', which he attributed to the moon being in opposition to Saturn. Showing a commitment to his art that fellow Society members surely admired, he cast a horoscope to see if he was well enough to attend. Satisfied with the result, he went to Gresham College at 1 p.m., and later went on to the White Hart. He left no record of what was discussed, only that the following day his bowel movements were restored to their former regularity.[29]

Within two years, the Society was firmly established with forty members. Ashmole was appointed steward, establishing a level of organization later developed by the Royal Society, founded at the same address in 1660.[30] Under Ashmole, promotional programmes were organized to raise the astrologers' profile. Bulstrode White-locke, who was made Commissioner of the Great Seal in 1648, was approached to see if he would become official patron.

An annual sermon was given at St Mary Aldermary, in the hope of establishing the art's theological respectability. The strategy did not work. In 1649 and 1650, the preacher was Robert Gell. In the published version of his 1650 sermon, sold by the publisher of Culpeper's astrological works, Nathaniel Brooke, Gell complained of 'the obloquy and reproach that some men have cast upon this Sermon, and the Preacher of it. That it had neither head nor tail. That in it I had defended Conjurers and Jugglers. That I held the influences of the stars so powerful that they inforced a man to sin.'[31]

Around 1650, Nicholas Culpeper delivered his own lectures to the Society, on the subject of medical astrology. Despite his relative youth – he was in his mid-thirties – he openly attacked the astrological élite who practised the horary method, even though many of them, including Lilly, were presumably in the audience. He urged them to turn their skills to practical use, in particular physic. 'Man was made not only for speculation,' he said, 'but also for practice; speculation brings only pleasure to a man's self; it is practice which benefits others.' He also rounded on those who did not pass on their astrological expertise to others. 'Of all the men in the world,' he said, 'I hate a drone most, that sucks sweetness of other men's labours, but doth no good himself; and will as soon teach Physick or Astrology to an Oak, as to a creature the center of whose actions is terminated in himself. Surely, surely, If God had not made the nature of man communicative, he would not have made one man to stand in continual need of another.'[32]

Despite Nicholas's arguments, speculation remained the astrologers' chief preoccupation. They were not supposed to discuss political matters, because the membership held such a combustible mix of views. Nevertheless, the Society's drones were abuzz with conjecture about the fate of the King and the government. Lilly led in the publication of a welter of almanacs and pamphlets prognosticating on the ever more uncertain near future.

The astrologers had plenty of material to work with. The Society's first meeting coincided with a decisive change of mood in the aftermath of the war. A split had opened up between Parliament and the army. Its cause was superficially administrative: finding a way of demobilizing the New Model Army after its great victory over the royalists. There was unrest in the ranks that soldiers would be dismissed without back pay – some were owed as much as forty-three weeks' worth. There was also the issue of legal liability for acts performed in combat, a crucial consideration in the aftermath of a civil war. In March 1647, a petition circulated through the ranks calling for these problems to be addressed, a draft of which came into the hands of a group of MPs who were visiting the army generals to draw up plans for demobilization. The petition was a measured statement of reasonable grievances posing no political threat, but once in the hands of Parliament it took on the appearance of a threat. MPs passed a furious 'Declaration of Dislike' labelling those who backed the petition, which included many of the army's leading officers, as 'enemies of the state'. Any hope of Parliament and its army working together to negotiate a post-war settlement was thus destroyed.

Parliament's paranoia may partly have reflected a recognition that, in such a constitutional vacuum, its control over the army was tenuous. But other concerns were at work, which intermingled with the astrologers' own activities. Through the city, all sorts of alien ideas were being discussed: not just prophetical speculations about the future of the King, but of the monarchy itself. Radicals nurtured in the independent churches of Coleman Street and elsewhere were beginning to talk of such revolutionary ideas as equality and democracy. Such views led to them being called the 'Levellers', giving them a distinct political identity.

At around the time of the army's petition, a Leveller pamphlet was leaked by an informer to an MP, 'who was pleased to call it a scandalous, and seditious paper'. It was written by, among others, the two leading Levellers, John Lilburne and Richard Overton, who were currently held in the Tower of London on charges of sedition. It was an explosive document, and its contents already well known through the capital after being read out from the pulpit at St Mary Spital, next to Nicholas Culpeper's house. It challenged the post-war Parliament to reshape the nation: overhaul the corrupt prison system, introduce a form of social security to help the poor, enforce the hearing of legal cases in English rather than Latin, and uphold religious toleration. Most daringly of all, it insisted that the House of Commons act as 'the supreme authority of this nation', being the representative body of the people.[33]

Most MPs were appalled by this unsolicited promotion. The House of Commons was now under the sway of the Presbyterians, a group of religious disciplinarians who wanted nothing to do with such a religious and political free-for-all. They wanted the King restored to his throne, ruling over a Commons with its privileges protected, and a Church reorganized along Scottish lines. A nascent form of this arrangement already existed in parts of London. In August 1645, an 'Ordinance of the Election of Elders' had made provision for twelve religious councils of elders or 'classes' to rule over London's churches in place of the bishop. Their introduction was haphazard, and the fourth classis was not formed until November 1646. The wood turner Nehemiah Wallington was among its members, and to him and his fellow elders the loose, Leveller talk in London's alley churches and taverns was anathema. It released a 'flood of errors and schisms', Wallington wrote in his journal, turning worshippers away from faith to the exercise of 'brain knowledge', which left 'little or nothing of holiness of life'.[34] One source of this 'brain knowledge' was the irrepressible John Lilburne, who was using his sojourn in the Tower to consult the archives stored there. These included the City's charters and other official documents, and on the basis of his researches he launched a blistering attack on London's government, identifying it as part of the same establishment that was holding back reform.

In response to such threats, the City fathers threw their support behind Parliament, a position bolstered by citizens electing a Presbyterian Common Council and by the setting up of a new Militia Committee, which put the Trained Bands, the most powerful military force outside the control of the army, at Parliament's disposal. Thus City and Parliament were once again seen as playing 'as two strings set to the same tune'.

This delicately poised situation was then transformed on 2 June 1647 by the army gaining control of the King. He was taken by a junior officer, apparently to pre-empt an attempt by Parliament to bring him to London. When it heard the news, Parliament fell into a state of panic, sitting all night, and even voting to strike the 'Declaration of Dislike' from the Commons journal.

Meanwhile, the army, under Sir Thomas Fairfax's leadership, conducted a rendezvous of all its forces near Newmarket, the result of which was a 'Solemn Engagement', read out to all the regiments. This was a more political document than previous petitions, an early warning that Leveller rhetoric was beginning to penetrate the rank and file. It promised that the army would disband, or fulfil any service required of it, once its demands had been met, and its enemies in Parliament had been dismissed, which amounted to a call for a purge of leading Presbyterians. To back up its demands, the army embarked on a menacing march towards London, and from temporary headquarters in St Albans, just twenty miles away from the capital, issued impeachment proceedings against eleven MPs, the first step in what looked like a military coup.

Then, on the brink of confrontation, the mood changed. The army withdrew reassuringly to Reading, where a series of proposals for a new constitution were drawn up calling for voting reform, biennial parliaments, a 'Council of State' to replace the Privy Council, religious toleration embracing bishops and presbyteries alike, and the restoration of the King. These 'Heads of Proposals' were discussed in Parliament on 20 July, and favourably considered. The King himself seemed ready to accept them.

But London was in uproar. There was widespread anger and confusion in the streets, radicals clashing with 'reformardoes' (demobbed soldiers), Presbyterian elders with fiery apprentices. When members of the Militia Committee met at the Guildhall on 23 July 1647, a group of young men threatened to 'hang their guts about their ears' if they proceeded.

Three days later, a crowd invaded the House of Commons and

proceeded to rough up pro-army MPs, throwing excrement into their faces. Once the protesters had disbursed, nearly sixty soiled members, together with a contingent of lords and the Speakers of both Houses, crept out of the capital and took refuge with the army.[35]

Colonel Edward Massey, who had led a parliamentarian brigade during the campaigns of the early 1640s, marched through the capital drumming up support to defend the city against Fairfax's forces. A Presbyterian preacher prophesied the New Model Army's downfall at the hands of a righteous God: 'The Lord shall make their Colonels like Oreb and like Zeeb, and their Commanders like Zebah and Zalmunna,' he proclaimed, citing the biblical campaigns of Gideon on behalf of the Israelites. Nicholas Culpeper was among the crowd listening to the sermon and, like many, was unconvinced. The same 'rabbi' (a common derogatory term for ministers) had previously doled out 'Anathemas by wholesale to people of all ranks and qualities' for their failure to support the war, he recalled three years later. Nicholas lamented how such 'Billingsgate Rhetoric' had become 'as frequent in the City Pulpits as Atoms in the Sun'.[36]

On 3 August, fifteen thousand New Model Army troops formed up in a line that stretched a mile and a half across Hounslow Heath, west of London, ready to be inspected by the two exiled Speakers of Parliament together with around a hundred MPs and fourteen peers. Two days later, the members were escorted back to Parliament, and the army mustered on Hyde Park. On 7 August, it paraded along Cheapside with flags and drums, putting on a display of martial discipline and ceremony that impressed citizens exhausted by years of protest and upheaval and left its opponents floundering.

In September, Fairfax set up his headquarters at Putney, a village on the banks of the Thames. With so many soldiers within such easy reach of their London stronghold, the Levellers stepped up their efforts to infiltrate the ranks. Many of their members were ex-soldiers, people like Nicholas Culpeper who had served in earlier campaigns. They understood the resentments of officers and soldiers who felt sidelined by parliamentary politicking and exploited by the continuing shortfall in their pay.

The agitators' efforts were rewarded on 18 October 1647 when a group of five 'London agents' in the cavalry presented Fairfax with a *Case of the Army Truly Stated*. Coming directly from within the army's ranks, such a political, even mutinous, document caused alarm. The *Case* was not about pay and conditions: it was a wholesale attack on the leadership for betraying the principles for which the war had been fought. The generals were accused of allowing the continuation of oppressive monopolies, taxes, and excise duties, and even of planning to restore the King with his veto over Parliament intact. It demanded not only that such policies be abandoned, but that instead the army actively promote a wholesale political revolution, with biennial parliaments voted for by all freeborn men. It called for liberty of conscience, the confiscation of Church lands, and the settlement of all backpay through the liquidation of the City stocks and shares that had gone to royal favourites. Picking up a Leveller preoccupation, the *Case* also called for the codification of all law into plain English, to be made accessible to the public by being published in a single, cheap volume – a call that in coming years would be precisely echoed in a medical context by Nicholas Culpeper.

Fairfax, an heroically fair and open-minded general, responded to the *Case* with characteristic circumspection. He preferred to deal with controversy through consensus rather than confrontation, and referred the matter to the army council for discussion. Oliver Cromwell, Fairfax's deputy as well as an MP, was more forthright. In a speech to the House of Commons, he disassociated himself and the army leadership from it completely. However, a committee set up to consider what punishment the perpetrators should face merely required that they explain themselves. The agitators refused even to do that, instead producing a completely different document, *An Agreement of the People*. This dispensed with criticisms of the army generals, but replaced them with a yet more forthright call for political revolution.

In late October, the army council, which represented the ranks and officers of each regiment as well as the senior leadership, convened a series of meetings, to be held every Thursday at Putney's tiny church of St Mary. The meetings were originally called to discuss army policy, but the council, which had developed an unmilitary taste for debate and discussion, allowed the proceedings to be overtaken by the agenda set out in the *Agreement*. Political ideas stretching back to the time of the Greek republic and forward to the French Revolution were beamed in through the stained glass windows and projected upon the debating table. They covered issues never before aired in such an open and influential forum: democracy, religious tolerance, freedom of the press, universal male suffrage – the entire agenda of modern Western democracy.

Controversy reigned from the reading out of the first article of the *Agreement*. It observed that 'the People of England' were 'very unequally distributed by Counties, Cities, & Burroughs, for the election of their Deputies in Parliament'. It therefore called for the boundaries of each MP's constituency to be redrawn according to the number of inhabitants.[37] Henry Ireton, Cromwell's son-in-law and a leading figure in the army, wondered if this meant every man, regardless of whether he owned property or paid taxes. If so, it would create an 'exception' to the political norm. Confining the vote to property owners was, in his view, 'original and fundamental, and beyond which I am sure no record does go'. 'Not before the conquest,' interjected Nicholas Cowling, one of a number of Levellers who had been allowed to attend the meeting. He was referring to the Norman Conquest of 1066. Before then, many Levellers argued, England had been democratic, everyone having the same 'birthright' to participate in the running of their community. The invasion by 'William the Bastard' had destroyed this by laying the 'Norman Yoke' of aristocratic oppression upon English shoulders, with vast tracts of prime land being handed over to his henchmen, and legal proceedings being conducted in French, so that locals could not understand them.

'We judge that all inhabitants that have not lost their birthright should have an equal voice in elections,' the Leveller Maximilian Petty told the Putney debaters. Colonel Thomas Rainsborough, one of the most radical members of the army leadership, developed this theme:

> I think that the poorest he that is in England hath a life to live, as the greatest he; and therefore truly, sir, I think it's clear, that every man that is to live under a government ought first by his own consent to put himself under that government; and I do think that the poorest man in England is not at all bound in a strict sense to that government that he hath not had a voice to put himself under.[38]

Though it is not known if any members of the Society of Astrologers participated directly in the Putney debates, they certainly helped shape its agenda. Lilly, Booker, and possibly Culpeper were visited by Levellers and army agitators, desperate for guidance on the accelerating 'revolution' (the word acquired its political meaning at exactly this time).[39] Richard Overton asked Lilly to cast a horoscope on 'whether, by joining with the agents of the private soldiery of the Army for the redemption of common right and freedom to the land and removal of oppressions from the people, my endeavours shall be prosperous or no'.[40] Lilly's reply is unrecorded. Nevertheless, he and the other astrologers knew that, whatever the charts said, something exciting and new was forming out of the speculation ventilating into the city streets. The poet John Milton, soon to serve as Parliament's Latin Secretary, captured the mood when he described London as having become 'a city of refuge, the mansion-house of liberty':

> The shop of war hath not more anvils and hammers working, to fashion out the plates and instruments of armed justice in defence of beleaguered truth, than there be pens and heads there,

sitting by their studious lamps, musing, searching, revolving new notions and ideas wherewith to present, as with their homage and their fealty, the approaching Reformation; others as fast reading, trying all things, assenting to the force of reason and convincement.[41]

LESSER CELANDINE
(PILEWORT)

Ranunculus ficaria

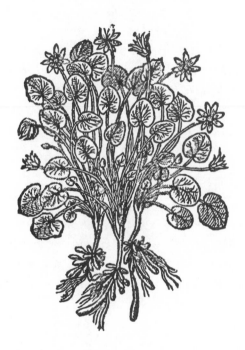

I wonder what ailed the Ancients to give this the name of Celandine which resembles it neither in Nature nor form: It acquired the Name of Pilewort from its Virtues, and it being no great matter where I set it down, so I do set it down at all, I humor'd Dr Tradition so much as to set it down here.

This Celandine then or Pilewort (which you please) doth spread many round, pale, green Leaves set on weak and trailing Branches which lie upon the ground, and are fat, smooth, and somewhat shining, and in some places (though seldom) marked with black spots, each standing on a long Footstalk among which rise smal yellow Flowers, consisting of nine or ten small narrow Leaves, upon slender Footstalks very like unto a Crowfoot, whereunto the Seed also is not unlike, being many smal ones set together upon a Head. The root is made of many small Kernels like grain of Corn, some twice as long as others, of a whitish colour with some Fibres at the end of them.

It groweth for the most part in the moist corners of Fields, and places that are near water Sides, yet will abide in dryer grounds, if they be but a little shadowed.

It Flowereth betimes about March or April, is quite gone in May, so as it cannot be found until it spring again.

Here's another Secret for my Country Men and Women, a couple of them together: Pilewort being made into an Oil Ointment or Plaster readily cures both the Piles or Haemorrhoids, and the King's Evil, if I may Lawfully call it the Kings Evil now there is no King.

With this I cured my own Daughter of the King's Evil, broke the Sore, drew out a quarter of a pint of Corruption, and cured it without any Scar at all, and in one Week's time.

The Lesser Celandine is not related nor even very similar to the Greater Celandine, hence Culpeper's puzzlement at the 'ancients' giving it that name. It is called Pilewort because its knobbly tubers resemble haemorrhoids, which it was used to treat. This is an example of the 'Doctrine of Signatures', according to which the medicinal value of certain herbs was divinely signalled by their resemblance to the conditions they treated.

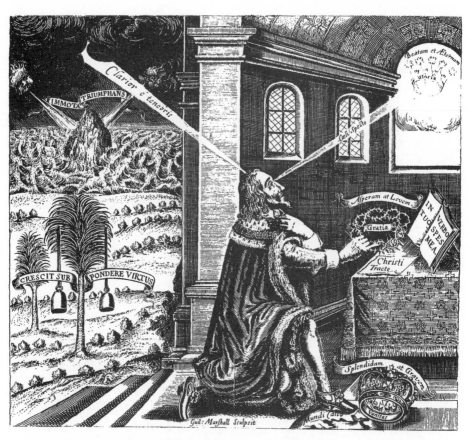

King Charles the pious martyr, as depicted in the Royalist apologia Eikon Basilike,
or 'The Portraiture of His Sacred Majesty in his Solitudes and Sufferings'.

he great drama that had been prefigured in Lilly's prophecies, was approaching its conclusion. The chicken of the Eagle had flown (Prince Rupert had been forced to leave England), the White King had been assaulted before and behind (Charles had surrendered), and the fiery trigon had turned retrograde (the Stuart dynasty was finished). In the process, over eighty thousand soldiers had been killed on the battlefield, and at least a further hundred thousand had died of disease – a greater proportion of the population of England and Wales than died in either of the twentieth century's World Wars. Civilians, too, had endured their share of trauma, suffering sieges, conscription, the commandeering of their houses and livestock, sacking and plundering by soldiers denied their pay, and swingeing war levies. Never before had death and taxes so lethally combined.[1]

Since his capture, Charles had remained serene in the conviction that he was indispensable to any negotiated settlement, a view confirmed by the pains taken by the various opposition factions to offer terms. He felt no need to take sides. MPs, soldiers, Presbyterians, and Independents were all traitors, and he could dally with the devils in any way he chose. As Nicholas later put it, Charles was an 'alchemist' whose aim was to 'sublimate all Treaties into air'.[2] This was to be his approach into the winter of 1647.

During that time he was held at Hampton Court under voluntary parole, a mixture of deference and confusion leaving him virtually unsupervised. On 11 November, on the pretext of having received death threats, he left. He had told a group of Scottish commissioners that he would go north to Berwick, but decided to go south instead, to the Isle of Wight, where he expected a sympathetic reception from the governor and easy access to the Continent.

The governor, horrified and perplexed at the unexpected appearance of his visitor, proved less than welcoming and put the King under guard at Carisbrooke Castle. Nevertheless, like the previous royal gaolers, he allowed Charles enough latitude to receive visitors, who continued to flock with yet more proposals.

Charles resumed his alchemical negotiations as if nothing had happened. He appeared close to accepting a settlement with Parliament while making encouraging overtures to the army. Then, behind the backs of both, he struck a secret deal with the Scots known as the Engagement, in which he promised to support Presbyterianism for three years, during which time a permanent religious settlement would be renegotiated. On 27 December, the Engagement was signed, wrapped in lead, and buried in the castle gardens to await a safe time for its collection, and Charles set about trying to get off the island. Unfortunately for him, at the moment he was preparing to rendezvous with a small boat at Newport, a nearby harbour on the River Medina with navigable access to the sea, the wind delayed his departure, and he found himself locked into the castle before he could escape. A crowd of women and boys led by a Captain Burley attempted to rescue him, but were easily overcome.

This episode marked the end of the relaxed manner of his detention. His guard was doubled, and a squadron was called up to patrol the Solent, the stretch of water between the island and the mainland. On 15 January 1648 Parliament passed the 'Vote of No Addresses', a self-imposed injunction to prevent further betrayals by pledging to 'make no further addresses or applications to the King', and to receive no further messages from him.[3]

There followed the incoherent series of military engagements that became known as the Second Civil War. The trigger was a series of rebellions that erupted across the country in the spring of 1648. Though the objective of the rebels was the King's restoration, their impetus was not royalism or even religion so much as desperation.

People were pinched by taxes and excise duties far higher than they had been under James or Charles and starved by a series of failed harvests. An army officer had noted a few months before that 'The poor did gather in troops of ten, twenty, thirty, in the roads and seized upon corn as it was carrying to market and divided it among themselves before the owners' faces, telling them they could not starve.' London was on a continuous emergency footing. Free corn and coal were being distributed to the poor. 'Necessity dissolves all laws and government, and hunger will break through stone walls,' proclaimed a pamphlet. Another admitted that even if elections had been held, 'the common vote of the giddy multitude' would be for the King.[4]

In the face of the army's undiminished military superiority, the uprisings were suppressed and a Scottish invasion, mounted under the terms of the Engagement, was annihilated by Oliver Cromwell in a series of engagements around Preston in Lancashire. Throughout, Charles was marooned on the Isle of Wight, reassuring himself and his followers of his continuing divine benefaction with regular exercises of the Royal Touch. This time, however, he did not have his personal physician to help him. Harvey's whereabouts during this period are unknown, but an application submitted by Charles to the House of Commons to have the doctor brought to the island was rejected.

In September 1649, Parliament responded to the army's victory by rushing back into the arms of its spurned monarch. An order was issued calling for the King to be released from Carisbrooke Castle and allowed to take up residence in the home of a sympathizer, William Hopkins, in Newport. At the Town Hall, a few tempting yards from the quayside, Charles met parliamentary commissioners, whom he flattered with yet more promises, while keeping an eye on the wind vane. 'The great concession I made this day – the Church, militia, and Ireland – was made merely in order to [further] my escape,' he confided to Hopkins. 'To be short, if I stay for a demonstration of their further wickedness, it will be too late to seek a remedy; for my only hope is that now they believe I dare deny them nothing, and so be less careful of their guards.'[5]

Army leaders and Levellers were appalled by Parliament's feeble dependency on the King, and agitated for the negotiations to be stopped. In a London tavern called the Nag's Head, they met to draft a manifesto that would bring the whole business to an end. The result was *A Remonstrance of His Excellency Thomas Lord Fairfax, Lord Generall of the Parliaments Forces*, which was presented to the army council in St Albans for discussion in early November. Though written in Fairfax's name, he had misgivings about the *Remonstrance*'s strident political tone, and its promoters faced stiff opposition.[6] However, all that changed on 15 November, when the Commons voted for the King to be 'settled in a condition of honour, freedom and safety, agreeable to the laws of the land'. The *Remonstrance* was finalized within a day, and presented to the Commons on the twentieth.

At first, the MPs might have wondered what the *Remonstrance* was remonstrating about. Its opening sections are impenetrable, a series of long, tangled sentences strung together with qualifications and parentheses, page after page filled with subjects in search of their objects, pronouns abandoned by their verbs. The point of it all was not clearly stated until page sixty-two, when the reason for the circumspection becomes obvious; for what the army demanded was that 'the Person of the King may and shall be proceeded against in a way of justice, for the blood spilt, and the other evils and mischiefs done by him'. He was to be tried as a traitor, for which the only punishment was death.[7]

Thus an historic, even world-changing policy, one that laid the foundations for future political revolutions not only in England, but by example in France and America, found its first, faltering expression. It took that crucial step of making the King accountable, not to God, but to his subjects, and exposing him to the censure not just of his conscience, but of the law. Yet this momentous alteration was born more out of exasperation than principle. Even after the Second Civil War, few called for the end of the monarch, and fewer still for the end of monarchy. The *Remonstrance* itself wanted Charles replaced, though by parliamentary election rather than line of descent, as his heir Prince Charles was listed among the 'delinquents' who should also face exemplary punishment.

Events after the publication of the *Remonstrance* moved swiftly, though it is unclear exactly who steered them. Oliver Cromwell's joint role as MP and victorious military leader put him in a commanding position, but he remained in the north, mysteriously detained from being able to have a direct hand in the King's removal. Fairfax, a military man with a dislike for politics, disapproved of the whole business and wanted nothing to do with it. So it was left to the more militant sections of the army council, notably Cromwell's son-in-law Henry Ireton, who had led the drafting of the *Remonstrance*, to take the initiative. Ireton ordered two radical officers to the Isle of Wight to assume command of the King's detention.

On 1 December, the army arrived in London. While Parliament debated the King's answer to the parliamentary commissioners in Newport, seven thousand troops were drawn up for review in Hyde Park, a mile from Westminster, to concentrate the minds of the MPs. The threat did not have its desired effect. On 5 December, after sitting for twenty-four hours, the Commons passed a motion accepting the King's terms as the basis for a peace settlement. Later that day, Ireton met with sympathetic MPs and tried to persuade them to organize a dissolution. When he failed, he decided upon a more military solution.

The MP Bulstrode Whitelocke was at the House the following day. He found his way blocked by a soldier, Colonel Thomas Pride, who was standing at the door to the chamber, picking out with the help of the veteran Independent Lord Grey of Groby those members whose names appeared on a list. Anyone who objected was dragged away by soldiers to a room called the Queen's Court, where they were left to cool off. Whitelocke was eventually allowed through, but was 'sad to see such doings' and had 'trouble in his thoughts whither he should continue his service in the Parlemt'. He eventually decided he would continue, the inveterate lawyer arguing under self-cross-examination that he should do so 'because there was no actual force upon himself, though there was upon others, & unless there were a particular force upon him, that he ought not to desert his trust'.[8]

Following what became known as Pride's Purge, Parliament was reduced to a 'Rump' of around two hundred MPs, less than half its original strength. It was reported that at times barely forty, the number needed for a quorum, attended. Feeble efforts were made to restore the excluded members, but the House was too weak to have any impact. The army council was now in command, and eager for action. It discussed a final draft of the *Agreement of the People* drawn up by the Leveller Lilburne. This was to provide the basis of the new constitution. John Goodwin of Coleman Street was among those invited to contribute to the discussions. Another was Hugh Peters, the minister of Salem, Massachusetts. Peters had returned to the old world to preach the benefits of a new one, free of kings and Catholicism. 'I have lived in a Country,' he told the Rump Parliament, 'where seven years I never saw beggar, nor heard an oath, nor looked upon a drunkard; why should there be beggars in your Israel where there is so much work to do?'[9]

The new *Agreement*'s most significant declaration was that Parliament should have 'the highest and final judgement concerning all natural [i.e. non-religious] things'.[10] Religion was to be left as a matter of individual conscience. Having laid out the foundations for a new, secular state, the council now had to consider how to dismantle the old one, which in the first instance meant deciding what to do about the King. After some last-minute agonizing, it resolved to appoint a committee to try Charles for treason. The final, least credible prediction of William Lilly's *Starry Messenger* was about to be realized.

As these developments were approaching their climax, Bulstrode

Whitelocke was among many who found the pressure unendurable, and he appears to have suffered a nervous breakdown. He was 'full of melancholy and apprehensions if not desire for death', he recorded in his diary on 19 December. In a desperate attempt to alleviate the symptoms, two physicians were called to let his blood, but still 'his melancholy did much overcome him'. He used his condition as an excuse to absent himself from the House, but he could not completely escape entanglement with the great affairs going on around him. He was now one of the legal commissioners for the Great Seal, and it was decided by the army leadership that he should be consulted on the proposed trial. The man who came to see him was Oliver Cromwell, who had returned to the capital and, Whitelocke noted, ensconced himself 'in one of the King's rich beds in Whitehall'.[11] Cromwell's views on the fate of the King at this time remain unclear, and he consulted Whitelocke on alternative strategies. Whitelocke would have urged any number of accommodations and compromises, but not the one that appears to have become fixed in Cromwell's mind by 26 December: that practical considerations outweighed legal legitimacy, and that one way or another, the King must die.

On 1 January 1649, the Commons passed an ordinance to set up a High Court to try Charles. It was rejected by the Lords, provoking the Commons to pass a vote on 4 January announcing 'that the people are, under God, the original of all just power'. Nominating itself the representative body of the people (meaning, since Pride's Purge, the nearest approximation), it declared 'whatsoever is enacted or declared for law by the Commons in Parliament assembled, hath the force of law, and all the people of this nation are concluded thereby, although the consent and concurrence of King or House of Peers be not had thereunto'.[12]

One hundred and fifty commissioners were enlisted to set up the court and establish its procedures. They first met on 8 January in the Painted Chamber of Westminster Palace. Of 132 by then appointed, only 53 turned up. There was not a single senior judge among them, which meant that John Bradshaw, Chief Justice of Chester, was forced to step up from relative legal obscurity to occupy the most prominent position in the impending trial: that of president of the court.

In a series of further meetings, all thinly attended, it was decided that during the trial the King should be lodged in the former house of Sir Robert Cotton, within easy reach of Westminster. It was also decided that the court's newly-appointed Sergeant-at-Arms, Edward Denby, should go through London with ten trumpets and two troops of horses to proclaim that hearings would begin on 20 January.

Speed was now of the essence. On Friday 19 January, Charles was brought in secret from Windsor to St James's Palace. The following day he was carried by sedan chair to Whitehall, then to Cotton House, the latter part of the journey conducted by water to avoid public attention. Meanwhile, the commissioners made last-minute arrangements for the trial. They finalized the wording of the charge, and made adjustments to the furniture in Westminster Hall, Bradshaw after some hesitation allowing the King's chair to be upholstered in crimson velvet.

William Lilly, writing after the Restoration and wanting to distance himself from the events about to unfold, recalled being in Westminster that January day. He unconvincingly claimed to be unaware of what was going on, it being his habit to take the short walk there from his home in the Strand 'every Saturday in the afternoon in those times'. Today, he 'casually met' Hugh Peters in Whitehall.

Lilly had seen Peters a few days earlier, while delivering a copy of his 1649 almanac to Lord Grey of Groby. Lord Grey had read to Peters a passage from the opening section: 'If we are not fools and knaves, we shall do Justice.' Now Peters revealed to Lilly the significance of this prognostication: Lord Grey was among the commissioners selected to try the King. Indeed, Peters was on his way to the trial at that very moment, and invited Lilly to join him.

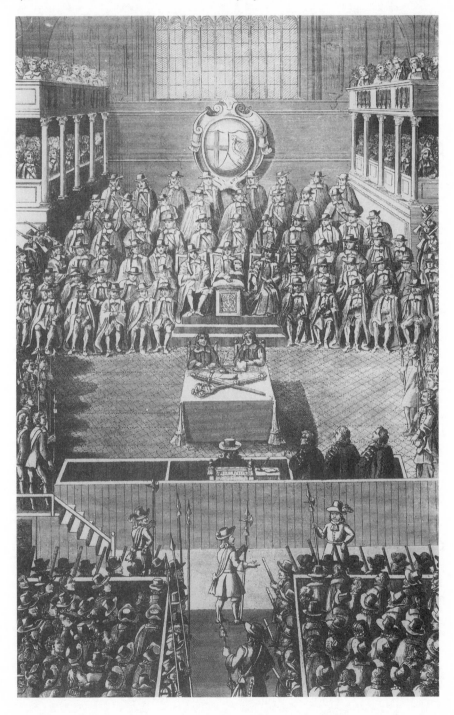

They arrived at Westminster Hall to find the commissioners, now numbering sixty-six, filing in. The two were 'permitted by the guard of soldiers to pass up to the King's Bench', to witness proceedings close-hand.

At 2 p.m. it was commanded that the Great Gate of the Hall be opened 'to the intent that all persons (without exception) desirous to see or hear, might come unto it'. Soon after, the King himself was brought in. 'After a stern looking at the Court and the People, in the Galleries on each side of him,' the official account of the proceedings records, 'he places himself in the Chair, not at all moving his Hat, or otherwise showing the least respect to the Court.' He was then addressed by Bradshaw, who sat at the centre of a dais running the width of the hall, upon which the commissioners sat on terraced benches. 'The Commons of England Assembled in Parliament,' Bradshaw announced, 'being deeply sensible of the Evils and Calamities that had been brought upon this Nation, and of the innocent Blood that had been spilt in it, which was fixed upon him as the principle Author of it, had resolved to make Inquisition for this Blood . . . and had therefore constituted that Court of Justice, before which he was then brought, where he was to hear his Charge, upon which the Court would proceed according to Justice.' The court solicitor, John Cook, was then asked to read out the charge. Charles tapped Cook on the shoulder with his cane, asking him to wait so he could say something, but Cook was told by Bradshaw to continue. (Lilly later noticed that the silver top of the King's cane fell off. The King seemed unable to pick it up off the floor, and waited for one of the court officials to retrieve it for him.[13])

The charge took some time to read out, as it contained a lengthy list of the King's alleged misdoings, naming each of the major engagements of the war, as well as several of the treaties he subsequently negotiated. Its conclusion, however, was stark: that he was 'guilty of all the Treasons, Murders, Rapines, Burnings, Spoils, Desolations, Damages and Mischiefs to this Nation acted and committed in the said Wars, and occasioned thereby'.

Charles's response was an emphatic denial of the court's jurisdiction. 'A King cannot be tried by any Superior Jurisdiction on Earth,' he declared. He therefore disrupted the proceedings by whatever means available to him. He constantly interrupted Bradshaw, and then indignantly protested whenever he himself was interrupted. He refused to answer the charges, or any of the questions put to him.

'I answer . . . so soon as I know by what Authority you do this,' he said during the trial's second day.

'If this be all that you will say, then, Gentlemen, you that brought the Prisoner hither, take charge of him back again,' answered the exasperated Bradshaw.

'I do require that I may give in my reasons why I do not Answer; and give me time for that,' Charles replied.

''Tis not for Prisoners to require,' came the response.

'Prisoners, Sir! I am not an ordinary Prisoner.'

It was after this exchange that Bradshaw charged Charles with contempt of court.

And so the trial continued. On the matter of the House of Commons having the authority to mount such a trial, the King pointed out that 'it is too well known that the Major part of them [MPs] are detained or deterred from Sitting'. On Bradshaw's claim to bring the charges on behalf of the people, he pointed out that 'you manifestly wrong even the Poorest Ploughman if you demand not his free Consent'.

In order to give the King time to change his mind, and allow a respite from his interjections, testimony was heard from other witnesses, most of them called to confirm the King's presence at the major engagements. This accumulation of evidence produced no change in the prisoner's disposition, and on 27 January he was formally given a final chance to answer the charges. Once again he refused. 'Do your duty,' begged the clerk of the court. 'Duty, Sir!' the King retorted. He had nothing to say about the charges, only the matter of the proceedings' legitimacy. 'You have written Your

Meaning in bloody Characters throughout the kingdom,' Bradshaw observed.

Charles asked to be heard by the Lords and Commons assembled in the Painted Chamber, a request that took the commissioners by surprise. They withdrew to discuss the matter, and apparently faced some dissension, one commissioner threatening to call publicly for the King's request to be granted. The opposition was overcome, and the commissioners returned to announce that the King's request was denied and that the court would proceed to a judgment. The King still refused to remain silent. 'I would desire only one Word before you give Sentence,' he asked. 'I am not far from your Sentence, and your time is now past,' Bradshaw replied. After a further statement by Bradshaw, and a few more interruptions, the charge was read out again, and the sentence announced, 'That the said Charles Stuart, as a Tyrant, Traitor, Murderer and a Public Enemy, shall be put to Death by the severing of his Head from his Body.'

Another interruption:

'Will you hear me a Word, Sir?' the King asked.

'Sir, you are not to be heard after the Sentence,' Bradshaw replied.

'No, Sir?'

'No, Sir, by your favour, Sir. Guard, withdraw your prisoner.'

'I may speak after Sentence, by your favour, Sir, I may speak after Sentence, even. By your favour hold: the Sentence, Sir . . . I say, Sir, I do . . . I am not suffered to speak; expect what Justice other People will have.'

With that, the King was taken away, and the trial came to an end.

On 30 January 1649, Charles was taken to the Banqueting Hall in Whitehall, where fifteen years earlier almost to the day he had watched the antimasquers perform their own grotesque theatre. This time, he was the spectacle, his stage a scaffold built next to the hall, his audience a vast crowd that filled Whitehall. William Lilly was there, and Nicholas Culpeper was likely to have been.

William Harvey was probably not, his association with the King excluding him from the capital as a 'delinquent'.

Staples had been hammered into the scaffold floor in case the King continued with his defiance, and ropes were required to tie him to the block. In the event, he met his death with regal composure. He tried to make a speech, but could not be heard over the hubbub. He instead addressed his remarks to his friend William Juxon, the Bishop of London, who had been allowed to accompany him onto the scaffold. 'For the people, truly I desire their liberty and freedom as much as anybody whatsoever. But I must tell you that their liberty and freedom consists in having government, those Laws by which their Life and their Goods may be most their own,' he said. 'A subject and a sovereign are clean different things; and, therefore, until you do that – I mean that you put the people in that liberty as I say – certainly they will never enjoy themselves.'

When he had finished his speech, he surveyed the block.

'You must set it fast,' he told the executioner, concerned that it might wobble when he leaned upon it.

'It is fast, Sir,' said the executioner.

'It might have been a little higher,' the King complained.

'It can be no higher, Sir,' replied the executioner.

'When I put out my hands this way, then . . .'

The King, determined that even his demise should come from a royal command, indicated a sign to show when the executioner should strike. He then laid his neck on the block. The executioner leaned over to tuck some stray strands of hair into the King's cap.

'Stay for the sign,' the King reminded him.

'Yes, I will and it please your majesty,' replied the executioner.

After a pause, the King stretched out his hands, and the axe was brought down. The executioner held up the decapitated head and, following custom, shouted: 'Behold the head of a traitor.' The royal body was swiftly placed in a coffin and carried away.

According to one account, people surged around the scaffold with cloths and containers to catch the dribbling blood, which was taken 'by some as trophies of their Villainy, by others as Reliques of a Martyr'.[14]

The judicial killing of a king was an unprecedented, terrifying act, placing even those who had supported it in uncharted territory. A tremor passed through the country, across the seas, into the royal houses of France, Spain, and the German empire. The sun of the social order had been extinguished, the heart of the nation stopped. The astrologers gazed at the stars, searching for signs of a response. Lilly, despite his own predictions, could not suppress a quiver of shock. Elias Ashmole, a royalist, was distraught. All around, he saw portents of a cosmic convulsion, which he listed in his notebook:

> The Ducks hovering over the Scaffold & there abouts, when the King was put to Death.
>
> The Whale cast up at Dover & died the hour of ye King's Death.
>
> The bright star that night fal[len] over Whitehall.
>
> Blood upon Cloths in Gloucestershire:
>
> Of the maid at Alcester who was cured of the King's Evil who had extreme pain that very hour & minute that the King was beheaded, that the cloths were taken off, & one drop of blood issued from that place where her sore was.
>
> One that brag'd that he had the honour to bring the King to ye Scaffold was found murdered in Montgomeryshire, & his Eyes pickt out [by] Crawes.[15]

Bulstrode Whitelocke had absented himself from Westminster on the day of the execution, staying 'all day at home, troubled at the death of the King, & praying to God to keep his judgements from us'. A week later, he was ordered to bring the Great Seal of State to the House of Commons. He and his fellow commissioner Sir Thomas Widrington, both holding on to the purse that contained the seal, solemnly brought it into the Commons. 'The members being all silent', they laid it upon the table. An act was immediately passed, calling for its destruction. A workman who was waiting outside with his tools was then brought in '& upon the floor he brake the old Seal in pieces'.[16]

Charles's head had barely time to reach the scaffold floor before Peter Cole, a publisher of radical books and pamphlets, was at the Stationers' Hall, preparing to register a transcript of the trial and the speech Charles had given on the scaffold. He discovered that a royalist writer, John Playford, had got there first. Spurred on by the commercial as well as the journalistic impulse, he put aside all political differences and cut a deal to publish jointly Playford's edited transcript. It appeared within two weeks under the title *King Charls his Tryal* at Cole's bookshop, at the sign of the Printing Press in Cornhill.[17]

Cole had been apprenticed in political activism as well as bookselling. His master had been John Bellamy, a member of the Common Council for Cornhill at the time it started to supplant the Lord Mayor and Aldermen in the government of the City. Bellamy had risen to the rank of Colonel in the parliamentary army during the Civil War, and had also led a challenge to the Stationers' Company monopoly on the licensing of English books.[18]

Cole had gained the freedom of the Stationers' Company in 1637 and teamed up with Benjamin Allen, who had been apprenticed to John Bellamy at the same time as Cole, to publish a new edition of Clowes's *A Prooued Practise for all Young Chirurgians*, concerning burnings by gunpowder. Part of the attraction of the work for Cole may have been Clowes's introduction, in which he railed against the 'scornful scanners' who had nitpicked through his previous works and defended those 'well disposed persons, who have with long and tedious labours published divers Books of Physic and Chirurgery in English' rather than Latin.[19]

Two years later, Cole published a biblical commentary by the

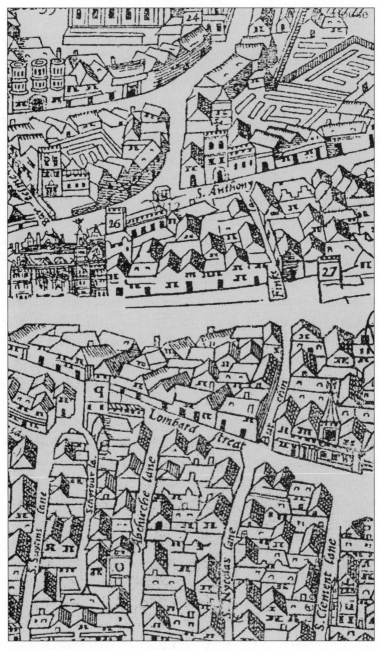

London's publishing district, Lombard Street and Cornhill (the main thoroughfare north of Lombard Street).

Puritan divine Richard Sibbes, who had died four years earlier. A
'J. G.' contributed a dedication. This is likely to have been John
Goodwin of Coleman Street, whose book *The Christian Engagement*
Cole would publish in 1641 (and who later complained to the Stationers' Company about Cole on some unspecified matter).[20] The
book was printed by Thomas Cotes, who had been William Attersoll's printer, and from whom Nicholas Culpeper had probably
collected the forty shillings inheritance left to him by Attersoll.[21]
These two links to Nicholas suggest that it may have been around
this time that he came into contact with Cole. Nicholas had just
left his apprenticeship and would have been receptive to working
in a print shop, humming with high technology and new ideas. A
reference to him at one stage being a 'compositor' indicates this
was the case.[22]

In the mid-1640s, Cole became seriously entangled with Parliament's attempt to crack down on the press, which for two years
had been virtually unregulated. Hostilities began with the discovery
of a slip of paper found behind the stall boards of shops and
scattered through the streets attacking the old guard of the parliamentary army. The House of Lords gave the Master and Wardens
of the Stationers' Company two days to find the culprit. It took
them a month to identify Nicholas Tew, who was found to have a
secret printing press in the basement of a house in Coleman Street,
where among incriminating papers the Company's searchers found
'divers scandalous books and pamphlets, and a letter for printing;
the letter thereof is very like the letter of the libel against the peers'.
Though neither the plates nor copies of the original leaflet could
be found, the same worn Dutch typeface used to print it was discovered in Tew's workshop. Tew refused to submit to an interroga-
tion by the officers of the Stationers' Company, and so was thrown
into the Fleet Prison on the order of two JPs.

The searchers also made another discovery, which from their
point of view was even more significant. Among the 'divers scandalous books and pamphlets' were several by the Levellers Richard

Overton and John Lilburne. These included *A Copie of a Letter Written by John Lilburne* attacking the MP William Prynne, the erstwhile martyr of Archbishop William Laud. Prynne, once censored, had turned censor. Still bearing the letters 'S. L.' for 'seditious libeller' burned into his cheeks, he called for the works of Independents like Lilburne to be suppressed. Tew also had copies of *Mans Mortallitie* by 'R.O.', probably Overton. It was about the nature of man as a rational being. Its subject matter was considered so controversial that, though it had clearly been produced in London, its title-page claimed it originated in Amsterdam, acclaimed by radicals and Independents as the home of free thought – the 'Town I exceedingly love and respect', as Nicholas Culpeper described it.[23]

This was not the first time the Stationers' Company censors had encountered Overton. Before his works were discovered at Tew's secret workshop, a press belonging to a Richard Overton was seized at Bell Alley near Finsbury, at the time a sparsely populated area north of the City wall used during the Civil War to muster troops. In March 1643, an order was issued that the press be restored to Peter Cole on Overton's behalf. However, Cole's own presses and material had been impounded by Parliament's Committee of Examinations as part of its attempted crackdown on unlicensed printing. On 20 June 1643, the Committee restored them to Cole, but, evidently suspecting that he was supplying unlicensed printers with equipment, demanded a bond that he would not 'remove the said presses or dispose of them without first acquainting this Committee and the Master and wardens of the Company of Stationers and have their consent thereto'. The bond was for £1,000, a sum so astronomical that it was designed to cripple Cole's business, if it was not a secretarial error.[24]

Cole continued to frustrate the authorities, jealously protecting his freedoms to publish from interference. The following year, he resisted an attempt by a warden from the Stationers' Company to search his premises. When one of his apprentices accused him of 'misuse . . . in beating him, not allowing him to go out, and thereby alluring him to desert', Cole defended himself on the grounds that he suspected the apprentice of informing against him 'concerning . . . treasonable and seditious books'.[25]

However, Cole was prepared to cooperate with the authorities when necessity required. In December 1644, and during the following year, he had several encounters with Thomas Edwards, who was spying on religious dissidents on behalf of the Presbyterian leadership in Parliament. The two first met at the shop of Ralph Smith at the sign of the Bible, which neighboured Cole's. Several people were there, arguing about 'Liberty of Conscience, and Tolerations', Edwards recalled, 'whereupon I spake against it, and Mr Cole Bookseller confessed he was against a general Liberty of Conscience by what he saw and knew; for he knew a company that were a Church, to which he had once thought of all other Churches to have joined himself a Member, who now deny the Scriptures to be the Word of God'. This was almost certainly not Cole's true opinion, and supports the suggestion that he was trying to deflect suspicion from himself and his radical writers, even gaining Edwards' trust so he could spy on him.

Following the encounter, Cole appears to have acted as an informant, visiting illicit gatherings on Edwards' behalf. At a later meeting, he reported to Edwards that he had gone 'on a Fast-day in the Evening to find these persons out, and found them playing at Tables'. Edwards said he would report the matter – 'acquaint Authority with it' and 'accordingly . . . it was given in to a Committee'. The following April, Edwards reported that Cole was involved in trying to 'help' Edwards 'to an unlicensed Book'. Edwards also paid a visit to Cole's shop, where they talked further about religious matters. Cole told Edwards 'That divers persons whom about 4 years ago he thought as godly as any, were now fallen to deny all things in matters of Religion, and held nothing, but laboured to Plunder men of their Faith . . . and some of them would come into his Shop, and had spoken fearful blasphemies.' The example Cole identified was one Clement Wrighter, whom Edwards elsewhere accused of having collaborated in *Mans Mortallitie*, the seditious tract found in the possession of Nicholas Tew.

In 1646, Edwards published *Gangraena, or, A catalogue and discovery of many of the errours, heresies, blasphemies and pernicious practices of the sectaries of this time*. It attacked the 'Mechanics preaching in Coleman Street' and in particular John Goodwin. It also revealed in embarrassing detail Cole's conversations with Edwards, which may explain why that year Goodwin applied to the Stationers' Company for Cole's entry for his sermons to be struck from the register.[26]

Cole was not to be deflected by such setbacks, and his coup with *King Charls his Tryal* established him as one of the most resourceful and opportunistic, as well as political, publishers in London. On the back of that success, he prepared immediately for the publication of his next headline-grabbing publication. A small advertisement appeared in the 27 August editions of several weekly newsletters, such as *The Moderate, A Perfect Diurnall*, and *Perfect Occurrences*. It read:

> There is come forth an excellent translation of the London Dispensatory made by the Colledg of Physitions in London, being that Book by which all Apothecaries in England are strictly commanded to make all their Phisick, With twelve hundred additions, wherein is shewed the Vertue and Operation of everie medicine, and every Simple. Printed for Peter Cole, at the Printing Presse in Corn Hill.[27]

The announcement marked one of the publishing sensations of a sensational century.

The royal physician William Harvey, now in his seventies, was out of a job. He had lost his principal patron and his post at

St Bartholomew's, though he continued as the College's Lumleian lecturer, in name if not in fact.

In 1650, he managed to obtain a licence to visit London to treat one of his patients, the widow of Sir Thomas Thynne. Soon after, he started to live openly at his brother Eliab's house opposite St Lawrence Poultry in the heart of the city. He recommenced his rounds, which he conducted, according to the gossip John Aubrey, in defiantly regal style, 'on horseback with a Foot-cloth to visit his patients, his man following on foot, as the fashion then was, which was very decent, now quite discontinued'. A foot cloth, also favoured by judges, was a richly embroidered blanket slung over the back of the horse that reached down to its hooves.[28]

Outwardly, Harvey may have appeared the same, but inwardly the death of his master the King had produced a profound change of heart. In *De motu cordis* he had written that 'all things do depend upon the motional pulsation of the heart'. But in 1649, following Charles's execution, he no longer believed that the heart was the 'framer of the blood', nor that it provided blood with its 'force, virtue, motion or heat'. By 1653, he was arguing that blood was 'the builder and preserver of the body and principal part wherein the soul hath her Session'; the heart, formerly the fountain of life, was 'erected for this end and purpose only, that it may by continual pulsation ... entertain this blood'. The idea that the heart serves the blood, which resides throughout the body, suggested an apt analogy to the idea that the King served the people, but Harvey could not bring himself to pursue it. The cosmic parallels that had been such a feature in *De motu cordis* were abandoned. The 'knowledge we have of the heavenly bodies', he pointed out, was so 'uncertain and conjectural' that their example 'is not hereto be followed'.[29]

Despite the heavens being so full of uncertainty and conjecture, the medical world remained virtually undisturbed by recent events. Returning to Amen Corner in 1650, Harvey found himself in surprisingly convivial company, surrounded by old friends.

The execution of the King had left a queasy atmosphere in London – literally, as there was an outbreak of a mysterious cholera-like disease which produced 'little skins ... the peeling of guts' in the excrement of sufferers. Nicholas's three-year-old son was struck down by the disease, 'which so puzzled the College of Physicians', and he treated it successfully with boiled mallows.[30]

Among some radical MPs, expectations for the new Commonwealth were high. 'Me thinks I see the kingdom of Jesus Christ begin to flourish, while the wicked ... do now perish and fade like a blown-off-blossom,' William Rowse wrote to the Speaker of the House of Commons.[31] But outside Parliament, the mood was very different. There were no triumphal marches, no mobs on the rampage. It was almost as if the capital's citizens, having provided the stage and setting for the grand finale, had looked away, hoping what they had not seen had not really happened. The College was only too happy to sustain this act of mass denial by reverting to its pre-revolutionary colours. Francis Prujean, a champion of the College's privileges and among those identified as papists in 1643, was elected President in 1650 and held the post for the next four years. Old faces that had been absent since the crises began reappeared around the Comitia room: Sir Thomas Cadyman, the former physician general of the royalist army, and Edmund Smith, one of the physicians-in-ordinary to the King during the war. They were joined by Charles Scarburgh, Harvey's assistant at Oxford and royalist soldier, who was admitted a candidate to the College in 1648, becoming a Fellow in 1650.[32]

With the old faces came the old methods. In the summer of 1649, the Comitia ruled that anyone advertising medical services would be punished. Soon after, a solicitor was appointed to prosecute unlicensed practitioners. And when Walter Charleton, who had failed to become a Fellow in the mid-1640s because of his royalism, reapplied for membership in April 1650, he was accepted.[33]

In some respects, the College's powers were now greater than ever. The Printing Act of 1643 had taken the licensing of medical texts from the hands of the Bishop of London and, formally at least, placed it in those of the physicians. In the midst of the Civil War, the College had been unable to exercise this power, but in 1649 the President and Censors began to make regular trips to Stationers' Hall, in the hope of overseeing the registration of approved titles.[34] The Stationers' Company, whose control over registration in theory could have conflicted with the College's, appears to have accepted the physicians' presence.

In one prominent area, however, the College remained dangerously exposed: control of the *Pharmacopoeia*. Following the botched publication of the first edition, relations with the College's publisher, John Marriot, had deteriorated to the point of open hostility. However, since the title was registered with the Stationers' Company in Marriot's name, the College was powerless to prevent him from producing countless new 'editions'. This he enthusiastically did, claiming each to be 'enlarged and corrected' when it was identical to the previous one.

Now the College decided it was ready to fight back. In June 1649, the Comitia approved for publication a new edition of its *Pharmacopoeia*, the result of two years' hard work. Once licensed, it would replace the first edition as London's official dispensatory, enabling the College to recover ownership of the precious title.

It was at this point that news broke of an English edition of *Pharmacopoeia*. Unknown to the College, at exactly the same time that it had embarked on its new edition of the *Pharmacopoeia*, Peter Cole had decided to commission a translation, and it was to Nicholas Culpeper that he turned.

Nicholas appears not to have sought the commission. His memoir mentions his surprise at being 'so unexpectedly taken notice of, as to be put upon the Translation of the Doctor's *Dispensatory*'.[35] He may have been proposed by a member of the Society of Apothecaries – though not in an official capacity, as he was still *persona non grata* at Apothecaries' Hall. It is more likely that, in the heat of the Civil War and Leveller activism, thoughts began to turn to the reform of medicine along with religion and law, and that he, together with fellow Coleman Street radicals, saw a translation of the *Pharmacopoeia* as a first step towards achieving this. Whatever the arrangement, the timing of the commission indicates that Cole had got wind of the College's plan to come up with a new Latin edition, and, ever the opportunist, had decided to register an English one at the same time.

When Cole had first suggested the idea, Nicholas was still recovering from the chest wound he had sustained at Newbury, and the injury was now exacerbated by his smoking. Nevertheless, he had thrown himself into the project with enthusiasm, being helped in drafting the manuscript by an amanuensis, William Ryves. He was still working on the text at the time of the King's execution in January 1649, and completed it some time in the summer of that year.

Few could have anticipated the nature of the work that finally appeared in Cole's shop in late August 1649 under the title *A Physical Directory*. For the physicians, its breathtaking cheek was only outdone by its disastrous effects. It was subtitled 'A Translation of the London Dispensatory made by the College of Physicians in London', but it was much more than that. The College had already conceded that an English edition of the *Pharmacopoeia* was inevitable, and would soon register its intention to provide one with the Stationers' Company (though none would be forthcoming for decades). What made Nicholas's book revolutionary and courageous, if not fool-hardy, was that, as the title-page promised, it included 'many hundred additions which the reader may find in every page marked with this letter A'. The College's *Pharmacopoeia* merely listed ingredients and recipes. It was intentionally mute on how they should be used. *A Physical Directory*, more than twice as long, was bursting through its margins with this valuable information. The physicians' secrets were out.

The book was an instant success. Within weeks of publication, smaller, cheaper pirated editions were in circulation. Spotting a

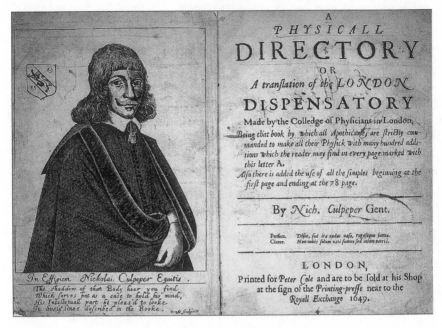

Portrait and Title-Page of Physical Directory

niche in the market, other publishers rushed out medical texts of
their own. The indefatigable book collector George Thomason, who
had not collected a single medical work before the appearance of
Nicholas's *Physical Directory*, quickly accumulated more than eighty,
all but five in English.[36]

Nicholas himself was heavily promoted as the book's author. A
portrait filled the page facing the frontispiece that was to introduce
nearly all his subsequent works. It gave him a striking resemblance
to John Milton and William Lilly, with the same long black hair,
dress, and pose, probably to align him with their Puritan affiliations.
The title-page proclaimed the work to be 'By Nich. Culpeper Gent.'.
He was evidently famous enough across the capital, and perhaps
beyond, for his name to be used without any mention of his medical
experience or biography, even though this was the first work
ascribed to him.[37]

The translation of such a technical work was no easy task, as

Nicholas acknowledged. Many of the medical terms used in the original had no obvious English equivalents. For example, the College insisted upon using antiquated measures such as the Roman 'cochlearium', which meant a spoonful, the spoon in question being that used to extract snails from their shells (*cochlea* is the Latin for snail). Identifying the colloquial English equivalents of the Latin names of ingredients was an even greater challenge. Nicholas was writing a century before Linnaeus developed a systematic method of botanical classification. Single names were used to identify different varieties of the same species; single varieties were often known by different names. To take an example from the list of thirty-three herbs beginning with 'A', 'Argentina' was identified by Nicholas as 'silver weed or wild tansy'. It is also known as prince's feathers, wild agrimony, goosewort, silvery cinquefoil, traveller's ease, traveller's joy and, botanically, *Potentilla anserina*. As Nicholas noted, it was also called 'wild' (as well as 'goose') tansy, but was not the same plant as 'Tanacetum', also known vulgarly as tansy, which was similar in appearance, but botanically unrelated and much stronger in its medicinal effects.[38]

There are many marginal notes in which Nicholas discusses the difficulties of translation, particularly when they gave him an opportunity to poke fun at the *Pharmacopoeia*'s august list of authors, which included William Harvey. Considering a subclause 'pro vehiculis Cordialium' at the end of the recipe for Moundeford's 'Aqua Cordialis' (a cordial), Nicholas translated *vehiculis* as 'mixture' on the grounds that he knew 'not what better word to give it, for their word *Vehiculum* signifies any thing to carry it in, even from a chariot to a wheelbarrow'.[39] He corrected several errors, usually, but not always, drawing gleeful attention to them. In the *Pharmacopoeia*'s recipe for *Potio vulneria, vulgo decoctum Scolpetarium*, which Nicholas translates as a 'Drink for wounded men', the recipe apparently calls for a song ('*canororum*'). Nicholas corrects it without comment to refer to crab shell ('*cancrorum*', '*cancri fluviatiles*', river crab or crayfish, being listed in the catalogue of simples or standard ingredients).[40]

He also pointed out many inconsistencies and absurdities, such as in the recipe for *Vigonia Oxycroceum (in quo nil croci) Prestantius*. 'In plain English', he wrote, this meant 'Vigo his more excellent Plaister of Vinegar and Saffron, in which is no Saffron'. 'Surely,' he added, 'the College quoted this receipt (which more properly might be called *Vigo* his nonsense) for Apothecaries to laugh at, not to make.'[41]

The notes are also full of advice on the best way of mixing the ingredients, and observations on the practical difficulties apothecaries faced in concocting some of the prescriptions, such as that for Fallopius' Allum-Water. '*Fallopius* invented this for an unction for the French pox,' Nicholas noted, 'but in my opinion it is but a childish receipt, for the Quick-silver [Mercury], will most assuredly fly out in the boiling.'[42]

However, these were not the additions that caused the medical establishment most concern. The physicians may not even have cared particularly about the hundred or so simples Nicholas added, drawn from such authorities as Galen and Dioscorides. He was merely updating the work to reflect medical fashion, which included the prescription of a variety of medicines not featured in the original *Pharmacopoeia*. Culpeper's clear and detailed guidance on the preparation of simples and compounds may even have been welcome, as it helped standardize practice among the apothecaries, who at the time had no official manual of methods, either from the College or the Society of Apothecaries. Indeed, this was one of the main causes of the continuing antagonism between the two organizations. The College Censors repeatedly upbraided apothecaries for failing to mix ingredients in what they considered to be the proper manner.

What really upset the doctors was that Culpeper revealed what the medicines in the *Pharmacopoeia* were for. From 'Acanthi', which Dioscorides recommended for ruptures and blisters, to Zingiberis, which 'helps digestion, warms the stomach, clears the sight, and is profitable for old men', he detailed the virtues of each simple, including those that he thought had none (which included sugar

cane and spinach). He did not censor the list. The most toxic
poisons were included, along with detailed instructions on how
such materials should be handled. When it came to the compounds,
he exposed even more of the physicians' secrets: providing easy-to-
follow recipes for each, complete with familiar English names for
the ingredients where possible, and adding a description of when
the concoction should be used.

Thus, in translating the book, Nicholas broke every rule in it.
But even this was not the worst of his sins. From the opening epistle,
Nicholas made it clear that his translation of the *Pharmacopoeia* was
not just, or even primarily, a medical work: it was a political one.
On the very first page of the book he placed a signed letter from
the 'Translator to the Reader'. Referring to the turmoils of the year,
and intermingling some technical terms to show off his knowledge
of medicine, he announced in the ringing tones of the pulpit, 'God
gave Tyrants in his Wrath, and will take them away in his Displeasure.' England had embarked upon a 'sad game' – republicanism
– in which all the other nations of Europe would soon find themselves participating:

> The Prize which We now, and They within a few years shall
> play for, is, THE LIBERTY OF THE SUBJECT: This is the part
> which some think is so sluggishly acted, but I am of [the]
> opinion will speedily be ended with a joyful *Plaudit* upon the
> English Stage. So far as I can see by the help of my Optic Nerves,
> (whether it be *Intromittendo Species*, or *Extramitendo Radios*, it
> matters not much) the Liberty of our *Common-Wealth* (if I may
> call it so without a Solecism) is most infringed by three sorts
> of men, *Priests, Physicians, Lawyers* . . . The one deceives men
> in matters belonging to their Souls, the other in matters belong-
> ing to their Bodies, the third in matters belonging to their
> Estates.

Of the three professions, the physicians were inevitably exposed as
the worst. They 'walk in the Clouds . . . their ways being not so

discernable to a vulgar view as the ways of the other two are; and that's the reason men are led by the noses (worse than beasts, as though oppression had already made them mad) by a company of proud, insulting, domineering Doctors'. Then, in a passage that echoed almost to the word John Aubrey's description of William Harvey, he wondered if it was 'handsome and well-beseeming a Common-wealth to see a Doctor ride in State, in Plush with a footcloth?'[43]

The reaction to the publication of the *Physical Directory* was swift and savage. The week it appeared, the newspaper *Mercurius Pragmaticus* ran a review condemning both author and work. The anti-parliamentarian newsletter was founded in 1647 by March-amont Needham. He was probably not the author of the unsigned article, as at the time he was in prison for sedition, and his inconstant loyalties, which a few years earlier had moved against the parliamentary cause in favour of the royalists, were now headed in the opposite direction. Whoever did write the review clearly knew of Nicholas, describing him as living 'about Moore-fields', a suburb neighbouring Spitalfields. He was dismissed as a 'figure-flinger', an astrologer, who lived 'upon Cousenage', in other words the Culpeper name, 'Cheating the poor People who had lost their Waistcoats, Aprons, Smocks'.

The reviewer dwelt particularly on the evolution of Nicholas's radicalism, which he claimed had passed through 'several degrees of *Independency*, *Brownism*, *Anabaptism*', the gamut of religious non-conformity. He was accused of having 'admitted himself of *John Goodwin's School* (of all ungodliness) in *Coleman-street*' after which 'he turns *Seeker*, *Manifestarian*, and now he is arrived at the Battlement of an absolute *Atheist*'. By 'two years drunken Labour', he had 'Gallimawfred the Apothecaries' Book into non-sense, mixing every Receipt therein with some Scruples, at least of Rebellion or Atheism, besides the danger of Poisoning Men's Bodies: And (to supply his Drunkenness and Lechery with a thirty shillings Reward) endeavored to bring into obloquy the famous Societies of *Apothecaries* and *Chyrurgeons*'.

The criticisms would continue, relentlessly pursuing the themes of venality, ignorance, and irresponsibility. Most also dwelt on drunkenness, reinforcing Nicholas's reputation as keen to 'make himself famous in Taverns and Alehouses', the cockpits of debauchery as well as the meeting-houses of rebellion.[44] Another critic accused him of writing for 'the acquiring of money from the Printers, for buying of Beer and Tobacco'. In his *Art of Simpling*, William Coles focused on the accusation that Nicholas had done the translation for money. He reprised the caricature of Nicholas as a 'figure-flinger' who had 'tumbled over' many books 'and transcribed as much out of them as he thought would serve his turn (though many times he were therein mistaken)'.[45]

Officially, the College's response to the *Physical Directory* was one of dignified silence. Unofficially, dissecting knives were drawn. William Johnson, the College's chemist, wrote a vitriolic personal attack added to the first publication that came to hand, a translation of an obscure medical work by the Italian physician Leonardo Fioravanti entitled *Three Exact Pieces*. Giving Nicholas a taste of his own medicine, Johnson accused him of being ignorant, arrogant, and even licentious. He was taunted for his failure to become an apothecary and for his terror of the College:

> Amen Corner . . .'tis a formidable place to you, for fear of dissection, for you never durst hitherto venture your approbation there before the Doctors' of your sufficiency in your trade you were bound to, and some while brought up in; And for your judgement in Physic, I know you dare not come thither to the test.

As for the book, the physicians, Johnson reported, regarded it with derision. 'Pray let me not trouble your weak brains with a relation of a Gentleman and Scholar's censure upon your Book,' Johnson snorted, suppressing guffaws, 'who perusing some passages in it in a Bookseller's shop, asked whether Culpeper made that obscene book or no, and being answered he did, replied truly Culpeper hath made Cul-paper, paper fit to wipe one's breeches withal.'

As a departing insult, Johnson argued that Nicholas would do well to heed not Hippocrates but Harpocrates, the Greek name for the Egyptian God Horus. Tradition depicted the deity as an infant with a finger held to his lips, representing the virtue of silence. Johnson went further, describing the child as having been born 'with one hand on his mouth, and the other on his members', and recommended Nicholas adopt a similar pose. Johnson's attack was not openly endorsed by the College, but it was signed 'From Amen Corner'.[46]

More clandestine methods were also set in motion to frustrate those associated with the book. Within a few weeks of its appearance, a warrant was issued for Peter Cole's arrest for sedition. The pretext was the publication of *King Charls his Tryal*, a work that had appeared ten months earlier and that had been properly licensed with the Stationers' Company.[47] Cole cut a deal with the authorities, offering to cooperate with their continuing efforts to close down the secret presses. But his collaboration was short-lived, if it was not a ruse. More warnings and warrants followed and would continue throughout the early 1650s.

Nicholas was subject to more direct pressure. In December 1650, an order was issued by the Council of State, the executive body which, under the presidency of Oliver Cromwell, ran the new Commonwealth government. The Council was to 'write to the mayor and aldermen of Cambridge to send up . . . Mr Culpeper in safe custody, and to approve of what they have done in restraining [him]'. Ten days later, Nicholas was in London before the Committee of Examinations, the parliamentary body that controlled the press. The same committee had earlier interrogated William Lilly about *The Starry Messenger*, but he had escaped prosecution. Neither the charges nor the outcome are recorded in Culpeper's case.

A few weeks later, Peter Cole was summoned. A complaint had been lodged concerning the translation of another College publication, *De rachitide*, 'On Rickets', by Francis Glisson. The original, in Latin, was an important work, arguably one of the first scientific medical texts on a specific disease. The translation was unofficial, attributed to a Philip Armin, but edited by Nicholas and published by Cole. This proved to be an uncharacteristic miscalculation on Cole's part, as it transpired that for the first time the College had thought to register the English as well as the Latin edition at the Stationers' Company. Furthermore, the registration was in the name of William Dugard, Parliament's official printer. Because of Dugard's involvement, the complaint was lodged by John Milton, who in 1649 had been appointed Latin Secretary by the Council of State.[48]

In the face of this intimidation, Nicholas and Cole did not falter. Within a year of publishing the first edition of the *Physical Directory*, a second was produced, with yet further additions to infuriate the physicians. Nicholas's tone had not moderated. Drawing on the language of the Levellers, he began a new introductory letter 'to the Impartial Reader' with an attack on 'William the Bastard', who, 'having conquered this Nation . . . brought in the Norman Laws written in an unknown tongue'. Since then, books had been published in French and Latin so that the 'Commonalty' could be 'kept in ignorance that so they may the better be made slaves of'.[49]

Though the physicians 'snarled' at him, and though the attacks had left him 'exceeding melancholy of complexion, subject to Consumptions and Chilliness of my Vital spirits', he produced a third edition the following year.[50] This time he began with a letter addressed not to the reader but to the physicians themselves. 'College, College, thou are Diseased,' he wrote. The cause was 'Mammon' (greed), the diagnostics or symptoms were 'seven miles about London, lay him in Prison: five pound a month for practising Physic unless he be a Collegiate; make a couple of crutches of the Apothecaries and Chyrurgions; Be as proud as Lucifer; Ride in state with a Foot-cloth; Love the sight of Angels [coins]; cheat the rich, neglect the poor'. The prognostics or outlook: 'pride goes before a

Fall'; the cure: 'Fear God; Do good to all; hide not your Talent in a Napkin.'

In this 1651 edition, he also explained why he had undertaken the work: 'I saw Ancient people coming to me, sick, and coughing, and crying out for the Lord's sake help us. I saw young Children ... desiring me to give them the grounds of Physic in their Mother Tongue.'[51] Now readers were coming to him as well, and in their multitudes. Peter Cole, a model for his successors in the publishing industry, was proving himself deft at combining a principled stand for press freedom with a more practical talent for selling books. Nicholas was now by far and away his most successful author, and he demanded more. More was forthcoming: a translation of selections from Galen, a translation of the latest guide to human anatomy by Johann Vesling. Nicholas also began to copy Lilly's practice of producing annual ephemerides or almanacs, the first being published by Cole in 1651. This contained lists of the positions and conjunctions of the heavenly bodies through the year, together with 'judgements' on what they might mean for the future of the country, which in the main consisted of an intensification of political revolution across Europe: the 'killing of kings ... subversion of kingdoms, terrible Strifes, Contentions and wranglings'.[52]

Later that year, Nicholas produced another almanac, together with *Semeiotica Uranica, or, An astrological judgement of diseases*, based on his lectures to the Society of Astrologers, about the links between astrology and physic. These were both published by Nathaniel Brooke, who thenceforth produced all Nicholas's astrological works, setting off an intense rivalry between him and Cole that would continue throughout Nicholas's career and beyond. The almanac was for 1652, and was even more apocalyptic about the political order than its predecessor. Anticipating a 'Year of Wonders', and prognosticating 'the ruin of Monarchy throughout Europe, and a Change of the Law', its main focus was a 'most terrible Eclipse of the Sun' due at 10.01 a.m. on 29 March, a Monday. Its occurrence in the tenth house, associated with royalty, meant the humbling of monarchy: 'Believe me ... before the effects of this Eclipse be over, the World shall see Princes are but men.' It also announced a change of religious government. 'The Law shall quite and clean be changed; when the Prince of Peace, the great Lawgiver, shall come in the Power of his Spirit, and dwell in our hearts, there shall be no more wranglings, no more going to Law.'[53]

In early 1652, Nicholas published a pamphlet with Brooke capitalizing on the growing anxiety about the eclipse. Entitled *Catastrophe Magnatum: or, the Fall of Monarchie*, it was clearly aimed at a wider audience than the almanac. It proclaimed the eclipse as laying the way for the 'Fifth Monarchy', the rule of Christ. As a prelude to this, there would be fire and plague – and democracy: 'the Government will come into the hands of the People'.[54]

As the day now billed as 'Black Monday' approached, apprehension intensified. The streets became littered with apocalyptic pamphlets and street hawkers sold cordials promising to reduce the eclipse's effects. The poor were said to be throwing away their few possessions, the rich to be loading their carts and heading for the hills. As the dawn of 29 March broke, 'hardly any would work, none stir out of their houses', except for the members of the Society of Astrologers, Nicholas presumably among them, who gathered to watch the event from the roof of Southampton House, off Holborn, to the west of the city.[55]

It was a black day for astrologers, but a cloudless one for the rest of the population, perfect conditions to witness a very partial eclipse that barely dimmed the brilliance of a glorious sky. In his defence, Nicholas could have pointed out that he had never predicted a 'black' Monday, more a 'ruddyish grey' one, his own calculations having shown that the moon would clip the edge of the sun rather than obscure it entirely.[56] But this was not enough to save him and the other members of the Society from a profusion of pamphlets that appeared within days ridiculing their prophecies. Most were targeted at Lilly. Nicholas was characterized as Lilly's 'ape', an appellation probably adopted to reinforce the view that

Cataſtrophe Magnatum:

⌊65

O R,

THE FALL OF *MONARCHIE.*

A *Caveat* to M A G I S T R A T E S, Deduced from the
Eclipſe of the S u n n e, *March* 29. 1 6 5 2.
With a Probable Conjecture of the Determination of the Effects.

By *Nich: Culpeper* Gent. Stud.in Aſtrol.and Phyſ:

D A N. 2. 21, 22.

*He changeth the times and the ſeaſons, he removeth Kings, and ſetteth up Kings : he
giveth wiſdome to the Wiſe, and knowledge to them that know underſtanding : he revea-
leth the deep and ſecret things, he knoweth what is in the darkneſſe, and the light dwelleth with him.*

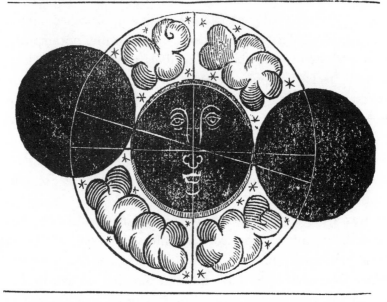

L O N D O N,
Printed for *T. Vere* and *Nath: Brooke* , in the Old Baily, and at the
Angel in Cornhil. 1 6 5 2.

in his writing Nicholas copied others. In one, entitled *A Faire in Spittle Fields*, Nicholas was mocked in lines of doggerel as 'the Vicar of St Fools' (the name of a country dance), who

> ... contradicts Physicians and the Schools
> And with a handful of conceited knowledge
> Dare challenge all the Doctors in the College.[57]

'Philastrogous' penned *Black Munday turn'd White*, sections of which also appeared under the title *Lillies Ape Whipt*. The anonymous author provided a detailed commentary upon the portrait of Nicholas's 'Brazen Face' that appeared opposite the title-page of the *Physical Directory*, apparently the real object of the attack. 'Philastrogous' drew particular attention to the 'dangling snakes' of his hair, 'a squeezing deglabing Countenance', and the coat of arms in the background, 'that we may take notice you are a Gentleman', a member of 'that ancient Family of the Culpepers, whose merits transcend the commendation of so weak a Pen'.[58]

Some considered the eclipse decisive in breaking the hold 'figure-flingers' had over the public. Certainly reputations suffered. Soon after the eclipse, a countryman came to Lilly's house in the Strand to consult on the theft of a purse. He found a turd on the astrologer's doorstep. 'Down came the profound Ass-trologer,' one of Lilly's critics reported, 'who opening the door came and seeing it in that shitten case, began to execrate and curse those beastly Knaves that did it; vowing if he did but know who did him that nasty trick, he would make them Examples of all such Rogues so long as they liv'd; Nay, quote the Countryman, if he cannot tell who beshit his door, he can as well be hanged as tell me who had my Purse, and so went his way.'[59]

But astrology, as its subsequent popularity shows, was not about prophesying events. It was about discussing, anticipating, hastening, even instigating them. Nicholas was explicit about this. 'Imagine what I write be every word false, what harm will it do Princes to prepare for the loss of a kingdom, though it never come?' he wrote in *Catastrophe Magnatum*. 'Is it not the way to teach them humility? I am sure they are proud enough. Were it not acceptable both before God and man, that they should leave off their TYRANNY?'[60]

ARRACH WILD & STINKING

Atriplex hortensis, olida

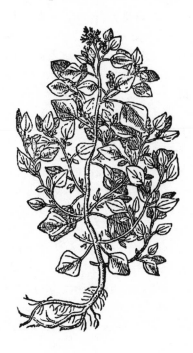

This hath small and almost round Leaves, yet a little pointed and without dent or cut, of a dusky mealy colour, growing on the slender Stalks and Branches that spread on the ground, with smal Flowers in clusters set with the Leaves, and small Seeds succeeding like the rest, perishing yearly, and rising again with its own sowing.

It smels like old rotten Fish, or somthing worse.

It grows usually upon Dunghills.

They flower in June and July, and their Seed is ripe quickly after.

The Works of God are given freely to Man, his Medicins are common and cheap, and easie to be found: 'tis the Medicines of the Colledg of Physitians that are so dear and scarce to find.

I commend it for an Universal Medicine for the Womb, and such a Medicine as will easily, safly, and speedily cure any Diseas therof, as the fits of the Mother, Dislocation or falling out therof; it cools the Womb being over-heated. (And let me tel you this, and I wil tel you but the truth, Heat of the womb is one of the greatest causes of hard labor in Childbirth) It makes barren women fruitful, it clenseth the Womb if it be foul and strengthens it exceedingly; it provokes the Terms if they be stopped, and stops them if they flow immoderately. You can desire no good to your Womb, but this Herb will effect it; therfore if you love Children, if you love Health, if you love Ease, keep a Syrup alwaies by you made of the juyce of this Herb and Sugar (or Honey if it be to clens the Womb) and let such as be rich keep it for their poor neighbors, and bestow it as freely as I bestow my studies upon them, or els let them look to answer it another day when the Lord shall come to make inquisition for Bloud.

Now spelled orache, the smell of this stinking plant comes from the leaves giving off ammonia, according to Grieve. 'The whole plant is of a most loathsome savour or smell,' wrote Gerard, adding that 'if any should chance to rest and sleep' upon it, 'he might had reposed himself among the chief of Scoggin's heirs', referring to John Scoggin or Scogan, Edward IV's famous court jester.[1]

ven in the absence of eclipses, Nicholas saw many dark days in the late 1640s and early 1650s. During this period, he may have moved from his tenement in the precincts of St Mary Spital to a new house in neighbouring Lollesworth Field, which was developed in 1649.[2] By August 1650, he was at 'Spittle-fields next door to the Red Lion', the famous address he would give in his subsequent publications, which would attract to its door the eminent and curious for decades to come. Here, he and his wife Alice raised a family that produced seven children. He makes few mentions of them, except in connection with the various medicines he used to treat their ailments. One suffered from an unspecified urinary complaint, another from the fatal cholera-like 'bloody flux' that struck in 1649, another, poignantly, from the 'King's Evil', scrofula.[3]

Only one of these children, Mary, survived to adulthood; but, despite such an appalling tally of losses, Nicholas's critics never used it as grounds to question his medical competence. This was not out of respect for his private life, but an acceptance that medicine could do little to diminish even this high level of child mortality, particularly in a city like London. However, it did inspire Nicholas to produce his second major medical work, a guide to midwifery entitled *A Directory for Midwives*.

Childbirth was a process fraught with dangers in the seventeenth century, but conducted according to a formal set of protocols designed to ensure the due observance of religious rituals as much as medical precautions. The recitation of prayers was as important as the provision of hot water and towels. The delivery room was

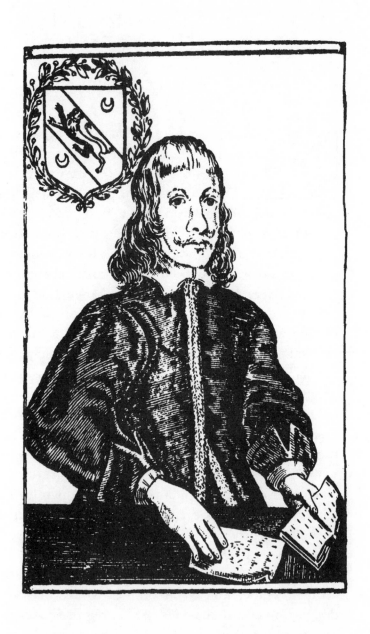

A DIRECTORY FOR MIDWIVES:

OR,

A Guide for Women,

In their ⎰ *Conception,*
⎱ *Bearing,* And
⎰ *Suckling their Children.*

Containing,

1. *The Anatomie of the Vessels of Generation*
2. *The Formation of the Child in the Womb.*
3. *What hinders Conception, and its Remedies*
4. *What furthers Conception.*
5. *A Guide for Women in Conception.*
6. *Of Miscarriage in Women.*
7. *A Guide for Women in their Labor*
8. *A Guide for Women in their Lying-in*
9. *Of Nursing Children.*

By *Nich. Culpeper,* Gent. Student in
Physick and Astrologie.

Exod. 1. 21.

*It came to pass, because the Midwives feared the Lord,
that God built them Houses.*

LONDON:
Printed by *Peter Cole,* at the sign of the *Printing-Pres*
in Cornhil, near the Royal Exchange. 1651

kept dark. Men were excluded. This was the only time a physician was prepared to devolve his responsibilities to another medical expert: the midwife. She was in command, attended by a group of 'gossips', including trainee midwives. As she performed external and internal examinations, and applied oils and ointments to ease the mother's pain and child's passage, devotions were read out and songs sung.[4] Physicians, performing the role of 'man-midwives', were, theoretically at least, summoned in cases of emergency, but this seems to have been rare.

Attempts had been made to bring midwifery under male control, but these had been successfully resisted.[5] However, following the Civil War, the midwives felt under threat, prompting a petition to Parliament. They complained that so many young men had been killed in the war 'before they had performed any thing to the benefit of Mid-wives' (i.e. fathered children) that their trade 'is now decayed'. 'We were formerly well paid, and highly respected, for our great skill and mid-night industry, but now our Art doth fail us, and little gettings have we in this age barren of all natural joys.'[6]

It was in this context, and against the background of 'myself having buried many of my children young', that Nicholas had cause 'to fix my thoughts intently upon this business' and to produce the *Directory for Midwives*. It was printed in pocket-sized octavo format, and written in an informal style, peppered with anecdotes and jokes so, as Nicholas put it in the preface, it 'should be for every one's good, and therefore within the reach of every one's purse'. It set out the theory of generation, birth and child-rearing, but omitted the practice of child delivery, including methods for performing such obstetric procedures as a podalic version for positioning the foetus in the womb. This was out of respect for the midwives' expertise and commercial interests, which he clearly rated above those of the doctors. For, Nicholas rhetorically asked of them, 'to whom doth the Practical part of [midwifery] belong, but to yourselves?'[7]

The bulk of the book dealt with the anatomy of the female and male sexual organs, the formation of the foetus in the womb, the causes of infertility, miscarriages, labour, lying-in, and nursing. It also included a handy list of Latin terms that midwives and mothers were likely to encounter if a physician intervened.

The *Directory* appeared in 1651, at the same time as another book on pregnancy and childbirth: *De generatione animalium* by William Harvey, his first major work since *De motu cordis*.

This was the only time that the work and ideas of Culpeper and Harvey would directly confront one another, and the contrast between them is striking. The *Directory* was dedicated to midwives, *De generatione* to the College. Nicholas encouraged the midwives to keep control of their practice, and not feel the need to 'call for the help of a man-midwife, which is a disparagement not only to yourselves, but also to your Profession'. According to Harvey (writing in Latin), 'the younger, more giddy, and officious Midwives are to be rebuked' for intervening too actively in the birthing process 'lest they should seem unskilful at their trade'. He considered it 'happier' for 'poor women, and those that dare not own their great bellies', to avoid using midwives altogether. This view would be widely endorsed, notably in *Observations in Midwifery* by Percival Willughby, the physician Harvey visited while with the King at Nottingham for the raising of the royal standard. *Observations in Midwifery* was compiled soon after the publication of *De generatione animalium* though was not published until 1863, when it proved highly influential. 'I know but Dr Harvey's directions and method,' Willughby wrote, 'the which I wish all midwives to observe and follow, and oft to read over and over again.'[8]

However, Willughby's injunction was misplaced. Harvey's book would be of very little use to a midwife as it contained only a few pertinent comments on human births based on his own obstetric practice tacked onto the end. *De generatione* is a scientific treatise, a masterpiece of the genre. But it is not a medical manual. Harvey spends the first 362 pages on the hen, examining through a series of 'exercises' every stage of development from the egg to the chicken.

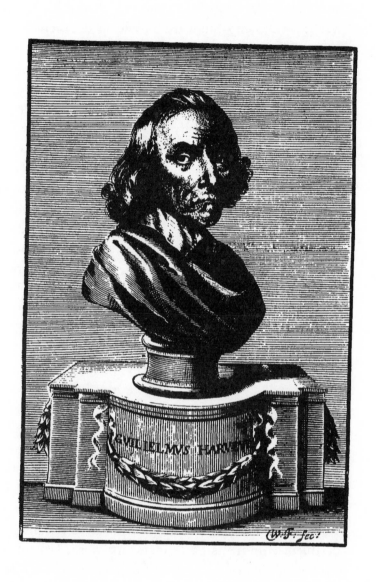

A N A T O M I C A L
EXERCITATIONS,

Concerning the   *871*

G E N E R A T I O N
Of Living Creatures :

To which are added Particular Difcourfes,
of *Births*, and of *Conceptions*, &c.

By *WILLIAM HARVET*, Doctor
of *Phyfick*, and Profeffor of *Anatomy*,
and *Chirurgery*, in the C O L L E D G E
of Phyfitians of *LONDON*.

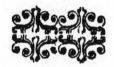

ottober 2 *LONDON,*

Printed by *James Young*, for *Octavian*
Pulleyn, and are to be fold at his Shop at the
Sign of the Rofe in St. *Pauls* Church-
yard. 1653.

He spends forty-seven pages watching the development of the ger-
minal spot or 'cicatricula' on the surface of the yolk. He observes
how it would dilate 'to the magnitude of a pea or lentil', then begin
to look like 'the eye of some small bird', then become part of
'a great Metamorphosis, and wonderful alteration' when the egg
'beginneth to step from the life of a Plant to the life of an Animal',
then begin to move, then sprout feathers, then bud legs, wings and
organs, then grow eyes (which until the tenth day 'stick fast in the
head . . . for if then you pluck them out, you shall find them black,
and bigger than beans'), then 'gently tumble and stretch out the
neck', then develop 'involutions of the brain' . . . and so on until,
three weeks later, the fully grown chick 'covets the freer air' and
'entereth into the world'.[9] At each stage of this process he quotes
the associated literature, mostly Aristotle and Fabricius, carefully
assessing what they say, and in many cases refuting it on the basis
of his own observations. In this respect, it is Harvey's work that
challenges authority, rather than Culpeper's. Having completed his
meticulous examination of the chicken, Harvey turns his attention
to 'viviparous animals', those that produce offspring in a living
state rather than in an egg. It is in this section, in an exercise
entitled 'History of the Generation of Hinds and Hoes . . . as the
example of all other Animals', that he sets out the results of his
lengthy experiments on the King's deer.[10]

Harvey peppers his work with examples of experimentation upon
himself, an impressive feature of his scientific work. For example,
in Exercise LVII dealing with 'certain paradoxes and problems', he
writes of pricking one finger with a needle, then another with the
same needle after it had been contaminated with poison from a
'spider's tooth', to show how the flesh could detect toxicity and
repair the damage. As proof that he took his own medicine, he also
describes how, when drinking an infusion of antimony 'in a vomit'
(an emetic), 'it is very strange . . . though we neither distinguish it
by taste, nor find any disgust in it, either swallowing it down, or
returning it back again, yet there passeth a censure upon it by the

stomach, which discerns between what is useful and prejudicial, and so provokes to Vomit'.[11]

When looking at human birth, he draws upon extensive personal experience, and quotes a number of novel cases, concerning such matters as 'a certain Servant-Maid being gotten with Child by her Master' who 'to hide her knavery came to London in September, where she lay in by stealth: and being recovered again, returned home: but in December following, a new birth (for she had a Superfoetation [a conception occurring while a foetus is already developing in the womb]) did proclaim the crime which she had cunningly concealed before'. On another occasion, he was brought some 'black little bones' produced by a mother following a successful birth, which Harvey identified as the residue of a previous abortion.[12]

Nicholas and Harvey both tried to dispel some of the many myths that surrounded pregnancy and birth. It was widely believed, for example, that the womb was made up of seven chambers, males developing in the three right-hand chambers, females in three left-hand chambers, and hermaphrodites in the middle. Nicholas dismissed this as anatomically 'childish'. He also rejected the idea that infertility was a sign that a woman was diabolically possessed, and that the seed from the right testicle produced male babies and the left female.[13]

Nicholas also promulgated a number of myths, but even Harvey was not completely immune from doing the same – for instance holding to the notion that the right testicle produced male babies. He has been credited with the dictum '*Ex ovo omnia*', everything from an egg, since the inscription appeared in a picture on the frontispiece of *De generatione*. In 1870, Thomas Huxley, the champion of Darwinism, struggled to show that this proved 'our great countryman Harvey' had thus laid to rest the myth of 'spontaneous generation', the ancient belief that some creatures emerge spontaneously from the medium in which they are discovered, such as flies from cow dung. Hopeful signs could be found in Harvey's assertion that all animals and plants spring from what he terms a 'primordium vegetale', 'a phrase which may nowadays be rendered "a vegetative germ"; and this, he says, is "*oviforme*" or "egg-like"'. But as Huxley had regretfully to admit, 'he does, more than once, use language which is consistent only with a full belief in spontaneous or equivocal generation'. Indeed he does, remarking, for example, that animals 'proceed' not only from their own kind, but 'are spontaneous, and the Issues of Putrefaction'.[14]

Harvey also subscribed to the notion that the foetus is nourished in the womb by the amniotic fluid surrounding it, which it ingests via the mouth. Only the thinner fluids, Harvey believed, permeate via the umbilical cord. In fact, Harvey seemed to be uncharacteristically confused when it came to the function of the navel. In the anatomical lectures he gave at the College in the 1630s, he puzzlingly pronounced that women experienced 'sexual pleasure through [the] umbilicus'.[15] Nicholas seemed to be better informed on this subject. In his *Directory for Midwives*, he identified the umbilical cord as the vessel through which the foetus was nourished from conception to birth, and he gently mocked the popular notion that the cord of a baby boy cut longer resulted in a bigger penis, because, if that were so, 'all Women laboring with Child would complain of Midwives' cutting them so short.

As for the source of female sexual pleasure, he knew it to be the clitoris. 'In form it represents the Yard of a man,' he wrote, 'and suffers erection and falling as that doth; this is that which causeth lust in Women and gives delight in Copulation; for without this a Woman neither desires Copulation, or hath pleasure in it.' Furthermore, where Harvey considered lust necessary but loathsome, and sex an activity that women 'suffer' rather than enjoy, Nicholas embraced it as a natural and welcome part of the reproductive process.[16]

There is another notable contrast in Harvey's and Nicholas's works. Where *De generatione* is strewn with dissections and vivisections, from the examination of the womb of a pregnant deer to the discovery of a large nerve in an ostrich penis, the *Directory for*

Midwives contains what must surely be one of the earliest manifestos for animal rights. It appears in a digression from the subject of the behaviour of children, which (writing at a time when he was surrounded by a young family) he considered to be ruled by pride, the 'first sin' committed by Adam and 'so bred in the bone, that 'twill never out of the flesh' – an echo of William Attersoll's views. This same pride induced 'the learned Rabbis [i.e. priests] of our Age' to set humans above the animals, on the grounds that 'no creature is rational but Man'. 'A few creatures (as Horses, and Oxen, and Asses, and the like) . . . may not be so rational as their Masters,' Nicholas concedes, but why? Because, he argues, they are driven to madness by enslavement. 'A Bird that hath been brought up in a Cage will fly into the Cage again though you take him out and set him on the further side of a Table; but a Bird that was brought up in the Woods, and so knows what liberty is, if you shut him in a Cage he will go near to die for madness. The reason is because the first knows not what liberty is, but by bondage is . . . deprived of reason.'[17]

The *Directory* deals with a number of other controversies arising from the study of sex and childbirth. For example, on the subject of the hymen, some authorities claimed it did not exist, others that it could only be broken by sexual intercourse. Nicholas argued that it could be ruptured in numerous ways other than intercourse, 'especially in young Virgins, because it is thinnest in them'.[18]

Harvey's *De generatione* enjoyed respectful critical reception, and, after the appearance of an English edition in 1653, became widely read. It was 'full of excellent learning and observation', wrote one critic, despite Harvey's failure to explain how an embryo managed to form 'without any sensible Corporeal Agent, by mere Imagination, not of the brain, but of the Womb'. Another, while detecting some anatomical errors, acclaimed it a 'golden book'.[19] It was for this he was later called the father of obstetrics, even of midwifery.

Nicholas's *Directory* had a much harder time. It was wildly popular, running to four editions in a decade, and spawning a pirated edition that appeared within months of its publication. However, in 1656 a rival midwifery manual appeared entitled *The Compleat Midwifes Practice*, apparently written by four anonymous midwives. In the introduction, it surveys the existing literature, most of which it considers 'wretched', but reserves special condemnation for the *Directory*, which it describes as 'the most desperately deficient of them all'. The familiar criticisms were trotted out, principally that Nicholas had written it 'for necessity', money, for otherwise 'he would certainly have never been so sinful to have exposed it to the light'. On the face of it, such a criticism was damning, coming from the midwives Nicholas had flattered with a dedication in his *Directory*. However, there are several indications that it was, ironically, commercially motivated. Firstly, it appeared in a preface written by, among others, Thomas Chamberlen, a member of a family of 'man-midwives' thwarted in its efforts to take control of midwifery practice. Secondly, an enlarged edition published in 1680, which repeated the same criticisms, also contained 'a further Discovery of those Secrets kept close in the Breast of Mr Nich. Culpeper', and claimed to be based on 'the experience of your English Viz . . . Mr Nich. Culpeper'.[20]

Nicholas was not put off by such criticisms. Now at the height of his popularity, he used the *Directory* to advertise his next work, a manual to instruct the readers of the *Directory* 'in the knowledge of Herbs before I am half a year older'. As authors often do, he missed the deadline. But when the promised work appeared a year later, it did not disappoint. It proved to be one of the most popular and enduring books in publishing history, perhaps the non-religious book in English to remain longest in continuous print.[21] It was called *The English Physitian*, though it became better known as *Culpeper's Complete Herbal*, and offered the reader 'a Compleat Method of Physick, whereby a man preserve his Body in Health, or cure himself, being sick, for three pence charge, with such things only as grow in England'.[22]

The layout of *English Physitian* is very simple. The main section is a directory of English medicinal herbs, from Adder's Tongue to Yarrow, describing for each their appearance, where they could be found, when they should be picked, their medicinal 'virtues and use', and their 'astrology'. This was followed by a section entitled 'Directions' containing instructions on how the herbs should be prepared and applied.

It was for the astrological sections, usually the briefest and often absent, that the *English Physitian* became best known, certainly within the botanical world. Agnes Arber, who in 1912 wrote what is considered to be the definitive history of herbals, consigned Nicholas's to a 'backwater' of superstitious texts. Confusing the *English Physitian* with the *Physical Directory*, she wrote that 'in the seventeenth century, England became badly infected with astrological botany' and identified Nicholas as its 'most notorious exponent'.[23] The *English Physitian* certainly contains a strongly astrological element, introduced to provide a way of explaining the actions of different herbs. It also added to what would now be called the 'holistic' aspect of Nicholas's herbal medicine. For him, 'Sickness and Health were caused Naturally (though God may have other ends best known to himself) by the various operations of the Macrocosm'. In other words, the human body, the 'epitome' of creation, acted as a sensitive instrument picking up disturbances in the cosmos.[24] This had important implications for the approach to medicine set out in the *English Physitian*. In particular, it meant that treating disease was not really a matter of 'curing' the body, returning it to some pristine state of health, so much as adapting it to an ever-changing environment. The body, like the heavens, was a flux, and the sort of physic set out in the *English Physitian* is about keeping it in balance. To this extent, it is an astrological work.

But this does not mean that the *English Physitian* is, as Arber assumed, a mystical work. Those who were interested in such matters as macrocosmic influences and occult forces, 'who study Astrol-

THE
Englifh Phyfitian:
O R
An Aftrologo-Phyfical Difcourfe of the Vulgar Herbs of this Nation.

Being a Compleat Method of Phyfick, whereby a man may preferve his Body in Health; or cure himfelf, being fick, for three pence charge, with fuch things only as grow in England, *they being moft fit for Englifh Bodies.*

Herein is alfo fhewed,

1. The way of making Plaifters, Oyntments, Oyls, Pultiffes, Syrups, Decoctions, Julips, or Waters, of all forts of Phyfical Herbs, That you may have them readie for your ufe at all times of the yeer.
2. What Planet governeth every Heib or Tree (ufed in Phyfick) that groweth in *England.*
3. The Time of gathering all Herbs, both Vulgarly, and Aftrologically.
4. The Way of drying and keeping the Herbs all the yeer.
5. The Way of keeping their Juyces ready for ufe at all times.
6. The Way of making and keeping all kind of ufeful Compounds made of Herbs.
7. The way of mixing Medicines according to *Caufe* and and *Mixture* of the *Difeafe,* and *Part* of the Body *Afflicted.*

By *Nich. Culpeper,* Gent. Student in *Phyfick* and *Aftrologie.*

L O N D O N:
Printed by *Peter Cole,* at the fign of the Printing-Prefs in Cornhil, near the Royal Exchange. 1652.

ogy, or such as study Physic Astrologically', were directed to Nicholas's work on astrological medicine, *Semeiotica Uranica*. The main readership was the 'vulgar', not meant pejoratively, but referring to those who could not read Latin and did not have formal medical training, in particular women, the mothers, sisters, ladies, and maids whom Nicholas acknowledges in numerous entries as the main providers of non-professional healthcare.[25] Reflecting this, the book is designed to be highly practical, more so than any other herbal – botanical, astrological, or otherwise. It was written in simple, accessible language. It combined Nicholas's own, obviously extensive experience of herbs with information drawn from more than forty authorities. It provided a handy index of diseases, making it easy to find which herb treated a given ailment. In prescribing treatments, it took into account the availability of ingredients, which might vary according to location, season, and budget. Though many herbs were identified for treating very specific and sometimes relatively rare conditions, a selection of easy, cheap remedies was recommended for the most common complaints, which, judging by the number of times they were mentioned, were agues (fevers, including malaria), coughs, dropsy (swellings), inflammations, 'pestilence' (plague or other epidemical diseases), problems of the liver, spleen, and menstruation, ulcers, vomiting, and wounds (domestic injuries such as cuts, rather than injuries sustained in battle).

To add to the book's 'vulgar' appeal, it cost three pence, the price of a pound of sweet almonds.[26] The price was prominently featured on the title-page, to prevent the book being sold for more. At the time it appeared, there were two other important herbals in English, Thomas Johnson's 'very much enlarged and amended' 1633 edition of John Gerard's *The Herball or Generall Historie of Plantes*, and *Theatrum botanicum: The theater of plants*, by John Parkinson (1567–1650), published in 1640 by William Attersoll's old publisher Thomas Cotes. Nicholas thought Johnson's work inferior to Parkinson's, an opinion that may have been coloured by Johnson's loyalty to the crown. The apothecary had received a doctorate in medicine by royal mandate at Oxford in 1643 (he had never studied at university). He had also fought for the King, dying in 1644 during a royalist engagement to relieve the besieged fortified mansion of the Catholic Marquis of Winchester.

The Parkinson and Johnson herbals, both of which Nicholas acknowledged as sources for the *English Physitian*, were large, lavishly illustrated, and therefore extremely expensive, 'of such a price, that a poor man is not able to buy them', as Nicholas put it. They were also very rare. In 1682, one library valued its first edition of Parkinson's *Theatrum botanicum* at £2 15s. 0d., Nicholas's *English Physitian* at two shillings.[27] Cheap editions were never produced. 'Why forsooth?' Nicholas asked. Because of 'the old threadbare Pleas, It would do people harm' to give them access to pharmaceutical information. 'It is a wonder they will suffer Cutlers to sell Knives, for fear children should cut their fingers and men their throats.'

What made the *English Physitian* unique, however, was not its price, but its style: irreverent, funny, bawdy, angry – vulgar. Nicholas squirted invective at the rich, criticizing the 'wantonness [of] the Gentry', at Catholics, accused of suffering from bad breath as a result of 'maintaining so many Bawdy Houses by Authority of his Holiness', and, inevitably, at the physicians, who 'suck out the Sweetness of other Men's Labors and Studies'. He even poked fun at his own readers. Of the 'furious biting Herb' crowfoot, he wrote that it grows 'very common everywhere, unless you run your Head into a Hedge', and added that the herb had names 'almost enough to make up a Welshman's Pedigree' – a reference to snobs claiming Welsh descent, which became fashionable in the Tudor era after Henry VII, for political reasons, discovered his own Welsh roots.[28]

One section of the book, however, breaks with its practical and populist tone. It is the entry for wormwood, which in the preface he mysteriously promises his astrologically-minded readers will provide the 'Key of all'. Wormwood contains absinthium, the active ingredient of absinthe, which is an hallucinogenic. The entry for the herb in the *English Physitian* reads as though it was written under its influence. 'Pride was the cause of Adam's Fall,' Nicholas writes, reverting to a favourite theme. 'Pride begat a Daughter, I do not know the Father of it unless the Divil, but she christened it, and call'd it Appetite, and sent her Daughter to taste these Wormwoods.' He identifies it as a herb ruled by Mars, which is confirmed by its discovery around 'Martial' places, 'for about Forges and Iron Works you may gather a Cart load of it'. Of its virtues, he writes that 'it helps the evils Venus and her wanton Girls produce' – an aphrodisiac, in other words. And being ruled by Mars, the planet opposite Venus in terms of its astrological influence, it does this 'by Antipathy'.

There follows an astrological drama between Mars and the other heavenly bodies. In one scene, a confrontation erupts between Mars and Venus: 'he asked her what the Reason was that she accused him for abusing Women, he never gave them the Pox, in the Dispute they fell out, and in anger parted'. Later, he meets her again 'as drunk as a Bitch', and he prescribes wormwood, an 'Antipathetical Cure' – bitterness set to provoke sweetness.

'Come Brother Jupiter,' the entry continues, 'thou knowest I sent thee a couple of Trines to thy Houses last night, the one from Aries, and other from Scorpio, give me thy leave by Sympathy to cure the poor man by drinking a draught of Wormwood Beer every morning. The Moon was weak the other day, and she gave a man to terrible mischiefs, a dull Brain, and a weak sight, Mars lays by his Sword and comes to her, Sister Moon saith he This man hath anger'd thee, but I beseech thee take notice he is but a Fool, prithee be patient, I will with my Herb Wormwood cure him of both Infirmities by Antipathy, for thou knowest, thou and I cannot agree; with that the Moon began to quarrel; Mars (not delighting much in Womens Tongues) went away, and did it whether she would or no.'

These ravings could be taken at face value as an example of the sort of 'rational' account for an herb's virtues provided by astrological physic, a 'Pattern of a Rule to the Sons of Art, rough cast', as Nicholas puts it. However, the 'pattern' does not fit in with any of the formulations set out in the *Semeiotica Uranica*.

One possibility is that the wormwood entry is an allegory on the theme of bitterness, the herb's best-known quality. Perhaps it is about the bitter feelings of a bitter man, now in his mid-thirties but already glimpsing death, forced to feverish work by the demands of his public, publisher, and purse, the object of legal and personal attacks by a resurgent élite, and out of favour with the new political rulers, who daily betrayed the democratic, parliamentary values he had fought and nearly died for. On 7 November 1652, the day after Nicholas completed the *English Physitian*, the MP Bulstrode Whitelocke had received an early intimation of just how wrong the revolution had gone while taking a walk through St James's Park with Oliver Cromwell. Cromwell, frustrated by political dithering and in-fighting, was on the threshold of reverting to Charles's tactic of dissolving Parliament, a first step towards becoming Lord Protector. As they passed along the avenues of poplars and limes, Cromwell complained bitterly about how MPs 'design to continue themselves & to get into offices, & ways of profit, & the pride & corruption of many of them'. 'What if a man should take upon him to be King?' Cromwell suddenly asked Bulstrode. Whitelocke was appalled. He would prefer a Stuart king, he said, his candour rewarded by Cromwell exiling him to Sweden.[29] Nicholas would have been equally appalled, perhaps more so, and his portrayal of a belligerent Mars, who 'loves to be fighting, and is the best friend a Soldier hath', suggests a struggle in his own mind between the decisive violence of war and the corrupting compromises of peace. 'Why should men cry out so much upon Mars for an Infortune?' he asks rhetorically.

There may also be a personal dimension to his words on wormwood, suggested by anomalies in the tone, which is bitter about women, almost misogynistic. It recalls a passage from the Bible: 'For the lips of an adulteress drip honey, and her mouth is smoother than oil:/But her end is bitter as wormwood, sharp as a two-edged sword.'[30]

Does the argument between Mars and Venus, in which she accuses him of 'abusing Women', and he accuses her of being 'as drunk as a Bitch', reprise one Nicholas had had with his wife Alice? This particular passage was probably written while he was away from London, staying in a house he owned or borrowed in Chesham, Berkshire, a day's journey west of Spitalfields.[31] Perhaps he had taken refuge there from a failing relationship, weakened by ill-health and his 'consumption of the purse', which had wasted her fortune as well as his. Alice may also have found another man.

By 1653, Nicholas's own health had taken a sharp turn for the worse, his war wound combining with consumption, probably induced by his smoking, to force him to his sickbed. As he lay there, a twenty-four-year-old raven-haired royalist Rosicrucian called John Heydon took up residence in the house. He claimed to be descended from Hungarian kings and Elias Ashmole described him as 'an Ignoramus and a Cheat'. Having abandoned a career in law, Heydon had decided to study the fashionable art of making 'alchemical' medicines, though, as events would demonstrate, more for their commercial than their therapeutic qualities.

What Heydon was doing in Spitalfields at this time is unclear. Perhaps he had heard that Culpeper was interested in chemical remedies and hoped to draw on his knowledge.[32] He later claimed that Alice had lured him there with 'letters of Love', she 'hearing of this Gentleman that he was an Heir'.[33] Whatever the reason, it is certainly possible that Alice, facing penury as her consumptive husband approached death, had decided to anticipate the inevitable and secure a future for herself and their one surviving daughter, Mary. Alice was resourceful, independently-minded, 'a wife at her own disposing'.[34] Nicholas would find himself increasingly at her own disposing, too. It was Alice who would do more than anyone to make his name as the greatest herbalist of the age, and a great deal to ruin it.

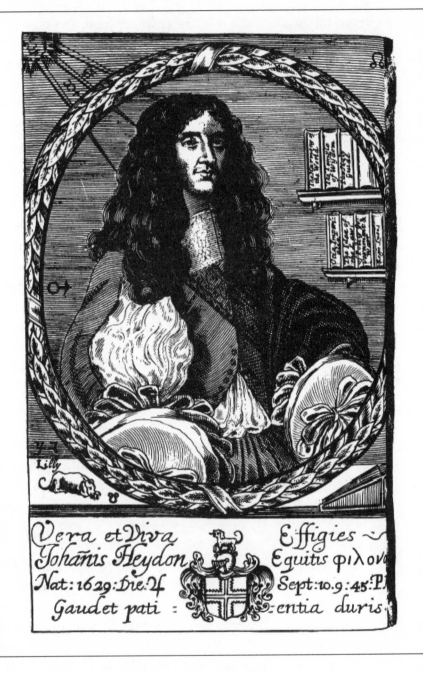

Vera et Viva   Effigies
Johañis Heydon   Equitis φιλοv
Nat: 1629: Die: ♃   Sept:10.9:45:P
Gaudet pati :   :entia duris

Lilly

The Wise-Mans Crown :
OR, THE
GLORY
Of the
Rosie-Cross.

SHEWING

The Wonderful Power of Nature,
with the full discovery of the true *Cælum Terræ*,
or first Matter of Metals, and their Preparations into incredible Medicines or Elixirs that
cure all Diseases in Young or Old : With the
Regio Lucis, and holy Houshold of *Rosie Cruci-
an* Philosophers.

Communicated to the World
By JOHN HEYDON, Gent.
A Servant of GOD, and Secretary to Nature.

Ἔις ἱμί τις ὁρίων ἰωτοὸης ἴςω. (i. e.)
He that looketh upon my Books, let him learn to be religious.

LONDON:
Printed for the Author ; and are to be sold by
Samuel Speed at the Rainbow in
Fleetstreet. 1 6 6 4

By the winter of 1653, Nicholas's illness had reduced him to a 'Skeleton, or Anatomy'.[35] He was writing feverishly, dictating to his amanuensis William Ryves, with Peter Cole and Nathaniel Brooke ready at the foot of the bed to snatch each page as it was finished. To satisfy their demands, he was in the throes of completing a second edition of his *Semeiotica Uranica* for Brooke and translations of other medical works for Cole.[36]

It was too much. On 10 January 1654, aged thirty-seven, he died at his home in Spitalfields, next door to the Red Lion. His wasted corpse was interred in the 'New Church yard of Bethlehem', an annexe to the cemetery of Bedlam mental hospital, 'where he desired to lie'. It was a popular burial place for Independents, a place to rest beyond the control of the ecclesiastical authorities.

Soon after his death, a rumour spread that Nicholas had been poisoned by the physicians. Not even his friends took this seriously, but if the doctors had resorted to such a desperate tactic to silence him, it failed. He was even more prolific dead than alive. In the coming years, his name would be attached to hundreds of works of all kinds and provenances: from a treatise on fevers to a book on makeup: *Art's Masterpiece, or the Beautifying Part of Physick.* In 1661 alone, nearly twenty works appeared featuring his name. He even continued to issue annual almanacs.[37]

Behind this flourishing trade in posthumous productions were a few pirates, but mostly Nicholas's publishers, Cole and Brooke, engaged in a furious competition for his literary legacy, at the centre of which stood Alice Culpeper. Within weeks of Nicholas's death she teamed up with John Heydon, soon to become her second husband, and a Dr Freeman to sell the miraculous chemical potion 'Aurum Potabile' under the Culpeper name. Aurum Potabile, or gold liquor, was a favourite among alchemists, who claimed it to be a 'Universal Remedy for all Diseases, for its chief aim is to exhilarate the heart and vital spirits, which supply the Microcosm, as the Sun doth the Macrocosm'.[38]

A handbill duly appeared on the streets advertising the 'Virtues, Use, and Variety of Operations of the True and Phylosophical AURUM POTABILE, Attained by the Studies of Doctor Freeman, and Doctor Culpeper, and left with his Widow, and administered by a Physician in her House near London'. This was the first time Nicholas's name had appeared with the title 'doctor' – it was a promotion he had scrupulously avoided in life. Dr Freeman was probably William Freeman, originally from Bedford, who described himself as a 'student in physic and astrology, and more occult science'. He, too, was unlikely to deserve the title the pamphlet gave him.[39]

Alice, who had probably produced the handbill, was unconcerned about such niceties. Her immediate concern was publicizing her potion, and to achieve this she turned to Peter Cole. Cole had started registering further titles in Nicholas's name, including seven translations from Latin works by important continental medical writers. Only one was actually by Nicholas, so to add credibility to his claim that they were authentic, Cole apparently offered to help publicize Alice's Aurum Potabile in return for her endorsement of works he published as being by Nicholas.

For the plan to work, Alice needed to keep firm control over the use of her husband's name. But in May 1655, it began to slip from her grasp. Nathaniel Brooke rushed out a work entitled *Culpeper's Last Legacy*, containing an assortment of medical treatises, including a work on disorders of the brain and nerves. An introductory letter, bearing Alice's name, testified that 'the Copy of what is here printed . . . was delivered to my trust among [Nicholas's] choicest secrets upon his death-bed'.[40] Whether this letter was forged, or genuine but written before Alice had come to her agreement with Cole, it produced a furious denial from her. A few months later, a work entitled *Mr Culpepper's Treatise of aurum potabile* appeared which opened with an attack on Brooke signed by Alice in which she accused him of publishing 'a hodge-podge of indigested Collections, and Observations'. Nicholas had left seventy-nine books of 'his own making, or Translating, in my hands', she claimed, and these, together with a further seventeen 'completely perfected' and ready for the presses, would be published exclusively by her and Nicholas's 'much Honoured Friend' Cole.[41]

The credibility of this announcement was undermined by the very work it introduced. Despite the claim of the title, the treatise on Aurum Potabile was certainly not Nicholas's. He had ridiculed those who promoted Aurum Potabile and the philosopher's stone as cure-alls.[42] The work was not even published by Cole, though he did supply a small essay that was bound into the back. It is completely out of keeping with Nicholas's style and medical philosophy, as his supporters noted. 'There is nothing more false then that he made it,' wrote one 'Tantarara Tantarara Philaretes', who had managed to see the original manuscript, 'as is manifest by the copy, which was never writ by his hand.' He accused Alice of behaving 'not much unlike the [whore] of Babylon who with her curious golden Potion, hath endeavoured the delusion of many people'.[43]

The author was probably Heydon. He was a keen alchemist and increasingly active in Alice's publishing ventures. But whoever the author was, the book served its purpose, attracting the attention of the desperate and curious, including the distinguished physician John Ward. He was a fan of Nicholas's herbal and visited the famous Spitalfields address to find out more about its author. He was rewarded with a sample of the liquor, which Alice 'did highly commend ... both inwardly and outwardly applied, an incomparable restorative as she said without any corrosive medicine to prepare it' (which was untrue, as 'aquafortis' – nitric acid – was used to dissolve the gold). 'She was a very ingenious woman,' Ward noted.[44]

By 1659 Alice's rift with Nathaniel Brooke appears to have been mended, for that year he published a memorial volume entitled

Culpeper's School of Physick that included an interpretation of Nicholas's birthchart by John Gadbury, a preface signed by a 'R.W.', and an unsigned memoir. It had been registered at the Stationers' Company in Heydon's name.[45] The following collection of medical fragments, however, may have included some lines by Culpeper, but very few. One section lists remedies featuring the baked head of a cat, the 'pizzle [penis] of a hare', 'a great over-grown Toad', even 'a young Puppy, all of one colour, if you can get such a one' which to cure gout was to be cut 'in two pieces through the back alive' and laid 'hot to the grieved place'.[46] Not since the translation of the *Pharmacopoeia Londinensis* had the Culpeper name been attached to such a catalogue of implausible ingredients.

Soon after the publication of the *School of Physick*, Alice fell out with Heydon, who later accused her of engineering his wrongful imprisonment. He spent two years in gaol on unrecorded charges, and after his release published *The Holy Guide, leading the way to unite art and nature.* This vindictively revealed the secret recipe for 'Culpeper's' Aurum Potabile, which included a small quantity of gold and a great deal of urine from a 'healthy man drinking Wine moderately', sealed in a gourd and set in horse dung for forty days, before being repeatedly distilled. In the same work, he describes Alice as 'Dr Culpeper's late wife', though she was still alive (he continued with the policy of denying Alice in a later work, announcing that 'I have hitherto kept myself unmarried and free from the company of a woman'). A few years later, she applied for and was granted a licence to practise as a midwife. Peter Cole was among those who signed her testimonial.[47]

Nicholas himself might have become lost in the midst of so many rifts and reconciliations, claims and rebuttals, had it not been for his ghost. This odd entity appeared in the back of *Mr Culpepper's Treatise of aurum potabile,* in a short treatise signed by Peter Cole entitled 'Mr Culpeper's Ghost Giving Seasonable Advice of the Lovers of his Writings'. The work contained what was purportedly Nicholas's personal, posthumous message to his readers, though 'whether any person brought it from the Elysian Fields ... or whether he delivered all this in an Apparition; or whether Spirits can write' Cole would not say for fear he should be 'counted a Conjurer, and one that had familiarity with Spirits'.[48]

The ghost's message was filled with foreboding. He urged Culpeper's readers to 'make hay while the sun shines, while the Liberties of a free Common-wealth last among them. For let them assure themselves, that if God ... shall cast again the Tyrannical Yoke of King-ship upon the Neck of the English Nation, they shall be deprived of all those blessed Opportunities they now enjoy, to improve their Understandings.' If monarchy and the aristocracy were to be restored to power, then the censures suffered by Prynne, Bastwick, and Burton would be 'but Fleabitings' compared to what was to come. For that reason, he offered a 'word to the wise' to 'buy these books while you can get them, study them well, and keep them warily', the books being helpfully listed at the front of the treatise, all of them published by Cole.[49]

Culpeper's ghost's pessimistic mood proved to be prescient, as well as commercially astute. In the years following Nicholas's death, London sank into a mood of despondency and stagnation. The wood turner Nehemiah Wallington, ever alert to portents, noted a number that occurred in the summer of 1654. A ship moored in the Thames called the *Mary*, bound for Barbados, caught fire, broke its moorings, and floated downstream, reaching within a stone's throw of the tinder-dry houses perched on London Bridge, before becoming marooned on a ledge, where seven barrels of gunpowder stored in the hold exploded, 'blowing the ship out of the water and breaking slates and windows for hundreds of yards along the south side of the river'. Thirteen people were killed. The following day a 'careless' gunner caused another ship, the *Amity*, to blow up, killing the cabin boy, who had just gone into his cabin to fetch some oranges and lemons he had brought back for his mother.[50]

On midsummer's day, 24 June, Nehemiah walked past the conduit's head in Gracechurch Street. In honour of the season, it would usually be decorated with 'flowers, bows, and garlands' as it spouted fresh water drawn from the springs of Finsbury. Today it was draped in mourning clothes as it dripped, 'with two long pieces hanging down at each end with a piece of paper written thus: the cause of this our mourning is our exceeding want of water which formerly we have enjoyed'. Water-bearers paraded around the conduit, carrying tankards upside-down 'in a doleful manner, saying at every corner of the conduit: "It is not for bread nor for beer we mourn, but we mourn for water".'

Closer to home, affairs were no better. Like Nicholas, Nehemiah had only one surviving child, his daughter Sarah. In 1647, she had married John Houghton, a journeyman turner from Bedfordshire, and in 1650 they moved to Fulham, a village to the west of London. By 1654 Houghton was facing financial ruin, and in late July/early August a heavily pregnant Sarah appeared at Nehemiah's door in Eastcheap 'both weary and lame, which made my heart yearn and my bowels with compassion to turn within me'. She was persuaded to return to Fulham, but a week later Wallington heard that Houghton had left for Cornwall. Nehemiah brought her home, where she gave birth to a son, and fell so ill she could not attend the christening.[51]

For Nehemiah, these events were not accidents but punishments, signs of divine displeasure at the compromised, corrupt 'Commonwealth' that had emerged out of the Civil War. The 'godly reformation' for which he had fought had turned into a 'pretence'.[52]

The signs were no better for William Lilly. Throughout the 1650s, he faced one prosecution after another. In 1652, Parliament ordered that his almanac for that year be called in. Lilly tried to fool the investigating commissioners by submitting six copies printed with offending passages removed, but he was found out and committed to prison. He had spent thirteen days in Newgate before Bulstrode Whitelocke, using his parliamentary contacts, managed to engineer his release.[53]

In 1655, in a case with similarities to the witchcraft charges brought against Nicholas in 1642, Lilly was accused by an Anne East of taking half a crown to tell her the whereabouts of 'ten waistcoats, of the value of five pounds' belonging to her husband. Since visiting Lilly, Mrs East claimed to have become bewitched. She 'could not rest at nights, but was troubled with bears, lions and tigers, &c'. The case was seized upon by Presbyterians as well as royalists as further evidence of astrological corruption. Among the critics was Alice Culpeper's estranged husband, John Heydon, who lambasted the 'journeyman traitors' for their 'nativities, Almanacks, and monthly Predictions verses and observations'.[54]

Lilly continued with his astrological career, but more privately. He settled at his country seat in Surrey, where he acquired neighbouring plots of land, which, in gratitude for past services, he settled on Bulstrode Whitelocke's son, Carleton. There he and Elias Ashmole would experiment with magical paraphernalia, such as the crystal given by Arthur Dee to Nicholas in 1640, which Lilly had bought from Alice during a visit to Spitalfields in 1658.[55]

As for Whitelocke himself, he returned from Sweden to continue as one of the Commissioners of the Great Seal in Parliament, which was now reduced from a purged 'Rump' to a 'Barebones' collection of appointees. Unable to stomach the legislation being ratified by the Great Seal, he resigned his commissionership, but not his parliamentary seat, which he continued to occupy with some discomfort, hoping that he might steer Cromwell's policy in a more positive direction. It was a period, he noted in his diary, that saw the 'decline in his health and strength, & likewise in his fortune'.[56]

The fortunes of others were better. By 1654, William Harvey was safely ensconced at Cockaigne House, his brother Eliab's smart new home in Broad Street. In February of that year, 'a noble building of Roman Architecture (of Rustique work with Corinthian pilasters)' was opened at Amen Corner to accommodate a new library. It had been paid for by an anonymous benefactor whom President Prujean now revealed to be Harvey. Two years later, the 'munificent old man' laid on a lavish banquet for the Fellows, at which he handed over deeds bequeathing his ancestral estate to the College in perpetuity and surrendered to his friend Dr Charles Scarburgh the Lumleian lectureship, an office which he had held for forty years.[57]

Now in his late seventies, Harvey suffered from gout and was often to be seen on the 'leads' or balcony of Cockaigne House with his feet in a bucket of water. He would sit there even in winter 'till he was almost dead with Cold, and betake himself to his Stove', the extremes in temperature apparently alleviating his symptoms. On 3 June 1657, he awoke at about 10 a.m. to find he could not speak, a 'dead palsy' having taken his tongue. He summoned, not a fellow physician, but his apothecary, a Sambroke of Blackfriars, who (in violation of College rules) let the blood in his tongue, but to no effect. He died soon after, his passage helped, according to his old Oxford friend Dr Scarburgh, by a powerful draft of opium. It was claimed he left an estate worth £20,000.[58]

Three years later, Charles II was 'restored' to the throne. A new regime of tight censorship was immediately enforced, announced, as Whitelocke noted in his diary, with a bonfire of banned books, including those of John Milton and John Goodwin of Coleman Street. The vindication of Culpeper's ghostly prophecies was too much for Peter Cole, who had presumably penned them. On 4 December 1665, after publishing a broadsheet listing the Bills of Mortality for previous plague years, he hanged himself at his warehouse in Leadenhall. He was buried in the unconsecrated 'pit' in the East Yard of St Peters-upon-Cornhill, near his old bookshop. His estate, which he had bequeathed to the children of his brother Edward, was 'forfeit by his suicide', half going to the King to help pay for his new palace at Greenwich, half to Lord John Berkeley and Sir Hugh Pollard.[59] Nicholas's books would have suffered the same fate had Cole not signed the titles over to another publisher.

WORMWOOD

Artemisia absinthium/pontica

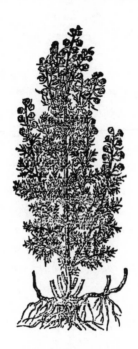

Common Wormwood I shall not describe, for every Boy that
can eat an Eg knows it.

Roman Wormwood; And why Roman, seeing it grows
familiarly in England? It may be it was so called because
'tis special good for a stinking Breath, which the Romans
cannot be very free from maintaining so many Baudy
Houses by Authority of his Holiness. The Stalks are slenderer
and shorter than the common Wormwood by one foot at
least; the Leaves are more finely cut and devided than they

*are but somthing smaller; both Leaves and Stalks are hoary;
the Flowers of a pale yellow colour, it is altogether like the
common Wormwood, save only in bigness, for 'tis smaller;
in tast, for 'tis not so bitter, in smell, for it is spicy.*

*It groweth upon the tops of the Mountains (it seems 'tis
aspiring) there 'tis Natural; but usually nursed up in Gardens for the use of the Apothecaries in London. Time. All
Wormwoods usually Flower in August, a little sooner or
later.*

*Will you give me leave to be Critical a little? I must
take leave; Wormwood is an Herb of Mars, and if Pontanus
say otherwise he is beside the Bridg. I prove it thus: What
delights in Martial places is a Martial Herb, But Wormwood delights in Martial places, (for about Forges and Iron
Works you may gather a Cart load of it) Ergo it is a
Martial Herb. It is hot and dry in the first degree, Viz.
Just as hot as your Blood and not hotter: It remedies the
evils Choller can inflict on the Body of man by Sympathy.*

*It helps the evils Venus and her wanton Girls produce,
by Antipathy; and it doth somthing else besides; It clenseth
the Body of Choller (and who dares say Mars doth no
good?) It provokes Urine, helps Surfets, Swellings in the
Belly; it causeth an Appetite to meat, because Mars rules
the Attractive faculty in Man: The Sun never shone upon
a better Herb for the yellow Jaundice than this is . . .*

*You say Mars is a Destroyer, mix a little Wormwood an
Herb of Mars with your Ink, and neither Rats nor Mice
will touch the Paper [that] is written with it, and then
Mars is a Preserver*

*I was once in the Tower [of London] and viewed the
Wardrobe, and there was a great many fine Cloathes (I
can give them no other title, for I was never neither Linnen
or Woollen Draper) yet as brave as they looked, my opinion
was, the Moaths might consume them (yea Henry the eighth
his Codpiece) . . . This Herb Wormwood being laid amongst*

Cloathes will make a Moath scorn to meddle with the Cloath, as much as a Lyon scorns to meddle with a Mouse, or an Eagle a Fly.

The Grave equals all men, and therefore shall equal me with the Princes, until which time the Eternal Providence is over me; then the ill tongue of a pratling Priest, or of one who hath more Tongue than Wit, or more Pride than Honesty, shall never trouble me. Wisdom is justified of her Children; and so much for Wormwood.

Wormwood, *Artemisia absinthium*, is a byword for bitterness. 'He hath filled me with bitterness, he hath made me drunken with wormwood,' says the Bible's Book of Lamentations. When Hamlet watches the play dramatizing his stepfather's murder of his father, he whispers as an aside, 'That's wormwood, wormwood.'

Absinthium, derived from the dried leaves and flowering tops of the plant, is a powerful stimulant used in a variety of alcoholic drinks. In the nineteenth century, the word 'absinthism' was coined for those addicted to such substances. The symptoms were restlessness, vomiting, vertigo, tremors, and epileptic convulsions during which the addict might bite his tongue, pass water, and foam at the mouth.

Richard Mabey notes that the Russian name for the herb is 'Chernobyl'.[1]

or nearly twenty years – since debauchery and ignorance had destroyed good manners – rowdy demagogues and disgruntled riff-raff had set a blazing torch to the suffering state and had made all things foul with sword and fire, with terror and grief, and with the blood of the innocent. At last the full course of the divine plan had been completed and as from a funeral pyre the phoenix arose.' Thus began the entry in the annals for the Comitia Majora Extraordinaria held at the College of Physicians to celebrate the restoration of the monarchy.

Charles's heir, also Charles, the boy William Harvey had entertained in a bush on the battlefield at Edgehill, had returned from exile to reclaim his throne on 25 May 1660. More than a decade of continuous emergencies had left the nation politically exhausted, and there was almost universal relief at the prospect of a return to normality.

The College's rapture at the monarch's homecoming urgently needed to find some form of material expression. Dr Baldwin Hamey, the doctor who had treated Harvey's dying brother, offered his prize possession, a sample of 'very fine unicorn's horn', which was mounted in gold. On 3 September 1660, the President, Dr Edward Alston, presented it to the King together with an 'elegant speech', and was knighted on the spot. Sir Edward rushed back to Amen Corner to describe to the waiting Fellows that the King had taken the gift 'with a smile and promised to look after us and our art'.[2]

Carpe diem became the College's motto: embrace the moment.

Two decades of pent-up rage at the 'unskilful illiterate and unlicensed practisizers of Physic' and frustration with the 'renewed
frauds abuses and deceipts of divers Apothecaries, Druggists and
others', combined with excited anticipation at a new age of order
and respect, was the perfect recipe for a new charter, under which
the Fellows flattered themselves with the title of the 'King's College
of Physicians' and powers that extended across the profession and
the land.³ They also wanted the right to license all medical texts
confirmed, so they could recover control over future editions of
Culpeper's translation as well as any other texts that compromised
their commercial secrets.

The King gave the new charter his personal seal of approval within
days of its completion. All that was required for it to become law was
the Great Seal of State. In the fondly remembered era of Charles I's
personal rule, this would have been a formality. But in these early
days of the Restoration, the King was keen not to stir up too many
old controversies, and so he insisted the matter be referred to Parliament. The College took the news phlegmatically and set up a committee to promote the charter's progress. To ease the way, it decided to
allow the automatic admission of royal physicians who were not
Fellows as *sociorum supernumerariorum*, supernumerary members,
and introduced a new category of honorary fellowship, which had
the benefit of not only providing income (Honorary Fellows had
to pay £20 to join), but attracted courtiers such as the Privy Councillor the Marquis of Dorchester, useful allies in the coming struggles.⁴

The finances, legalities, and patronage in place, the College could
confidently expect its own imminent restoration as sovereign of the
medical world. But it was not to be. The new charter received its
first reading in the House of Commons on 19 April 1664. It received
a second reading, after which it was referred to a Committee of
forty-six members, and was never heard of again.⁵

The failure was in part due to the College's treatment of the
apothecaries. In its depositions to Parliament, it had accused them
of fraud and 'deceipts'. The College had even threatened their mon-

opoly of dispensing by claiming for its members the right to make and sell their own medicines. When the apothecaries objected, the College's reaction was incomprehension. How could they be so 'unmindful of the benefits for which they were indebted to us?' the Fellows protested.[6]

As it was put by the medical historian Harold J. Cook, the Society of Apothecaries had discovered a 'self-confident and serious tone' which left the College completely bemused. The cause, in part, was Nicholas Culpeper.

Nicholas's books were selling better than ever. There was a hiatus in 1660, the year Charles II took over the throne, but in 1661 more editions of his works appeared than ever before, and they continued to appear in profusion during 1662, 1663, and 1664. Along with his works came countless others, offering cheap and simple remedies in the vulgar tongue, many attributed to him, even though not a word of his was to be found in them.[7] He was so popular that he was even used to promote official public health policies. In 1665, the year of the Great Plague, the Lord Mayor of London had to resort to using Culpeper's name alongside Sir Walter Raleigh's to get citizens to pay attention to a pamphlet on methods of avoiding infection.[8] Thanks to this epidemic of popular works, medical knowledge that just twenty years before had been beyond the reach even of the middle classes was now easily accessible. Patients could come to apothecaries direct, seeking one of Nicholas's recommended treatments, and the apothecaries could draw on all the academic authority of his translation and annotation of the *Pharmacopoeia* without having to refer to physicians. None of this was explicitly acknowledged. A state of collective amnesia overcame the medical world when it came to Nicholas. Even his own works began to deny him. In new editions of the dispensatory and the herbal, all the references to tyranny and monopoly, and to greed and snobbery, were removed. But his influence was none the less potent for that.

As well as the spread of medical understanding, another factor stood in the College's way. On 28 November 1660, a group of twelve men met at Gresham College after a lecture by Christopher Wren, then Gresham Professor of Astronomy and later the architect of St Paul's Cathedral. They decided to found 'a College for the Promoting of Physico-Mathematical Experimental Learning', which would practise what had become dubbed the 'new philosophy'. This emphasized the importance of observation, experimentation, and measurement, rather than books, to understanding how the natural world works. The body they created became the Royal Society, and would include among its early members not only such scientific luminaries as Wren and Robert Boyle, but also some of the most senior members of the court, including the King himself.

Physic was one of the primary areas of interest for these new philosophers, some of whom set up laboratories to investigate new chemical remedies, which they believed to be more effective than herbal ones. A leading and eloquent champion was Marchamont Needham, founder of the newspaper that had lambasted Nicholas's translation of the *Pharmacopoeia*. Needham argued that old remedies were out of date, as they were being used to treat new diseases spread by 'venereous and scorbutic ferments' (i.e. by sex and scurvy, associated with poor living). 'There is no way to redeem our Profession,' he argued, 'but by setting the whole frame of Physick upon a new foot of Operative and Experimental Philosophy.'[9] With that end in mind, he and thirty-four others drew up a proposal for a Society of Chemical Physicians, which was endorsed by some of the most powerful men in the land, including the Archbishop of Canterbury and the Duke of Buckingham, John Sheffield. Buckingham was proving to be as keen a court operator as his predecessor, the royal favourite of James I and Charles I, George Villiers, 'for whether you take him in the Chymical, or in his Politick capacity,' wrote Needham, 'he appears no less in either; and yet he can be greater, if he please, because with so rare a Wit and other Abilities of mind, seated in a comely Body, I know not what he may effect in Philosophy and Polity, by plying his Laboratory at Home, and another at Court.'[10]

Sensing a dangerous rival, the College immediately launched an attack. It branded these 'chemical' competitors 'empirics' – which indeed they were, since they based their findings on empirical knowledge rather than academic learning. Continuing its policy of refusing its critics the dignity of a public response, it once again co-opted William Johnson, its own chemist and the man elected to attack Culpeper, to do the job on its behalf. One of the central criticisms the chemists levelled against the College was that it was an unscientific institution, the effectiveness of its remedies and methods demonstrated by reference to ancient texts rather than modern methods of observation and experimentation. Johnson countered by pointing out that the College had accepted a limited number of chemical remedies, and had listed them in the *Pharmacopoeia*. 'These fellows do by chemistry, just as our fanatics do in religion, cry it up zealously, but with a manifest design to pull it down; both being equally ignorant, and both enemies to the truth,' he wrote, harking back to the association of medical with religious heresy that had been a feature of the attacks on Nicholas.[11]

Johnson's attack provoked a pamphlet war worthy of the early 1640s, polarizing opinion between the scholastic College and the scientific chemists. The impulse on both sides was commercial as much as philosophical – the control of a monopoly on the one hand, the sale of new patent remedies on the other; as the stakes became higher, so did the matters of principle each side proclaimed.

The unexpected beneficiary of all this was William Harvey. Both sides now claimed him as their own. He was 'our Hippocrates', according to Needham. George Thomason, who wrote a stinging attack against the 'dross' promoted by the College, dismissed its anatomy lectures as a 'Theatrical business . . . for the entertainment of any rude fellows', but acknowledged 'the Invention of the Circulation of the Blood by industrious Doctor Harvey is highly to be commended', even though it had led to no reform in the physicians' therapeutic practices. Johnson responded by drawing the completely opposite conclusion. Harvey's discovery was made at the College, and Thomson was simply ignorant of the advantages 'this discovery hath brought to Man-kind, in order to the cure of Diseases, both Internal and External'. As the pitch of the debate rose, so did Harvey's status.[12]

In 1665, the Great Plague spread through London, marking the period when the College would reach its post-Restoration nadir. Though it drew up the official policy for dealing with the epidemic, the Society of Chemical Physicians openly posted their own bills around the streets offering alternative remedies. Amen Corner was evacuated, and a thief broke in and forced open the locked chest in Harvey's library, stealing around £1,000 of silver that had been collected as a fighting fund for the College's continuing struggles to get its charter ratified. Shortly after, Francis Prujean, the veteran Elect and one of the College's most effective champions, died, and within the year Amen Corner was destroyed in the Great Fire.

However, the College's day was about to come.

Early on the morning of Monday, 2 February 1685, King Charles II awoke feeling ill. He fetched from his private closet some of Goddard's drops, a secret remedy concocted by Jonathan Goddard. Goddard had been Cromwell's physician, but had maintained royalist sympathies. He had also been an enemy of Nicholas's, apparently dismissing him as a 'foulmouth'd impudent scribbler'.[13] The miraculous properties ascribed to his drops had enabled him to survive the change of regime unharmed, and, as well as becoming a member of the Royal Society, he had managed to sell the recipe for his drops to the King for a reputed £6,000.[14] But on this occasion the drops did not work, for when Lord Thomas Ailesbury, the gentleman of the bedchamber, awoke, he found the King deathly pale.

At 8 a.m., the barber-surgeon Edmund King was called to give

Charles his morning shave. He was about to begin when Charles suffered a series of convulsions. King performed an emergency phlebotomy, letting sixteen ounces of blood from a vein in Charles's right arm. Dr Scarburgh, Harvey's old friend and successor as Lumleian lecturer, was now Charles's personal physician. He arrived with other members of the royal medical team and decided upon 'scarification deep enough to effect a fuller and more vigorous revulsion', and 'cupping', the application of heated cups to the skin, which, upon cooling, would draw blood through the wounds. By these means, a further eight ounces of blood were drawn, using instruments that may have been Harvey's, Harvey having bequeathed all his surgical equipment to Scarburgh in his will.

Next, Scarburgh prescribed a series of medicines designed to draw out 'impurities' from the King's stomach and 'rid his whole nervous system of anything harmful to it': an antimonial emetic (the same remedy sold by John Evans of Gunpowder Alley, before he was stopped by the College Censors) to provoke vomiting, and a series of enemas (one comprising over a pint of liquid, injected into the rectum) to force the evacuation of the bowel. The King's hair was cut off so that a blistering agent could be applied to the scalp, and a red-hot cauterizing tool pressed to his skin to cause it to blister. These efforts produced two hours of agonized convulsions, followed by a period of semi-conscious calm. In the evening, 'in their object of diverting and withdrawing the humours from his head, and at the same time to give strength of his loaded brain', the doctors applied noxious plasters to the soles of Charles's feet to draw the humours down, and gave him a powder made from the root of white hellebore to promote sneezing. With that, the King was given a light broth for sustenance, a laxative made from manna (the sugary sap of the ash tree *Fraxinus ornus*) 'to keep his bowels active', and a decoction of barley, almonds, and liquorice to counteract scalding by his own urine, which was likely to result from the use of so many blistering agents. Then he was left to rest for the night.

The following day, Tuesday, Charles grew stronger and the treatments gentler. He was given a soothing julep (syrup) of black cherry, lime flowers, lily of the valley, and 'prepared pearls'. On Wednesday afternoon, the King relapsed. The doctors applied one of the *Pharmacopoeia*'s rarest medicines, 'the skull of a man that was never buried, being beaten to a powder and given inwardly'.[15]

Thursday morning disclosed another recovery in the King's condition, and the afternoon another relapse, leading the physicians to suspect an 'ague' or fever, as a malarial outbreak was currently at large in London. Relieved at reaching a diagnosis, they prescribed a treatment new to English medicine, cinchona or Peruvian Bark. Cinchona, from which comes quinine, had only recently been introduced to the *Pharmacopoeia* and was controversial because of its unpleasant side effects when taken in large doses. The King was at first reluctant to take it, and the Queen, along with her physician, tried to stop it being given to him; but the opinion of the physicians prevailed, and it was administered.

The drug did not have its anticipated effect, and the King's condition deteriorated. He now seemed close to death. In a last attempt to save him, the physicians reverted to their panaceas and administered crushed bezoars, stones from the intestines of the wild Persian bezoar goat.

The King died, according to Scarburgh, 'on February Sixth soon after noon, towards the end of the fifty-fourth year of his age'. That afternoon, Charles's brother was proclaimed King James II.[16]

The notable feature of the physicians' treatment of the King's final illness, other than the pain it inflicted, was that it was so orthodox, based on the principles of Galen. The nearest their patient came to any chemical or modern remedy was the use of Goddard's drops and the Peruvian Bark. Otherwise, the doctors had stuck more or less rigidly to the principles of humoral physic and the medicines listed in their *Pharmacopoeia*.

Nevertheless, the outcome of their ministrations was entirely favourable. It marked the moment of their own, longed-for restoration. James II rewarded the physicians with honours (money had been promised, but honours were cheaper) and the ratification of their new charter, restoring and extending the powers they had craved for half a century. Prosecutions of unlicensed practitioners recommenced in earnest, and the control of medical publishing was implemented with speed. It was as though the clock had been turned back twenty years: the 'revolution' had turned full circle. There was just one annoying difference. Nicholas Culpeper's *English Physitian* continued in print, and would remain in print for centuries to come.

EPILOGUE

William Harvey is acclaimed in the annals of medical history as, to quote some typical examples, the 'brightest ornament', 'in every respect worthy of his public reputation', to be classed 'with our Shakespeares and our Miltons', simply 'immortal'.[1] Nicholas Culpeper, on the other hand, is dismissed as an 'arch herbalist and quack salver'.[2]

But Nicholas was no more an 'arch herbalist' than the learned Fellows of the College of Physicians. They, like he, based most of their medicines on herbs, and continued to do so for centuries. A small number of 'chemical' remedies were included in the *Pharmacopoeia*, but only under sufferance. As for 'quack salver', treatments based on ground-up human skulls, the gall stones of Persian goats, and the scarification of the patient's skin were suspect even then, and certainly no more credible than Nicholas's preferred preparations, such as a decoction of common groundsel to soothe the stomach, or oil of bay-tree berries to calm convulsions.

Even the assumption that the physicians were on the side of science, and Nicholas of mysticism, is wrong. Some College Fellows became members of the Royal Society and its informal antecedents. But the College itself was ambivalent about science in medicine, because it challenged its own authority to set the standard by which medical knowledge should be judged. That ambivalence survives to this day. 'Evidence-based' medicine – the idea that medical practice should be based on scientific evidence (such as randomized trials) – is still considered controversial by some doctors. Many see it as an infringement of their clinical freedom, limiting their right to choose, and compromising their responsibility for the way they treat their patients.[3]

Culpeper was no scientist. But he did believe in some sort of scientific basis for medical knowledge, believing, hoping that astrology might provide it. Medicine, as he put it, required the attendance not just of 'Dr Experience' and 'Dr Tradition', but also of 'Dr Reason'. It was the latter who personified the scientific ideal, and who he claimed was absent from the learned deliberations of the College.

But the College did have its Dr Reason: William Harvey. Harvey showed how the rational study of human physiology and disease – indeed any natural phenomenon – should be done: objectively, experimentally, empirically, diplomatically, opulently, fraternally. For science to succeed, it had to be conducted under the controlled conditions of state patronage, upon the laboratory bench of professional loyalty.

This approach became the model for the Royal Society, and it produced splendid results, as the forthcoming contributions of the Society's most distinguished alumnus and president, Sir Isaac Newton, showed. But there was a cost. Modern science is often portrayed as having been born of a democratic impulse. But at this early stage of its development, it was decidedly élitist. The Royal Society was not set up to address social concerns but to satisfy aristocratic curiosity. Its members were called the 'virtuosi', and many saw themselves engaged in producing new forms of occult knowledge.[4] One of the chief reasons Marchamont Needham championed a reformed physic based on the new philosophy was because the 'common methods and remedies are every where to be had in print', and the man responsible for that was Nicholas Culpeper.[5]

F. N. L. Poynter, one of the most influential medical historians of the late twentieth century and one of the decipherers of Harvey's almost indecipherable lecture notes, wrote in 1972 that Culpeper 'had far greater influence on medical practice in England between 1650 and 1750' than Harvey.[6] By translating and annotating the

Pharmacopoeia, he consolidated the apothecaries' position in the frontline of healthcare, from where they would go on to become the general practitioners of today. By writing the *English Physitian* or *Herbal* he established the principle of the public right to know. He made medical knowledge widely accessible to ordinary people for the first time, and their appetite proved to be inexhaustible. New editions, under various titles and in various versions, have been published nearly every decade from the beginning of the eighteenth century to the end of the twentieth, as many as six or seven a decade in the late eighteenth and early nineteenth centuries.[7] It became one of the most popular medical books in Colonial America, where many of Nicholas's Puritan brethren probably appreciated its political message as much as its medical one. As late as 1770, doctors in Boston, Massachusetts, tried to set up a College of Physicians of their own, but found their efforts frustrated by the conviction among 'every plain honest country gentleman and judicious citizen that reading Culpeper's English Physician enlarged' provided them with all the medical knowledge they needed.[8]

Whether or not Nicholas saved many lives is debatable; but whether or not the discovery of the circulation of the blood, or indeed any medical knowledge from that period, saved many lives is similarly open to question. Most medical historians agree that mortality rates stayed at the same level for at least a century after Harvey's *De motu cordis* and Culpeper's *Herbal* appeared.[9]

What Culpeper did was challenge the principle that medical knowledge belonged solely to physicians – indeed that expert knowledge of any sort belonged to the experts. He helped to reveal a division that has yet to heal, between orthodox and alternative medicine, between professional expertise and personal empowerment. He would probably have deplored many of the practices that currently take place in the name of 'alternative medicine' – he would have considered Chinese or Indian remedies, for example, as being out of place in a northern European or northern American clime. But he would recognize the current controversies over medicine as the same ones he was engaged in 350 years ago: self-help versus expert consultation, education versus advice, community values versus commercial interests, simple natural remedies versus complex artificial compounds.

Medicine has, of course, made great strides in the last 350 years. Doctors now enjoy a high degree of trust among their patients. Most people exercise more control over their care, and, thanks to the principle of informed consent, have more awareness of their treatment than ever before. However, in an age of genetic manipulation, ethical committees, health scares, and intensive care, when every personal problem can be seen as a medical condition, when increasing scientific complexity makes secrets of every medical advance, and the Internet makes each available to everyone, the struggles of Harvey and Culpeper during the Civil War are as relevant as ever. Their story is a timely reminder of the issues at stake, of the political, philosophical, as well as emotional impact of a science that dabbles intimately with our personal lives.

NOTES

ABBREVIATIONS

OED	*Oxford English Dictionary*, second edition (Oxford, 2002)
CJ	*Commons Journal*
LJ	*Lords Journal*
Annals	*Annales Collegii Medicorum*, Royal College of Physicians. Translations taken from transcripts, ref. MSS 2289–97
HMC	Historical Manuscripts Commission
CSP	*Calendar of State Papers*
BL	British Library
GL	Guildhall Library
STC	*A Short-Title Catalogue of Books Printed in England, Scotland, & Ireland 1475–1640*, second edition (Bibliographical Society, 1986)
CLRO	Corporation of London Records Office
PRO	Public Record Office
RCP	Royal College of Physicians
TT	Thomason Tracts, British Library
LMA	London Metropolitan Archives

TANSY

1 Mabey, *Flora Britannica*, 369.
2 Grieve, *The Modern Herbal*, entry for Tansy; see also Richard Bradley, *The Country Housewife and Lady's Director* (1736).
3 The number of clergy who held university degrees doubled from 1600 to 1640 to three-quarters. Hirst, *England in Conflict*, 34.
4 Attree, 'Sussex Colepepers', 65–74. The tradition concerning the roses is mentioned in Aubrey, *The Natural History and Antiquities of the County of Surrey*, iii, 185, and in Camden, *Britain*, i, 296.
5 Geoffrey Chaucer, *The House of Fame*, book iii, 1277.
6 Lloyd Prichard, 'The Significant Background of the Stuart Culpepers', 408.

7 'A Rolle of the severall Armours and furniture with theire names of the Clergie within the Arch Deaconry of Lewes and Deanery of South Malling', *Sussex Archaeological Collections*, iii, 225–7.

8 Copy of the Parish Register of Ockley transcribed from the originals by Mr Malden in 1916, currently held by Briony Thomas of Ockley, to whom I am most grateful for information relating to the history of the village for this period.

9 Attersoll, *The Neuu Couenant*, 142.

10 The terminology is confusing because of the way periods of time were reckoned. 'Tertian' meant every three days, counting the first incident of fever as day one, a day of remission as day two, and the next incident as day three. 'Quartan' similarly counted the onset as day one, two days of remission as days two and three, and the next incident as day four. In modern terms, each type of malaria is distinguished by the type of parasite that causes it. Tertian malaria of the benign (i.e. non-fatal) form probably then suffered in England is produced by *Plasmodium vivax*, quartan by *Plasmodium malariae*, and quotidian probably by multiple infections of tertian. Ward, 'The Effect of Malaria upon the Diffusion of Disease', 193–6. See Dobson, *Contours of Death and Disease*, 319–20.

11 See Dobson, *Contours of Death and Disease*, 312 ff.

12 Ibid., 387; transcript of Ockley parish register.

13 Gerard, *Herball* (1971), 162.

14 G. E. Corrie, *Sermons by Hugh Latimer* (Cambridge, 1844), 534, quoted in Thomas, *Religion and the Decline of Magic*, 209.

15 Examples cited in Thomas, *Religion and the Decline of Magic*, 218 ff.

16 Thanks to the Revd Roger Dalling, former vicar of Isfield, for this information. The Ouse has since been canalized, and the surrounding fields drained.

17 Attersoll, *Historie of Balak*, A4^v–A5^r.

18 Puritans 'are best thought of as representing a distinctive strain of piety within the broad protestant establishment', Woolrych, *Britain in Revolution*, 41.

19 Attersoll, *The Neuu Couenant*, 142.

20 Ibid.

21 Attersoll, *Commentarie vpon the Epistle of Pavle to Philemon*, ¶5^r.

22 Attersoll, *Historie of Balak*, A3^v.

23 *DNB*, 'William Attersoll'.

24 Attersoll, *The Neuu Couenant*, 247.

25 According to the *OED*, the word comes from the late Greek παῖς, 'orig. a child's word'.

26 Numbers 14: 2, 16: 1.

27 Attersoll, *A Commentarie vpon Moses*, A4^r, 63; *A Commentarie vpon Saint Pavle*, 163.

28 Attersoll, *A Commentarie vpon Moses*, 136, 131–2, 135–6.

29 Ibid., A3^r.

30 Attersoll, *A Commentarie vpon Saint Pavle*, 189.

31 Culpeper, *Life*, C^r; Fioravanti, *Three Exact Pieces*, 14.

32 Attersoll, *A Commentarie vpon Moses*, 1165.

33 Article seventeen of the Thirty-Nine Articles, the statement of the Church of England's doctrine ratified in 1571, states that 'Predestination to life is the everlasting purpose of God, whereby (before the foundations of the word were layd) he hath constantly decreed by his counsell secrete to us, to deliver from curse and damnation, those whome he hath chosen in Christe out of

mankynde, and to bring them by Christe everlasting salvation' (Church of England, *Articles*, 11). The difference between mainstream Protestant opinion and the Puritans over this issue was whether God had simply chosen who would be saved, or decided both who would be saved and who would be damned. Attersoll subscribed to the latter form, so-called 'double' predestination.

34 Ibid., 132, 134.

35 Culpeper, *English Physitian*, 54.

36 Attersoll, *The Neuu Couenant*, 177.

37 *Chenopodium olidum*, or orrach, belonging to the goosefoot family.

38 Culpeper, *English Physitian*, 49.

39 *Salvia sclarea*, a member of the dead nettle family,

40 Culpeper, *Life*, C–c2. There are some discrepancies between different editions of *Culpeper's School of Physick*; some, for example, do not mention his education. It seems that later editions were abbreviated.

41 Venn, *Alumni Cantabrigiensis*, Cambridge, 1927, entries for Attersoll and Nicholas Culpeper.

42 Monardes, *Ioyfull Nevves*, f38r [i.e. f39r], *ii^v.

43 'Philaretes', *Work for Chimny-sweepers*, Aiii^r; Culpeper, *Life*, C7^r; *CJ*, i, 469; Vaughan, *Directions for Health*, 81; see Rive, 'Tobacco in England', 1–12.

44 James I, *A Counterblaste to Tobacco*, C3^r, A3^v, C3^r.

45 Rive, 'Tobacco in England', 5; Hirst, *England in Conflict*, 55.

46 James I, *Planting of tobacco*.

47 Food prices nearly doubled between 1580 and 1620 according to the 'Phelps Brown' index, generally accepted as reliable, particularly for southern England. See Outwaite, *Inflation*.

48 'Philaretes', *Work for Chimny-*

sweepers, Aiii^r. Della Porta wrote of the plant's medicinal virtues, but did not provide a specific endorsement. See Porta, *Natural Magick*, 228; Hill, *The World Turned Upside Down*, 198–9.

49 Culpeper, *Physical Directory*, 47.

50 Charles I, *Tobacco*.

51 James I, *Planting of tobacco*; Charles I, *Venting of tobacco*.

52 Culpeper, *Life*, C^v. Where it can be independently confirmed, the *Life* is mostly accurate. The author of the memoir may be Nathaniel Brooke, publisher of the *School of Physick*. Jonathan Sanderson points out that Brooke wanted to demonstrate his claim over Peter Cole to be Culpeper's authorized publisher, and may have used the *Life* to demonstrate his closeness to the author; Sanderson, *Nicholas Culpeper and the Book Trade*, 40–1.

53 Sir John married twice and had five daughters who were alive in 1631, the time he wrote his will, just before Nicholas's elopement, but they all married. Sir John had an uncle, also Sir John, who had a son, also John, who had a daughter called Frances, born in Lewes. He also had grandchildren through the marriage of his daughter Charity to James Rivers, from a prosperous Kentish family, who lived in London. My thanks to Betty Shirley and the Shirley Association (www.shirleyassociation.com) for this information. There is no inquest for death by lightning relating to the period in the surviving records. See Hunnisett, *Sussex Coroners' Inquests*. The memoir also mentions a Sir Nicholas Astey as the friend who encountered Culpeper on the road soon after he had received the news of his lover's death. His identity also remains a mystery. My thanks

to Philip Bye, senior archivist at East Sussex Record Office for information on this subject.

54 Culpeper, *Life*, C2^{r-v}. In 'Publishing the Works of Nicholas Culpeper', Mary Rhinelander McCarl argues that the story of Culpeper's attempted elopement was 'an allegory for his overwhelming interest in alchemical researches'. The account is certainly colourful, but it is not in the form of an allegory, which is characterized by the heavy use of symbolism and mythic themes, none of which appear in the story.

55 Attersoll, *A Commentarie vpon Moses*, 132.

BORAGE

1 Richard Jefferies, *Nature near London* (London, 1883). Quoted in Mabey, *Flora Britannica*, 310.

2 Mabey, *Flora Britannica*, 310.

3 3 Henry VIII, c. 11, Goodall, *The Royal College of Physicians*, 1–2.

4 Clarke, *History of the Royal College of Physicians*, 79.

5 Goodall, *The Royal College of Physicians*, A^{v}–A2^{r}, 18–19.

6 32 Henry VIII, c. 42; Goodall, *The Royal College of Physicians*, 25–6.

7 Sanderson, *Nicholas Culpeper and the Book Trade*, 11.

8 Caius' silver caduceus is still at the Royal College of Physicians, in a display case next to the Censors' room; Friedlander, *The Golden Wand*, 87.

9 Cook, *Decline*, 66.

10 Geoffrey Chaucer, *Canterbury Tales*, Prologue, lines 413–46; Thomas Browne, *Religio Medici* (London, 1642), A^{r}.

11 Marlowe, *The Tragedie of Doctor Faustus*, I. i.

12 Dekker, *London Looke Backe*, B3^{r}.

13 Clark, *A History of the Royal College of Physicians*, 137.

14 Pelling, *Medical Conflicts*, 137.

15 Galen, *On the Usefulness of the Parts*, vi, 351–2.

16 Culpeper, *Galen's Art of Physic*, 5 ff.

17 Quoted in Porter, *The Greatest Benefit*, 77.

18 Needham, *Medela Medicinae*, 7–8; in 1559, the College threatened a doctor with imprisonment unless he withdrew the suggestion that Galen might have erred; he submitted.

19 Keynes, *Harvey*, 423–6.

20 Fuller, *Worthies*, Kent, 79; Keynes, *Harvey*, 5–6.

21 Harvey, *Lectures*, 96.

22 Underwood, 'The Early Teaching of Anatomy at Padua', 1–26.

23 Dekker, *The Wonderfull Yeare*, C4^{r}.

24 Culpeper, *Galen's Art of Physic*, 54.

25 Keynes, *Harvey*, 237, 434.

26 Harvey, *Lectures*, 42.

27 Goodall, *The College Vindicated*, 31 ff.

28 Fuller, *Worthies*, Kent, 79.

29 Harvey, *Anatomical Exercitations* (London, 1653), 24–5.

30 *Orders of the Hospitall of Bartholomew*, 2 ff; according to a rating of the wages of 'the best and most skilful workmen' living in London made 24 August 1588, a blacksmith and miller were worth £6 per annum including board and lodging. See *LJ* xxii, 197, quoted in Aughterson, *The English Renaissance*, 201–2.

31 *Annals*, iii, f1a.

32 McClure, *Chamberlain*, i, 367; HMC, *Salisbury*, 162.

33 *Annals*, iii, ff15a–16b; for the numbers of apothecaries, see Wall, *History of the Society of Apothecaries*, 17, 289. Only a selection of cases was mentioned in College Annals, and then only in summary; a 'Book of Examinations' contained the full

reports, but it was destroyed when the College was burned down in the great fire of 1666.

34 *Annals*, iii, f16b.

35 *Annals*, iii, f25b.

36 *CSP Domestic 1611–1618*, 536.

37 Urdang, *Pharmacopoeia Londinensis*, 25.

38 Ibid., 23; translation by Urdang.

39 *Annals*, iii, ff34b, f36b. Sanderson, *Nicholas Culpeper and the Book Trade*, 80.

40 Urdang, *Pharmacopoeia Londinensis*, 32.

41 Holinshed, *Chronicles*, 1349.

42 The evidence for him dissecting a human foetus is discussed in the introduction to Harvey, *Lectures*, 13, 76, and 98. The size of his father's colon is mentioned in his lecture notes (f26^v), as well as the 'large spleen' of his sister (f36^r), though it is unclear which sister, as the only to survive infancy, Anne, died in 1645. He had a half sister, Gillian, who died in 1639. For a survey of the animals he dissected, see Cole, 'Harvey's Animals', 106–13. A translation of the Latin report on the 152-year-old man, Thomas Parr, is reproduced in Keynes, *Harvey*, 222–5.

43 Keynes, *Harvey*, 194.

44 'I saw them [lungs] in the recently dead Δ, and before the *halter* had been loosened from those hanged': Harvey, *Lectures*, 170.

45 Ibid., 40. See chap. 'Melancholy Thistle' note 2 below for an assessment of Harvey's Latin.

46 Harvey, *Lectures*, 168, 155, 149–50, 137.

47 Ibid., 144.

48 Ibid., 53, 127. His lecture notes contain nothing on the uterus or vagina, presumably because dissections were invariably conducted on a male corpse. He mentions the 'horns of the uterus', the medieval term for structures which Gabriele Falloppia, a predecessor of Fabricius at Padua, had identified in his *Observationes anatomicae* of 1561 as the uterine tubes which now bear his name.

49 Harvey, *Lectures*, 28.

50 The dating of this lecture is a matter of controversy. Harvey's biographer Geoffrey Keynes assumed Harvey's lecture notes, which first mentioned his theory of the circulation of the blood, were for the period 16–18 April 1616 (see *Harvey*, 86); but this seems unlikely given the necessity of dissecting corpses in winter. Keynes based his dating on a transcript of the lecture notes made by the Royal College of Surgeons that omits marks on the title-page. These suggest that the notes were for the years 1616 to 1618. See the introduction to Harvey, *Lectures*, for a full discussion of the dating of the lectures.

51 Harvey, *Lectures*, 7.

52 Ibid., 42.

53 Aristotle, *On the Parts of Animals*, bk. 1, pt. 1.

54 Harvey, *Lectures*, 55, 124–5.

55 Ibid., 151 and note; Suetonius, *De Vita Caesarum*, 206, 225.

56 Harvey, *Lectures*, 27.

57 Ibid., 153–4. 'Membrana carnosa' literally means fleshy membrane; Harvey is referring to the *panniculus carnosus*, a thin, sheathlike layer of muscular fibres just beneath the skin.

58 Ibid., 167, 172.

59 Ibid., 214, 174–5, 34.

60 Ibid., 187.

61 For example, at the top of a new page of notes (f77^v), he writes: 'See how arduous and difficult [it is] to discern, either by sight or by touch, dilation or constriction and what is systole and what diastole'; this

suggests the audience was to be presented with a live specimen to inspect: *Lectures*, 186.

62 Harvey, *Lectures*, 185.

63 Ibid., 188.

64 Ibid., 179.

65 Adrian Desmond and James Moore, *Darwin* (London, 1992), 314.

66 Harvey, *Lectures*, 174, 202.

67 Ibid., 214.

68 Ibid., 215.

ANGELICA

1 *CSP Venetian*, 1623–5, xviii, 620.

2 *CSP Domestic*, James I, 1623–5, ii, 505.

3 HMC, 13th Report, Appendix, pt. 7, 2–6.

4 John Nichols, *The Progesses &c. of King James the First* (London, 1838), iv, 1037. Quoted in Keynes, *Harvey*, 144.

5 Eglisham, *A Forerunner of Revenge*, 8.

6 Lockyer, *Buckingham*, 34.

7 Quoted in Hirst, *England in Conflict*, 108.

8 From Bishop Gilbert Burnet's account in his *History Of My Own Times*, quoted in *Munk's Roll*, 113; HMC, *Mar & Kellie*, 113.

9 HMC, *Mar & Kellie*, 225–6.

10 Eglisham, *A Forerunner of Revenge*, 8, B3^v–B4^r; *Iohn Lambe*, 4, 15; Keynes, *Harvey*, 152–3. HMC, *Mar & Kellie*, 225.

11 Razzell, *The English Civil War*, i, 48.

12 The notes of the inquiry are contained in HMC, *Thirteenth Report*, Appendix pt. 7, 1–8. The notes were found in the archives of the Earl of Lonsdale at Lowther Castle in Cumbria, and were the work of a 'Mr Lowther', probably John, MP for Westmorland, or his younger brother Richard, MP for Berwick.

13 *Munk's Roll*, i, 174; a Dr Moore was also cited as 'condemned' when the College Censors interrogated Dr Arthur Dee, son of Dr John Dee, for illicit practice in 1614, though whether condemned by the College or someone else is unclear. *Annals*, iii, f19b.

14 HMC, *Thirteenth Report*, Appendix pt. 7, 5.

15 Norman Moore, *The History of the Study of Medicine in the British Isles* (Oxford, 1908), 97–106, quoted in Keynes, *Harvey*, 138 ff.

16 Hacket, *Scrinia Reserata*, 222. A fontanel is now used to describe the gaps in an infant's skull, but then referred to an opening in the skin created using instruments such as cauterizing irons to provide an aperture for the discharge of humours. See Woodall, *The Surgeon's Mate*, 7.

17 BL MS Sloane 395B, f1; Keynes, *Harvey*, 37.

18 Gee, *The Foot out of the Snare*, R–R2.

19 RCP SR 318; Devon, *Issues of the Exchequer*, 350. There is no evidence to support the idea that Harvey acted in league with Villiers or, indeed, Charles I to poison James, but it may have been considered possible that such an accusation would be made given Harvey's failure to intervene to stop James being prescribed unauthorized medicines. Such a pardon would be necessary to limit any damage done to his reputation.

20 Taylor, *A Fearful Summer*, A3^r.

21 Ward, 'Diary', entry for 3-2-1664. The biological cause of plague epidemics such as that of 1625 has become a subject of debate among historians of medicine, the latest opinion throwing doubt on whether they were bubonic caused by the infective agent *Yersinia pestis*;

alternative suggestions include an haemorrhagic disease possibly caused by a filovirus, the sort responsible for more recently identified diseases such as Ebola. See Scott, *Biology of Plagues*, 389–94.

22 Dekker, *A Rod for Run-aways*, A2^v.

23 Herring, *Certaine Rules*, A3^r; Attersoll, *A Commentarie vpon the Fourth Booke of Moses*, A4^r.

24 *Annals*, iii, f108b–109a.

25 *Orders to be vsed in the time of the infection.*

26 *Orders heertofore conceiued and agreed* [p. 2].

27 *The Four Great Years of the Plague.*

28 The apothecary William Shambrooke made this quantity. The number of doses is calculated on the basis of one dram of Mithridate per dose. See Wall, *History of the Worshipful Society of Apothecaries*, 34, 221; Culpeper, *London Dispensatory*, 131.

29 Wall, *History of the Worshipful Society of Apothecaries*, 34.

30 *A Generall or Great Bill for this yeere of the whole number of burials* (London, 1625). There were around nine hundred communicants in Harvey's parish. See Liu, *Puritan London*, Appendix 1, 217.

31 Quoted in Keynes, *Harvey*, 149.

32 Most of what follows is quoted in Seaver, *Wallington's World*. References are given for the original manuscripts. GL MS 204, 407–8; Wallington, *Historical Notices*, I, xvi–ii.

33 Dekker, *A Rod for Run-aways*, B^{r-v}.

34 Rappaport, *Worlds within Worlds*, 49–53; Pearl, 'Change and Stability in Seventeenth-century London', 3–34.

35 BL Add MS 21,935 (called 'A Bundle of Mercies'), ff8^r–10^r, 1r; Seaver, *Wallington's World*, 153.

36 Montagu, *Appello Caesarem*, a3^v.

37 Wallington, *Historical Notices*, i, 12–13.

38 GL MS 204, 505; Seaver, *Wallington's World*, 31.

39 John Donne, *Devotions Upon Emergent Occasions*, ed. John Raspa (Oxford, 1987), 24–5, quoted in Wear, *Knowledge and Practice*, 331 ff.

40 Wallington, *Historical Notices*, I, xviii.

41 Porter, *Greatest Benefit*, 197; MS Ashmole 423; Lilly, *History*, 44.

42 *Munk's Roll*, 178; *Annals*, iii, f14b. The Sanders interrogated by the Censors and Patrick Saunders may have been the same person. Though a candidate, i.e. a probationary member, there is no record of Saunders's admission to the College as a Fellow.

43 BL Add MS 40,883, f149^r.

44 GL MS 204, 417.

45 GL MS 204, 431–2.

46 Dekker, *The Black Rod*, B^v–B2^r; *A Rod for Run-aways*, A4^v.

47 BL MS Sloane 1457, f11^v; Seaver, *Wallington's World*, 47.

48 BL MS Sloane 1457, f12^r.

49 Wallington, *Historical Notices*, i, 16–22.

50 Ibid., 13–14.

51 Harvey, *Anatomical Exercitations*, 53 ff.

52 Keynes, *Harvey*, 196, 202.

53 Ibid., 196–201.

54 Maynwaring, *Religion and Alegiance*, 20.

55 Charles I, *By the King. A proclamation for suppressing of false rumours touching Parliament* (London, 1629).

56 Woolrych, *Britain in Revolution*, 88.

57 Crawfurd, *The King's Evil*, 72–3.

58 James I, *A Speech to the Lords and Commons of Parliament at White-Hall, on Wednesday the XXI. of March. Anno 1609* (London, 1609).

59 Allen, *Cheirexoke*, 8.

60 Charles I, *By the King. A*

proclamation for the better ordering of those who repayrr to the Court for their cure of the disease called the King's Evill (London, 1626).

61 Keynes, *Harvey*, 210–12.

62 The quotes for this section are drawn from Whitelocke, *Diary*, 73–6.

63 Keynes, *Harvey*, 204–5; *Annals*, iii, f133b.

64 Spalding, *The Improbable Puritan*, 50.

BALM

1 Culpeper, *Pharmacopoeia Londinensis*, 21.

2 *OED*.

3 Culpeper, *Life*, B4^r, C2^v; Galen's *Art of Physick*, pp 58–9; Tobyn, *Culpeper's Medicine*, p 26.

4 Six editions of *The Anatomy of Melancholy* appeared within thirty years of its first publication.

5 Bod MS Ashmole 226, f156. The identification of Foreman's Burton with the author of *The Anatomy of Melancholy* is discussed in Traister, 'New Evidence about Burton's Melancholy?', 66–70.

6 Burton, *Anatomy of Melancholy*, 'Democritus to the Reader', 52, 59, 76.

7 Rosemary Weinstein, 'London at the Outbreak of the Civil War', in Porter, *London and the Civil War*, 31–41; Howell, *Londinopolis*, 350; Lithgow, 'The Present Surveigh of London', 542.

8 Lilly, *History*, 22–7.

9 Johnson, *Herball*, 1515–16.

10 Schofield, *Ralph Treswell*, 79–82, 22, 25–6, and plate 11.

11 Razzell, *English Civil War*, 175; Wall, *History of the Society of Apothecaries*, 63–4, 317–18.

12 Shakespeare, *Romeo and Juliet*, V: i: 37–48.

13 See, for example, Maud Grieve, *Culinary Herbs and Condiments* (London, 1933), entry for Apple (Bitter). She gives 1½ teaspoons (just over two drams) as a fatal dose. This was not the only occasion when one of Harvey's prescriptions was to be publicly questioned. In 1619, he had been consulted by the wealthy city merchant Sir William Smith, who was suffering from a bladder stone. Harvey examined Smith and diagnosed a small stone which could be treated using a secret remedy of his own, for which he would charge £50 per year for as long as Sir William avoided having an operation to remove the stone. In the event, Sir William needed the operation, and a huge stone was removed. He later died, perhaps of complications arising from the operation, owing a quarter's payment to Harvey (£12 10s.), which on his deathbed he forbade his son and heir to pay. Harvey, possibly under the sway of a litigious lawyer, decided to sue for the amount, which resulted in a damaging case lasting over two years. The records of the case are in the Public Record Office, Chancery: Entry Books of Decrees and Orders, Ref C 33/141, and summarized in Keynes, *Harvey*, 115–20.

14 *Annals*, iii, ff130b, 133b, 138a.

15 Wall, *History of the Society of Apothecaries*, 221.

16 *Annals*, iii, ff149b–150a.

17 Ibid., ff19b, 20b, 21a.

18 The only record of the proceedings in the Star Chamber between the physicians and the apothecaries is contained in a manuscript at the Apothecaries' Hall entitled 'Briefs of Proceedings in Star Chamber ag[ains]t severall Members of ye Apoth[ecaries] Compa[ny]' (MS 8286). The above is based on the analysis of the manuscript's

contents made by E. Ashworth Underwood in Wall, *History of the Society of Apothecaries*, 277–97, 304.

19 Wall, *A History of the Society of Apothecaries*, 80, 285. According to the Court minutes, Culpeper's initiation took place on 14 November 1634. Simeon Foxe's attendance at the Apothecaries' Hall is not mentioned in the Society's official Court minutes, but described in the 'Briefs of Proceedings in Star Chamber' manuscript (MS 8286) mentioned above. The College Annals suggest the event took place on 20 September 1634, a few days before Foxe was elected President. The apothecaries first appeared before the Star Chamber on 17 November 1634, summonses being issued in the preceding two weeks. *Annals*, iii, ff146b–150a.

MELANCHOLY THISTLE

1 See Guybert, *The Charitable Physitian*, 65–7 for a list of items in a typical apothecary shop.

2 See the editors' introduction to Harvey, *Lectures*, 18, for an assessment of his Latin skills. The editors write: 'One gains the impression that Harvey was not fully a master of the Latin language, and that as certain thoughts and ideas occurred to him he found it much easier and quicker to express them in the vernacular rather than to search for Latin equivalents.' The standard of Latin in his published works is considered high.

3 Urdang, *Pharmacopoeia Londinensis*, 30.

4 The title is taken from the second edition of 1618 (*STC* 16773), slightly altered from the first edition of 1618

(*STC* 16772). The editions consulted are in the Royal College of Physicians library, refs 18370–1 and 18372.

5 Ward, *Diary*, 72.

6 Huntington Library, MS HAF Box 15(32). It should be noted that the term Mithridate was also used as a generic term for compound treacles. Cheaper versions were available that omitted the more expensive ingredients. In Guybert's *The Charitable Physitian*, 'I.W.', the translator, lists Treacle and Mythridate as costing from as little as 8*d*./ounce, compared to Confectio Alkermes, which cost 2*s*. 5*d*./oz. See p. 59.

7 Ward, *Diary*, 60.

8 Guybert, *The Charitable Physitian*, 45, 49.

9 The latter was the result of an attempt by the College to be as comprehensive as possible. Unfortunately, in listing the simples, the *Pharmacopoeia* did not provide any clear way of distinguishing synonyms from separate entries.

10 The College was referring to Jacque Dubois (1478–1555), also known as Jacobus Sylvius, who wrote books on Galen, Mesue, and Hippocrates. Urdang, *Pharmacopoeia Londinensis*, 58.

11 Johnson, *Iter plantarum*, A–B4.

12 GL MS 8200/1. Nicholas was bound to Drake on 1 March 1637.

13 GL MS 8200/1, 19 February 1638/9.

14 Culpeper, *English Physitian*, 226.

15 Smith, 'The London Apprentices', 151–2.

16 CLRO Reports of Court of Aldermen, 54, f267^v.

17 GL MS 3295/1, 30-4-1630; also 1-2-1629/30 and 3-2-1630/31; Seaver, *Wallington's World*, 116–17.

18 Culpeper, *Life*, B4^r–[B5^v].

19 The word is probably derived from

the Greek for a 'slight mania'; the term 'hypomania' is listed in the *OED* with this meaning.

20 Wall, *History of the Society of Apothecaries*, 306.

21 *Mercurius Pragmaticus*, 4–11 September 1649.

22 Stowe, *A Survey of London*, 275; Pearl, *London and the Outbreak of the Puritan Revolution*, 183.

23 Kirby, 'The Radicals of St Stephen's, Coleman Street', 100.

24 Calder, *The New Haven Colony*, 4–6.

25 *Annals*, 18 December 1627. Quoted in Keynes, *Harvey*, 152–3.

26 *Iohn Lambe*, 2; Thomas, *Religion and the Decline of Magic*, 412; Kirby, 'The Radicals of St Stephen's, Coleman Street', 107.

27 Quoted in Woolrych, *Britain in Revolution*, 81; Laud, *A Sermon*, 36.

28 Orr, 'Sovereignty', 474–90, esp. 479 ff.

29 *Annals*, iii, f151b.

30 Seaver, *Wallington's World*, 159–61.

31 Edwards, *Gangraena*, pt. 2, 31.

32 Goodwin, *Imputatio Fidei*, c^v, quoting Daniel 12: 4.

33 PRO SP 16/371/39. Quoted in Lindley, *The English Civil War and Revolution*, 38; Kirby, 'The Radicals of St Stephen's, Coleman Street, London', 114. On the matter of predestination, Goodwin appears to have been theologically closer to Laud than his Puritan associates, some of whom attacked him for heresy (Walker, *A Defence of the True Sence*, 55–6). However, he kept his published views vague so as not to alienate his congregation.

34 Liu, *Puritan London*, 83; Edwards, *Gangraena*, 124–5.

35 Steiner, *History of Guildford*, 13; Calder, *The New Haven Colony*, 1–31.

36 Quoted in Allen, *English Political Thought*, 475.

37 Lilly, *History*, 30–1.

38 Read, *Manual of Anatomy*, 186–7; *The Chirurgicall Lectures* (London, 1635), 24–5. 'The Paracelsian doctrine is full of difficulties, which he maketh more obscure by coining strange words . . . so that his discourses are but a kind of canting Philosophy.'

39 *Annals*, iii, f136b.

40 Read, *The Chirurgicall Lectures*, 78.

41 Clowes, *A Prooued Practise for all Young Chirurgians*, 142–3.

42 Culpeper, *London Dispensatory*, 165–6.

43 Culpeper, *Directory for Midwives*, 5, 55–6, 22, 186–7.

44 Read, *Physicall Secrets* (London, 1639), Introductory Letter; McCarl, 'Publishing the Works of Nicholas Culpeper', 243.

45 Culpeper, *Life*, C3^r. According to the memoir, Culpeper received his inheritance from Nathaniel Brooke, which was unlikely, as Brooke was seventeen years old at the time, and an apprentice. Perhaps Brooke's name was used to identify the address retrospectively. See Bodleian MS Ashmole 332, f42; McKenzie, *Stationers' Company Apprentices*, 45; for a biography of Brooke, Sanderson, *Nicholas Culpeper and the Book Trade*, 101 ff.

46 Culpeper, *Physical Directory*, 1650, B2^v; Attersoll, *Historie of Balak*, A5^r.

47 Sanderson, *Nicholas Culpeper and the Book Trade*, 43–4.

48 Culpeper, *Life*, C5^r–v; TT E487(3) 'Philaretes', *Culpeper Revived*.

49 Thomas, *Excavations at the Priory and Hospital of St Mary Spital*, 104b.

50 Walter Rowley, *A New Wonder, a Woman Never Vext* (London, 1632). Quoted in Thomas, *Excavations at the Priory and Hospital of St Mary Spital*, 104a.

51 Ian Roy, ' "The Proud Unthankfull City": A Cavalier View of London

in the Civil War', in Porter, *London and the Civil War*, 167.

52 Thomas, *Excavations at the Priory and Hospital of St Mary Spital*, 114b and tables 68–77.

53 See appropriate entries in Culpeper, *English Physitian*. In his *Theatrum Botanicum*, John Parkinson also reported finding Common White or 'Meadow' Saxifrage there. Lamb's conduit was named after William Lamb, a member of the Clothworkers' Company who financed its restoration in 1577. The conduit has long disappeared, but a street of that name now runs along its course.

54 See GL MS 8200/1, *Apothecaries' Court Minutes*, entry for 13 May 1644, which mentions Leadbetter holding a 'pair of indentures' (i.e. the two parts of the document) relating to Culpeper's bond.

SELF-HEAL

1 Johnson, *Herball*, 633.
2 See William Johnson, 'Friend Culpeper', in Leonardo Fioravanti, *Three Exact Pieces*, 9–15.
3 Culpeper, *Catastrophe Magnatum*, 10; *Semeiotica Uranica*, 182.
4 *Orders and Directions Together with a Commission for the better Administration of Justice* (London, 1630), 10.
5 *Decree of Starre-Chamber: Concerning Inmates, and divided Tenements, in London or three miles about* (London, 1636), C^v–$C2^v$.
6 See Keynes, *Harvey*, 202–4.
7 Quoted in Thulesius, *Nicholas Culpeper*, 40.
8 Culpeper, *School of Physick*, 263.
9 Culpeper, *English Physitian*, 'Groundsel'.
10 RCP MS 654, f356.

11 Culpeper, *English Physitian*, 'Poppy'.
12 Culpeper, *English Physitian*, 'Vine'.
13 Culpeper, *Directory for Midwives*, 99.
14 Culpeper, *English Physitian*, 255.
15 Clark, *History of the Royal College of Physicians*, 178; Wellcome MS 6172, John Ward, *Diary*, 2 February 1664, 563.
16 Culpeper, *Astrologicall Judgment of Diseases*, 175–6.
17 Arthur Dee, *Fasciculus Chemicus, abstrusæ Hermeticæ Scientiæ ingressum, progressum, coronidem, verbis apertissimis explicans* (Paris, 1631), translated by Elias Ashmole and published under the title *Fasciculus chemicus: or Chymical Collections. Expressing the ingress, progress, and egress, of the secret hermetick science, out of the choisest and most famous authors* (London, 1650).
18 *Mercurius Pragmaticus*, 4–11 September 1649; McCarl, 'Publishing the Works of Nicholas Culpeper', 228; Arber, *Herbals*, 262.
19 The Cavalier poet Richard Lovelace died in Gunpowder Alley in 1658, in what Anthony à Wood described as a 'mean lodging'. See *The Poems of Richard Lovelace*, 225.
20 *Annals*, iii, f156b.
21 Lilly, *History*, 63–75.
22 Whitelocke, *Diary*, 129; Lilly, *History*, 102–3. Lilly, writing towards the end of his life, dates this incident to 1643. He had a habit – unexpected in an astrologer – of being sloppy with dates. The evidence from Whitelocke's diary, which he updated regularly, indicates that Lilly was consulted in late 1641. Lilly also identifies the doctor as 'Prideaux'. Whitelocke refers to his doctor being 'Pridgeon', Prujean; see Whitelocke, *Diary*, 180.
23 Culpeper, *Semeiotica Uranica*, 16.
24 Culpeper, *Life*, $C7^v$–r.

25 John Fage (ffage, Phage) was apparently the owner of the copy of Culpeper's *Semeiotica Uranica* now in the Wellcome Library (shelfmark 19390/A), as his name is inscribed on the title-page, and a price of 2*s*. 6*d*. Culpeper describes Fage as being 'of Midhurst in Sussex'. Fage was author of *Speculum ægrotorum: the sicke-mens glasse*, a translation which Culpeper criticized, accusing him of 'mistaking the word Caedo to kill for Cado to fall: wherein the man most egregiously shewed his deficiency, both in Scholler-ship and Physick: yet this commendation ile give him, his heart was more free to do good then his braine was able'. The astrological case study relating to Fage appears in Culpeper, *Semeiotica Uranica*, 49–53.

26 Culpeper, *English Physitian*, 'Liverwort'.

27 The crystal is now on display in case H30 of the medical gallery, Science Museum, London, together with Culpeper's letter authenticating it, inventory numbers A127915 and 6; my thanks to Stewart Emmens, Assistant Curator of Public Health, for providing transcripts of Culpeper's letter.

ROSA SOLIS

1 Mabey, *Flora Britannica*, 125; *King's American Dispensatory*, entry for 'Drosera'.

2 Harvey, *Anatomical Exercitations*, 285–7.

3 Edward May, *A Most Certaine and True Relation*; Keynes, *Harvey*, 323–8.

4 Harvey, *Concerning the Motion of the Heart*, *.3^r–4^r, *.1^v–2r.

5 Keynes, *Harvey*, 279–80.

6 Harvey, *Anatomical Exercitations*, 397, 88.

7 Quoted in Woolrych, *Britain in Revolution*, 134.

8 W. C. Souter, 'Dr William Harvey in Aberdeen', *Aberdeen University Review*, 1631, quoted in Keynes, *Harvey*, 284–5.

9 Wallington, *Historical Notices*, i, 275–6.

10 *A Remonstrance of the State of the Kingdom*, 13–16, 20, 22.

11 Wallington, *Historical Notices*, i, 304–5.

12 Porter, *London and the Civil War*, 4.

13 Quoted in Hill, *World Turned Upside Down*, 22. Wallington, *Historical Notices*, i, 279.

14 GL MS 204, p. 472. Seaver, *Wallington's World*, 150–1.

15 *Annals*, iii, 209a; Cook, *Decline*, 101.

16 According to Rushworth (*Historical Collections*, i, 477) on 27 December 1641, the royalist supporter and soldier David Hide was first heard to use the term, threatening to 'cut the Throat of those Roundheaded Dogs that bawled against Bishops'. This origin is disputed, as it is elsewhere claimed that Queen Henrietta Maria first used the term to describe John Pym MP.

17 *A Letter from Mercurius Civicus to Mercurius Rusticus*, 18. Wallington, *Historical Notices*, i, 277–83.

18 Parker, *Lilly*, 84. Lilly does not explain why he was at Whitehall. He may have been with the Countess of Carlisle, sister of the Earl of Northumberland, who according to one report tipped off the House of the King's intentions. See Rushworth, *Historical Collections*, i, 477.

19 *An Exact Collection of all Remonstrances, Declarations, Votes, Orders, Ordinances &c which were formerly published either by the King's Majestie's Command, or by*

Order from One or both Houses of Parliament (London, 1643). Quoted in Wallington, *Historical Notices*, ii, 339.

20 D'Ewes, *Journal*, 381–3.

21 Rushworth, *Historical Collections*, i, 477.

22 D'Ewes, *Journal*, 383; Wallington, *Historical Notices*, i, 286–7; Rushworth, *Historical Collections*, i, 477.

23 *A Letter from Mercurius Civicus to Mercurius Rusticus*, 17. Wallington, *Historical Notices*, i, 285.

24 Quoted in Hill, *The World Turned Upside Down*, 22.

25 Porter, *London and the Civil War*, 11–12.

26 D'Ewes, *Journal*, 392; TT E201(7) *Diurnall Occurences*, 3–10 January 1642; Lawson Nagel, '"A Great Bouncing at Every Man's Door": The Struggle for London's Militia in 1642', in Porter, *London and the Civil War*, 71.

27 Wallington, *Historical Notices*, i, 289–90.

28 *The Petition and Resolution of the Cityzens of the City of Chester; The Petition of the Knights, Gentlemen, and Yeomanry of the Country of Devonshire*, A2ʳ.

29 2 Samuel 2; Wallington, *Historical Notices*, ii, 6 and 332; TT E134(17).

30 The history of the Artillery Ground is difficult to entangle at this time. It was claimed by the 'Society of the Artillery Garden', later known as the Honourable Artillery Company (which still exists), but the claim was disputed by the parish of St Botolph's. In 1591, it was recorded as being 'discontinued', but the Privy Council demanded that it be 'renewed, being a matter very requisite and necessary for the benefit of the common weal'. It appears that by the 1620s, it was once more in regular use. Thomas,

Excavations at the Priory and Hospital of St Mary Spital, 150b; *Acts of the Privy Council, 1591–1592*, 74.

31 PRO, SP 12/213/55. Quoted in Boynton, *The Elizabethan Militia*, 105.

32 *A Letter from Mercurius Civicus to Mercurius Rusticus*, 15.

33 *Mercurius Civicus*, December 1641. See Robert Ashton, 'Insurgency, Counter-Insurgency and Inaction' in Porter, *London and the Civil War*, 51.

34 Clarendon, *History*, ii, 75; CLRO, MS 86.5; *CSP Domestic, 1641–3*, 323; *Mercurius Aulicus*, 28 September 1643. See Nagel, '"A Great Bouncing at Every Man's Door"', 78.

35 Nagel, '"A Great Bouncing at Every Man's Door"', 79.

36 TT E202(28).

37 BL Add MS 37343 f8; Quoted in Spalding, *Improbable Puritan*, 82–3.

38 TT E240(3), E202(38), E202(39).

39 Harvey, *Anatomical Exercitations*, 418.

40 Harvey himself does not seem to have altered his practice substantially to reflect the implications of his theory. He continued to perform blood-letting, or phlebotomy, on a daily basis (see, for example, Keynes, *Harvey*, 327), but then it would remain common practice for centuries to come, long after Harvey's theory became orthodox.

41 Gauden, *Eikon Basilike*, 34.

42 TT E69(12).

43 Keynes, *Harvey*, 286–7.

44 Gardiner, *Civil War*, i, 14.

45 TT E240(49).

46 Keynes, *Harvey*, 194.

47 Aubrey, *Brief Lives*, in Keynes, *Harvey*, 432–3.

48 The portrait is now in the collection of the Scottish National Portrait Gallery, ref PG1244.

49 *A Letter from Mercurius Civicus to Mercurius Rusticus*, 13.

50 TT E242(2); Nagel, ' "A Great Bouncing at Every Man's Door" ', Porter, *London and the Civil War*, 83.

51 *CSP Domestic, 1641–3*, 369.

52 Ward, *Diary*, 415–17.

53 Lithgow, 'The Present Surveigh of London', 538–42; N. G. Brett-James, *Growth of Stuart London* (London, 1935), 292; Victor Smith and Peter Kelsey, 'The Lines of Communication: The Civil War Defences of London', in Porter, *London and the Civil War*, 117–44.

54 *CSP Venetian, 1642–3*, 257.

55 BL Add MS 40,883, f49r; Seaver, *Wallington's World*, 152.

BRYONY

1 Johnson, *Herball*, 869.

2 Grieve, *The Modern Herbal*, entry for 'Bryony'; Mabey, *Flora Britannica*, 132.

3 Culpeper, *Life*, C6^r LMA, John Cordy Jeaffreson (ed.), *Middlesex County Records* (Old Series), iii, 17 December 18 Charles I [1642].

4 About a fifth of those charged with witchcraft were men. See Gaskill, 'The Devil in the Shape of a Man', 145.

5 *Annals*, iii, f206a; Webster, *Great Instauration*, 309.

6 Cooke, *Decline*, 105; Clark, *History of the Royal College of Physicians*, 273–5.

7 GL MS 8200/1, *Apothecaries' Court Minutes*, 31 January 1642[/3].

8 Wall, *History of the Society of Apothecaries*, 331, 97.

9 1 Samuel 15: 23 ('witchcraft' is translated 'divination' in modern editions); *Mercurius Aulicus*, 10–17 August 1645; Jacobs, *Epistolae*

Ho-Elianiae*, 506 (dated 3 February 1646); Purkiss, 'Desire and its Deformities', 106–7.

10 Goodwin, *Anti-cavalierisme*, 5, 33.

11 Pearl, *London and the Outbreak of the Puritan Revolution*, 250.

12 See Thomas, *Religion and the Decline of Magic*, 409, 439.

13 Lithgow, 'The Present Surveigh of London', 537.

14 Ian Roy, ' "The Proud Unthankfull City": A Cavalier View of London in the Civil War', in Porter, *London and the Civil War*, 167.

15 TT E65(32), *A Letter from Mercurius Civicus to Mercurius Rusticus* ([London], 1643), 32.

16 Spalding, *Improbable Puritan*, 88; Whitelocke, *Diary*, 141.

17 Keynes, *Harvey*, 292.

18 Quoted in Hill, *The Intellectual Revolution of the Seventeenth Century*, 188.

19 Cook, *Decline*, 53.

20 Keynes, *Harvey*, 292–3.

21 Ibid., *Harvey*, 305.

22 Ibid., 291–3, 301; Lilly, *History*, 53.

23 BL Add MS 18980, f125.

24 Whitelocke, *Diary*, 145.

25 Rous, *A Brief Narrative of the Late Treacherous and Horrid Designe*, 13.

26 BL Add MS 40,883, f133v; Seaver, *Wallington's World*, 170; Wallington, *Historical Notices*, ii, 149.

27 *CJ*, iii, 316.

28 Money, *Battles of Newbury*, 11; Seaver, *Wallington's World*, 170.

29 *A Letter from Mercurius Civicus to Mercurius Rusticus*, 4.

30 TT E71(31), Saltmarsh, *A Peace but no Pacification*, [A4^v]. There is no record of Culpeper's enlistment. The evidence from Culpeper, *Life* (B7^v, C6^r) points to him having joined in 1643 and participating in the Newbury campaign. Given the proximity of his house to the Artillery Ground, his political sympathies, and his association with

London trade, it is likely that he joined the Trained Bands rather than became a regular in Essex's army. He was unlikely to have enlisted in the call-up of late 1642 prior to Turnham Green, making the late summer of 1643 the most probable time. It is upon this assumption that what follows is based.

31 William Attersoll, *A Commentarie vpon Moses*, A4^v; Livy, *The Romane Historie*, iii , bk. 23, 473.

32 TT E69(15), Foster, *A True and Exact Relation*, A2^r.

33 *Mercurius Aulicus*, 9 September 1643.

34 *A most certain, strange and true discovery of a witch, being taken by some of the parliament forces* (London, 1643), reprinted in Money, *Battles of Newbury*, 84–6. See also Diane Purkiss, 'Desire and its Deformities', 103–32.

35 The accounts that follow come mostly from Money, *Battles of Newbury*, 44–65; Gardiner, *Civil War*, i, 209–19 (Gardiner drew heavily on Money for his account of the battle); TT E69(2), *A True Relation of the Late Battell neere Newbery*; TT E69(10), Digby, *A True and Impartiall Relation*.

36 TT E69(15), Foster, *A True and Exact Relation*, B3–4.

37 Gardiner, *Civil War*, i, 205, 213.

38 Fuller, *Worthies*, 112.

39 Read, 'A Treatise of the First Part of Chirurgery', *Workes*, 20.

40 Clowes, *A Prooued Practise for all Young Chirurgians*, 4.

41 Hildanus, *Experiments in Chyrurgerie*, 31–3.

42 Gerard, *Herball*, 239.

43 *A Letter from Mercurius Civicus to Mercurius Rusticus*, 4.

44 Spalding, *Improbable Puritan*, 95.

45 Gadbury, *Collectio Geniturarum*, 142–3.

46 Acts 17: 6, 'Reconciliation of Man to God' in Denne, *Grace, Mercy, and Peace*, 23–4; see Hill, *The World Turned Upside Down*, 13.

HEMLOCK

1 Felter, *The Eclectic Materia Medica*, entry for 'Conium'.

2 TT E4(27); Lilly, *A Prophecy of the White King*.

3 See Hill, *The World Turned Upside Down*, 89.

4 TT E106(15).

5 Cressy, *Literacy and the Social Order*, 2; Houston, *Literacy in Early Modern Europe*, 121.

6 Quoted in Wolfe, *Milton in the Puritan Revolution*, 129.

7 Lilly, *History*, 103–4.

8 Goodwin, *Anti-cavalierisme*, A3^r–^{v}.

9 Lilly, *Prophecy*, 13.

10 TT E13(1), Lilly, *England's Propheticall Merline*, b3^r; b3^v.

11 Lilly, *Anglicus . . . 1645*, preface. Quoted in Geneva, *Astrology*, 47.

12 *Mercurius Britannicus*, 1643, quoted in Adair, *By the Sword Divided*, 144.

13 *Perfect Passages of each Daye's Proceedings in Parliament*, 6 to 13 November 1644; Money, *Battles of Newbury*, 188, 199.

14 TT E288(17), Lilly, *The Starry Messenger*, title-page.

15 Lilly, *The Starry Messenger*, 10–11.

16 Ibid., 3 ff.

17 Though in Lilly's time the zodiac was represented as a square, it is easier to think of it as two concentric circles. The outer circle is divided up into twelve segments of equal size (30 degrees), identified by a particular constellation or star sign (Aries, Taurus, Gemini, and so on). The inner circle is also divided into twelve 30-degree segments, the astrological houses, identified by

number. The position of the houses with respect to constellations (the inner circle with respect to the outer) is determined by the time of the episode being astrologically investigated (be it a birth, a burglary, the onset of an illness, an event, or, in the case of the 'horary' astrological technique used by Lilly, the time a question is asked). Put another way, the signs of the zodiac are tied to the rotation of the heavens, the houses to the rotation of the earth, the two becoming enmeshed by the timing of the event. When drawing up a scheme or chart, the position of the eight planets (sun, moon, Mercury, Venus, Mars, Jupiter, Saturn – Uranus, Neptune and Pluto had not been discovered in Lilly's time) with respect to both the signs and the houses is also noted. Each planet 'rules' both a star sign and a house (the sun rules Leo and the fifth house, the moon Cancer and the fourth house; the other planets rule two signs and two houses each). It is also 'exalted' (has a positive influence) in some signs, and is 'in detriment' (negative) in others. Its influence is further mediated by 'aspects', its position or angle with respect to the other planets: those in the same position or within eight or nine degrees of each other are in conjunction, those at 180 degrees (in opposite positions in the sky) are in opposition, those at 90 degrees to each other are in square and so on.

18 TT E50(27), Lilly, *Merlinus Anglicus Junior*, 9. This was the second, unexpurgated edition of the work. A first edition was published in April. See Geneva, *Astrology*, 177.

19 Lilly, *The Starry Messenger*, 21.

20 Wharton, *An Astrologicall Judgement*, 8–9.

21 Lithgow, 'The Present Surveigh of London', 536.

22 Whitelocke, *Diary*, 154.

23 BL Add MS 40,883 f148[v]; Seaver, *Wallington's World*, 124.

24 BL Add MS 40,883 f179[v]; Seaver, *Wallington's World*, 124.

25 Lilly, *The Starry Messenger*, *[v], *2[v].

26 Whitelocke, *Diary*, 167–8.

27 Josten, *Elias Ashmole*, 447, 451.

28 Bodleian MS Ashmole 423, f168.

29 Josten, *Elias Ashmole*, ii, 417–19.

30 See Thomas, *Religion and the Decline of Magic*, 361.

31 TT E568(15), Gell, *Stella Nova*, A3[v]. See Josten, *Ashmole*, ii, 492. A copy of Gell's sermon is at MS Ashmole 1239, art. VII.

32 Culpeper, *Semeiotica Uranica*, 'To the Astrological Phisitians of England', A3.

33 TT E392[19], *Gold Tried in the Fire, or the burnt petitions revived*, A[r]; Pease, *The Leveller Movement*, 158; Woolrych, *Britain in Revolution*, 355.

34 Folger MS V.a.436, 177, 449; Seaver, *Wallington's World*, 171.

35 Robert Ashton, 'Insurgency, Counter-Insurgency and Inaction: Three Phases in the Role of the City in the Great Rebellion', in Porter, *London and the Civil War*, 54–6.

36 Culpeper, *Physical Directory*, 1650, B2v; Gardiner, *Civil War*, iii, 278. Oreb and Zeeb were the princes of Midian, Zebah and Zalmunna the kings, defeated by the Israelite general Gideon; Judges 7: 42–8; 8.

37 *An Agreement of the People*, 2.

38 Quoted in Lindley, *The English Civil War and Revolution*, 152; on the Norman Yoke, see Hill, *Puritanism and Revolution*, 50 ff.

39 See Rachum, 'The Meaning of "Revolution"', 195–215.

40 Bodleian MS Ashmole 420, f267.

41 Milton, *Areopagitica*, 31.

LESSER CELANDINE

1 Ian Gentles, 'The Civil Wars in England' and Charles Carlton, 'Civilians', in Morrill, *The Civil Wars*, 106–7, 273.

2 Culpeper, *Ephemeris for the Yeer 1651*, H2ʳ.

3 Gardiner, *Constitutional Documents*, 356.

4 Hill, *The World Turned Upside Down*, 107–8.

5 Gardiner, *Civil War*, iv, 220–1.

6 CJ, vi, 76–7; see Woolrych, *Britain in Revolution*, 423–4.

7 *A Remonstrance of His Excellency Thomas Lord Fairfax*, 61.

8 Whitelocke, *Diary*, 225–6.

9 Wolfe, *Milton in the Puritan Revolution*, 36.

10 Gardiner, *Civil War*, iv, 277.

11 Whitelocke, *Diary*, 248; Gardiner, *Civil War*, iv, 283.

12 *CJ*, c6, 110–11.

13 Lilly, *History*, 148–150; *A True Copy of the Journal of the High Court of Justice*, 26 ff.

14 Ibid., 113.

15 Josten, *Elias Ashmole*, 485–6.

16 Whitelocke, *Diary*, 230. The Seal was Parliament's, not the King's, which had been broken up following the fall of Oxford in June 1646; see Spalding, *Improbable Puritan*, 111.

17 Barnard, 'London Publishing 1640–1660', 5–6.

18 Plomer, *A Dictionary of Booksellers and Printers*, entry for 'Cole'; Sanderson, *Nicholas Culpeper and the Book Trade*, 90.

19 Clowes, *A Prooued Practise for all Young Chirurgians*, ¶4ʳ; originally published in 1596, this was the third edition, dated London, 1637, 'Printed by M. Dawson, and are to be sold by Benjamin Allen & P. Cole'.

20 Sanderson, *Nicholas Culpeper and the Book Trade*, 93.

21 In Culpeper, *Life*, Culpeper is described as receiving the money from 'the two Executors at *Nathaniel Brook* his shop at the Angell in Cornhill' (C3ʳ). In 1639, Thomas Cotes had a bookshop 'at the signe of the Angel in Popes-head Alley', which led off Cornhill (see, for example, the bibliographic details for Francis Quarles, *Memorials vpon the Death of Sir Robert Quarles, Knight* [London, 1639], 'Printed by Thomas Cotes, for Nicholas Alsop; and are to be sold at the signe of the Angel in Popes-head Alley', and Francis Cockin, *Divine Blossomes* [London, 1657], 'printed by W.G. for E. Farnham, at the entrance into Popeshead-alley out of Cornhill').

22 Sibbes, 'Philippians'; *Mercurius Pragmaticus*, 4–11 September 1649.

23 Plomer, 'Secret Printing During the Civil War', 380–1; Culpeper, *Ephemeris for the Yeer 1651*, entry for June 1651.

24 Stationers' Company *Court Book*, C, f187ᵛ; *CSP Domestic*, Charles I 1641–3, xviii, 513 (there is a secretarial mistake in another section of the entry, which tends to suggest the '1,000*l*' mentioned should have read 100*l*, still a considerable sum); Sanderson, *Nicholas Culpeper and the Book Trade*, 92.

25 *CSP Domestic 1660–1661*, Charles 2, i, 380.

26 Edwards, *Gangraena*, 143–4, 114–15; Sanderson, *Nicholas Culpeper and the Book Trade*, 93.

27 TT E532(32) and (35).

28 Bodleian MS Aubrey 6; quoted in Keynes, *Harvey*, 436.

29 Harvey, *Anatomical Exercitations*, 281; Hill, 'William Harvey and the

Idea of Monarchy', 160–81; Keynes, *Harvey*, 350.

30 Culpeper, *Semeiotica Uranica*, 1655, 177.

31 Quoted in Coward, *The Stuart Age*, 244.

32 Cook, *Decline*, 116; Keynes, *Harvey*, 371; *Munk's Roll*, i, 234.

33 *Annals*, 4:20b, 22a–22b, 24b; Cook, *Decline*, 115.

34 See Sanderson, *Nicholas Culpeper and the Book Trade*, 69 ff, for the first detailed survey of visits by College officials to the Stationers' Hall.

35 Culpeper, *Life*, C6[r].

36 McCarl, 'Publishing the Works of Nicholas Culpeper', 236; Sanderson, *Nicholas Culpeper and the Book Trade*, 120–1.

37 Sanderson, *Nicholas Culpeper and the Book Trade*, 232.

38 Culpeper, *Physical Directory*, 1649, 28, 54. Argentina was not listed in the original *Pharmacopoeia*; it was one of many added by Culpeper. See below.

39 *Pharmacopoeia Londinensis*, 1618, 6; Culpeper, *Physical Directory*, 1649, 86.

40 *Pharmacopoeia Londinensis*, 20, see also entry in the *Catologus Simplicium* under 'Animalium partes'; Culpeper, *Physical Directory*, 102.

41 Culpeper, *Physical Directory*, 3, 20, 9, 310–11. 'Oxycroceum', literally sharp saffron, was the term used for a variety of compounds using saffron.

42 Culpeper, *Physical Directory*, 94.

43 Culpeper, *Physical Directory*, A[r–v]. Aubrey wrote his remarks after the publication of Culpeper's *Physical Directory*, so Culpeper did not get them from Aubrey, though the reverse may be the case.

44 Heydon, *The Holy Guide*, lib. 3, 143.

45 Mackaile, *Moffett-Well*, 170; Coles, *The Art of Simpling*, 77.

46 William Johnson, 'Friend Culpeper', in Leonardo Fioravanti, *Three Exact Pieces*, 9–15. Sanderson argues that Johnson's attack did not represent the College's view, as it was not mentioned in the College *Annals* nor was the book in which it appeared endorsed at Stationers' Hall by the College. However, many delicate matters went unrecorded in the *Annals*, and it was unlikely that the College would openly associate itself with Johnson's critique. See Sanderson, *Nicholas Culpeper and the Book Trade*, 72–3.

47 19 November 1649. *CSP Domestic, Commonwealth*, 1649–50, i, 555.

48 *CSP Domestic, Commonwealth*, ii, 454, 469; no first name or place of origin is given for 'Mr Culpeper', but he is identified elsewhere in the State Papers of this period as Nicholas. He was arrested with a Mr Harlackenden, possibly Richard Harlackenden of Essex, surgeon to the Essex Trained Band, PRO S/P28/227. *CSP Domestic, Commonwealth*, 1651, iii, 70. Sanderson, *Nicholas Culpeper and the Book Trade*, 68.

49 Culpeper, *Physical Directory*, 1650, B[r].

50 Culpeper, *Physical Directory*, B2[r–v].

51 Culpeper, *Physical Directory*, 1651, A[v], A2[r–v].

52 Culpeper, *Ephemeris for the Yeer 1651*, G4[v].

53 Culpeper, *Ephemeris for the Year 1652*, title-page, 15, 18–19.

54 Culpeper, *Catastrophe Magnatum*, 72.

55 Evelyn, *Diary*, iii, 63; Thomas, *Religion and the Decline of Magic*, 355; TT E656(9), 7–8.

56 Culpeper, *Ephemeris for the Year 1652*, 14.

57 TT E662(1), J. B., *A Faire in Spittle Fields*, 6–7.

58 TT E656(9), 'Philastrogous', *Lillies Ape Whipt*, 2.

59 *Lillyes Lamentation*, 2 November 1652; quoted in Parker, *Lilly*, 216.

60 Culpeper, *Catastrophe Magnatum*, 75.

ARRACH

1 Grieve, *The Modern Herbal*, entry for 'Arrach'; Johnson, *Herball*, 327.

2 See Thomas, *Excavations at the Priory and Hospital of St Mary Spital, London*, 150a, on the development of Lollesworth Field.

3 Culpeper, *Semeiotica Uranica*, 153, 77–8; *English Physitian*, entry for 'Lesser Celandine'.

4 See Sanderson, *Nicholas Culpeper and the Book Trade*, 168; Evenden, *The Midwives of Seventeenth-Century London*, 80 ff.

5 Since the sixteenth century, midwives had been licensed by the Church on the basis of testimonials given by clients, figures of standing in the community, and medical professionals. There was no formal apprenticeship, but they were expected to have served under a licensed midwife for a period of years, sometimes a decade or more, before applying for a licence. In the seventeenth century, the Chamberlen family made a number of attempts to set up a society for midwifery, but were suspected by some midwives of trying to establish a monopoly. See Aveling, *The Chamberlens*, especially 20–4.

6 *The Mid-wives Just Petition*, A2^v.

7 Culpeper, *Directory for Midwives*, 212, ¶4^r.

8 Harvey, *Anatomical Exercitations*, 488; Willughby, *Observations in Midwifery*, 119–20.

9 Harvey, *Anatomical Exercitations*, 81, 83, 85, 89, 101, 112, 118, 121.

10 Ibid., 396 ff.

11 Ibid., 349.

12 Ibid., 479, 480.

13 Culpeper, *Directory for Midwives*, 131, 112, 12, 56–7; Thompson, *The Wandering Womb*, 55.

14 Harvey, *Anatomical Exercitations*, 3, 514, 515; Keynes, *Harvey*, 351–2; Huxley, 'Address of Thomas Henry Huxley', 400a–b.

15 Harvey, *Anatomical Exercitations*, 358; Harvey, *Lectures*, 53. It is possible that Harvey was using the term 'umbilicus' as a polite term for clitoris, but this seems unlikely given that the notes were written for his own use, rather than for publication. In *Anatomical Exercitations* he refers to the clitoris, noting that it was absent from the genitals of deer: see p. 399.

16 Harvey, *Lectures*, 125, 127; Culpeper, *Directory for Midwives*, 48, 175, 28.

17 Culpeper, *Directory for Midwives*, 41–2.

18 Ibid., 29.

19 Ross, *Arcana Microcosmi*, 'Appendix'; Johannes ab Angelis, *Vindiciæ ab epistolica Theodori Aldes dissertatione, contra Gulielmum Harvæum* (Amsterdam, 1667), quoted in Keynes, *Harvey*, 358–9.

20 Bourgeois, *The Compleat Midwifes Practice*, A2^r-A3^v. For authorship of this work, see Evenden, *Midwives of Seventeenth-Century London*, 9. Bourgeois, *The Compleat Midvvife's Practice Enlarged*, title-page. Evenden takes the criticisms of the *Directory for Midwives* in *The Compleat Midwifes Practice* at face value, assuming them to be motivated by the political efforts of the female authors to attack medical patriarchy. This is unlikely, given Thomas Chamberlen's involvement.

21 The *Compleat Angler* has traditionally been awarded this accolade; however, it was published in 1653, a year after the first edition of *English Physitian*.

22 Culpeper, *English Physitian*, 1652, title-page. To be fair to Nicholas, the book possibly took longer than expected to appear because, as he put it, it had been left 'hanging longer in the Press than I imagined it would'.

23 Arber, *Herbals*, 247, 261.

24 Culpeper, *English Physitian*, A^v. The best and most comprehensive modern account of astrological medicine can be found in Graeme Tobyn, *Culpeper's Medicine*, pt. 3. Tobyn quotes Geoffrey Cornelius, who pointed out that two separate but frequently conflated 'approaches' existed in astrology regarding the way the macrocosm and the microcosm interact. The Aristotelian approach, characterized as 'celestial causation', saw celestial events such as a conjunction of stars as causing earthly ones. The Platonic approach, characterized as 'cosmic harmony', saw the macrocosm and microcosm as mirroring one another. Culpeper, like most astrologers, veered between the two approaches. However, they were not necessarily incompatible, as it depended upon the meaning of 'macrocosm'. If it was a set of occult or divine forces, more like the laws of physics, acting both upon the celestial and elemental spheres – the stars and the earth – the movements of the stars themselves could not be said to cause earthly events. Culpeper possibly subscribed to this view, though not consistently. See Tobyn, 135–7.

25 Culpeper, *English Physitian*, 1652, 242[i.e. 252]–53; Jones, *Genealogy of a Classic*, 195; Sanderson, *Nicholas Culpeper and the Book Trade*, 146–7. Examples of references to women providing physic can be found in the entries for 'Herb True-Love', to be found in every 'good Woman's Garden', and 'woodbine', which should be stocked in 'every Gentlewoman's House'.

26 Guybert, *The Charitable Physitian*, G3^r–H2^r.

27 Peter Elmer, *The Library of Dr John Webster*, Medical History Supplement, vi (London, 1986), quoted in Sanderson, *Nicholas Culpeper and the Book Trade*, 142.

28 Culpeper, *English Physitian*, 10, 202, 239, 56, 40. Dr John Dee was an example of the sort of 'Welshman' Culpeper was poking fun at. In a long family tree, he traced his descent back to the Welsh prince Roderick the Great.

29 Whitelocke, *Diary*, 281–2.

30 Proverbs 5: 3–4.

31 He identifies the property as his country seat in his ephemeris of 1653.

32 By the 1650s, English medicine was beginning to be influenced by medical theories of the alchemist Johannes Baptista van Helmont (1579–1644), who challenged traditional medicine derived from Galen, criticizing the use of compound medicines and practice of blood-letting. He also developed the idea, first promoted by Paracelsus, that illnesses could be treated using medicines derived from chemicals rather than herbs. Under the influence of the royal physician Theodore de Mayerne, the College of Physicians had partially accepted the idea of chemical medicines in 1618, but not their implications for Galenic medicine. English followers of Van Helmont, the 'Helmontians', became identified with the radicalism of the 1650s, raising the possibility that Culpeper may have been a supporter. Culpeper certainly subscribed to many of their beliefs

and attitudes, such as a preference for simple medicines over compound ones, the need to set up a system that did not rely on the charity of physicians to treat the poor, and an interest in astrology as well as alchemy. There are also translations of a number of Paracelsian and Helmontian works attributed to him, and in the memoir of his life, he was said to be 'not only for Galen and Hippocrates, but he knew how to correct and moderate the tyrannies of Paracelsus' (Culpeper, *Life*, C5^v). However, it seems likely that he was recruited to the cause retrospectively, not least so that his name could be used to promote the sale of chemical remedies. One of the keys to Culpeper's pharmacy was that remedies should be made from cheap, accessible ingredients using simple methods. Most chemical medicines required a great deal of skill, as well as access to a laboratory. For the influence of Paracelsus and Van Helmont on the medicine of the period, see Webster, *Great Instauration*, 274–8 *et seq.* and Wear, *Knowledge and Practice*, pt. 2.

33 Josten, *Elias Ashmole*, ii, 734; Bodleian MS Ashmole 2 f3; Heydon, *The Wise-Mans Crown*, A5^v.

34 Culpeper, *Life*, C5^v.

35 Ibid., B8^r.

36 Culpeper, *Culpeper's Astrologicall Judgment of Diseases*, A2^r.

37 See McCarl, 'Publishing the Works of Nicholas Culpeper', Appendix, 263 ff, for a calendar of the works written by, and attributed to, Nicholas Culpeper, identifying their publisher and year of publication.

38 Ibid., 239–41.

39 Bodleian MS Ashmole 1807, ff. 59a, 60a, 61–97.

40 Culpeper, *Culpeper's Last Legacy*, 'Master Culpepers Wifes Accompt', n.p.

41 Culpeper, *Mr Culpepper's Treatise of aurum potabile*, A3^v, A5$^{r–v}$. The treatise was published by George Eversden rather than Cole, though it did include a copy of Cole's testimonial to Culpeper, *Culpeper's Ghost*.

42 Culpeper, *London Dispensatory* B^r.

43 TT E487(2). Philaretes, *Culpeper Revived*, quoted in McCarl, 'Publishing the Works of Nicholas Culpeper', 240.

44 Ward, *Diary*, 4-6-1662, WMS 6170, i, 106–7; Heydon, *The Holy Guide*, lib. 5, 18.

45 McCarl, 'Publishing the Works of Nicholas Culpeper', 269.

46 Culpeper, *School of Physic*, 92, 132, 121, 88.

47 Heydon, *The Holy Guide*, lib. 5, 18, lib. 3, 123; Heydon, *The Wise-Mans Crown*, B2^v; Alice Culpeper's licence to practise midwifery was granted in 1665, GL MS 10,116/4; see Evenden, *The Midwives of Seventeenth-Century London*, 118–19.

48 Culpeper, *Culpeper's Ghost*, A3^v.

49 Ibid., 2, 4–5.

50 Folger MS V.a.436, 497–8, 312–15; Seaver, *Wallington's World*, 53, 56.

51 BL MS Sloane 922, ff145^v–7^v; Seaver, *Wallington's World*, 94–5.

52 BL MS Sloane 922 f173v; Seaver, *Wallington's World*, 172.

53 Josten, *Ashmole*, i, 628; Lilly, *History*, 135–6; Whitelocke, *Diary*, 280.

54 Heydon, *The Wise-Mans Crown*, C$^{r–v}$.

55 Science Museum, inventory number A127916.

56 Whitelocke, *Diary*, 393.

57 Keynes, *Harvey*, 397, 399, 403.

58 Aubrey, 'Brief Lives', in Keynes, *Harvey*, 431–7.

59 Sanderson, *Nicholas Culpeper and*

the Book Trade, 100–1; *The Four
Great Years of the Plague.*

WORMWOOD

1 Lamentations 3: 15; *Hamlet*, III.
  ii.175; Pharmaceutical Society, *The
  British Pharmaceutical Codex*, entry
  for 'Absinthium'; Mabey, *Flora
  Britannica*, 370.
2 *Annals*, iv, ff75b–76a; translation in
  Wall, *A History of the Society of
  Apothecaries*, i, 107–8. The entry is
  for the minutes of the Comitia
  meeting of 17 August 1660 to which
  the events of 3 September have been
  appended.
3 Goodall, *The Royal College of
  Physicians*, 66, 88.
4 Cook, *Decline*, 140, 143–4.
5 *Annals*, iv, ff83a–84a; *CJ*, viii, 546,
  548–9.
6 Wall, *A History of the Society of
  Apothecaries*, 109.
7 The collector George Thomason did
  not collect a single medical work
  before acquiring Nicholas's *Physical
  Directory* in September 1649. After
  that, he acquired 82, nearly all in
  English. See McCarl, 'Publishing the
  Works of Nicholas Culpeper', 236,
  253.
8 *The Orders and Directions of the
  Right Honourable Lord Mayor.*
9 Needham, *Medela Medicinae*, A8^r;
  Bolnest, *Medicina instaurata*
  Dedicatory Epistle, A5^r.
10 Bolnest, *Medicina instaurata*, A8^r.
11 Johnson, 'Agurto-Mastix', 18.
12 Thomson, *Galeno-pale*, 27; Johnson,
  'Agurto-Mastix', 25.
13 Quoted in Thulesius, *Nicholas
  Culpeper*, 172. Thulesius ascribes the
  quote to the 1650 edition of
  Culpeper's *Physical Directory*,
  though I have been unable to find
  it.

14 Cook, *Decline*, 54.
15 Culpeper, *Physical Directory*, 1651,
  34.
16 The account of Charles II's death is
  taken from Crawfurd, *The Last Days
  of Charles II*, 22–46 and 'Translation
  of Scarburgh's MS', 69 ff.

EPILOGUE

1 *Munk's Roll*, entry for Harvey;
  Aiken, *Biographical Memoirs of
  Medicine*, 298; Goodall, *The College
  of Physicians Vindicated*, 143.
2 Garrison, *An Introduction to the
  History of Medicine*, 209.
3 For the connections between
  College Fellows and the founding of
  the Royal Society, see Gillispie,
  'Physick and Philosophy', 210–25; a
  recent statement of the controversy
  concerning evidence-based medicine
  can be found in Sackett, 'Evidence
  Based Medicine', 71–3. For an
  example of scepticism about
  evidence-based medicine in the
  medical profession, see 'Evidence-
  Based Medicine, in its Place', 785.
4 See, for example, Stubbe,
  Campanella Revived.
5 Bolnest, *Medicina instaurata*,
  Dedicatory Epistle, A5^r. A great deal
  of controversy and literature
  surrounds the politics and religion
  of the 'new philosophy' – see, for
  example, Kearney, 'Puritanism,
  Capitalism, and the Scientific
  Revolution', 88–97; Solt,
  'Puritanism, Capitalism, Democracy,
  and the New Science', 18–29;
  Greaves, 'Puritanism and Science',
  345–68. In 'Some Spiritual
  Alchemies of Seventeenth-Century
  England', 293–318, Robert M.
  Schuler examines the connections
  between the new philosophy and
  occult knowledge such as

Rosicrucianism and alchemy, and the participation in the setting up of the Royal Society of figures such as Elias Ashmole.

6 Poynter, 'Nicholas Culpeper and the Paracelsians', 201–20. The manuscript reading room at the Wellcome Institute library, one of the biggest medical history collections in the world, is named in his honour.

7 Figures based on a survey of the catalogues of the British and Bodleian Libraries, and Library of Congress.

8 Quoted in Maier, 'Reason and Revolution', 241. For the influence of Culpeper's *English Physitian* in America, see Stetson, 'American Garden Books Transplanted and Native', 345–7.

9 The noted epidemiologist Thomas McKeown (1912–88) argued that an improvement in mortality rates in the eighteenth and nineteenth centuries was not due to medical advances. 'The population growth was not influenced by improved sanitation before about 1870,' he wrote, 'or by specific medical measures before the introduction of the sulphonamides in 1935.' He attributes the growth to improved nutrition (McKeown, 'An Interpretation of the Modern Rise of Population in Europe', 345). However, McKeown's thesis remains controversial. Razzell in ' "An Interpretation of the Modern Rise of Population in Europe" ', 5–17, suggested the introduction of the smallpox vaccine may have been a factor. This is reinforced by A. J. Mercer in 'Smallpox and Epidemiological-Demographic Change in Europe', 287–307.

ILLUSTRATIONS

BIBLIOGRAPHY

Adair, John, *By the Sword Divided* (Stroud, 1998).

Aiken, John, *Biographical Memoirs of Medicine in Great Britain* (London, 1780).

Allen, J. W., *English Political Thought, 1603–1660* (London, 1938).

Allen, Thomas, *Cheirexoke: The Excellency or Handy-work of the Royal Hand* (London, 1665).

Anon., *An Agreement of the People for a Firme and Present Peace, upon grounds of common-right and freedome* (London, 1647).

Anon., *A Briefe Description of the Notorious Life of Iohn Lambe* (Amsterdam, 1628).

Anon., *Decree of Starre-Chamber: Concerning Inmates, and divided Tenements, in London or three miles about* (London, 1636).

Anon., *The Four Great Years of the Plague* (London, 1665).

Anon., *Gold Tried in the Fire, or the burnt petitions revived* (London, 1647).

Anon., *A Letter from Mercurius Civicus to Mercurius Rusticus: or, Londons confession but not repentance* ([London], 1643).

Anon., *The Mid-wives Just Petition: or, A complaint of divers good gentlewomen of that faculty* (London, 1643).

Anon., *The Orders and Directions of the Right Honourable Lord Mayor . . . to be Diligently Observed and Kept by the Citizens of London, During the Time of the Present Visitation of the Plague* [London, 1665].

Anon., *Orders and Directions Together with a Commission for the better Administration of Justice* (London, 1630).

Anon., *Orders and Ordinances for the better government of the Hospitall of Bartholomew the Lesse* (London, 1652).

Anon., *Orders heertofore conceiued and agreed to bee published by the Lord Mayor and Aldermen of the citie of London* (London, 1625).

Anon., *Orders to be vsed in the time of the infection of the plague vvithin the citie and liberties of London* (London, 1625).

Anon., *The Petition of the Knights, Gentlemen, and Yeomanry of the Country of Devonshire* (London, 1642).

Anon., *The Petition and Resolution of the Cityzens of the City of Chester* (London, 1642).

Anon., *A Remonstrance of the State of the Kingdom* (London, 1641).

Anon., *A Remonstrance of His Excellency Thomas Lord Fairfax, Lord Generall of the Parliaments forces. And of the Generall Councell of officers held at St Albans the 16. of November, 1648* (London, 1648).

Anon., *A True Copy of the Journal of the High Court of Justice, for the tryal of K. Charles I* (London, 1684).

Anon., *A True Relation of the Late Battell neere Newbery, shewing the happy successe of his Excellencies forces against the cavaliers* (London, 1643).

Arber, Agnes, *Herbals: Their Origin and Evolution. A chapter in the history of botany 1470–1670* (Cambridge, 1986).

Aristotle, *On the Parts of Animals*, tr. William Ogle (reproduced at etext.library.adelaide.edu.au/a/a8pa/).

Attersoll, William, *A Commentarie vpon the Epistle of Saint Pavle to Philemon* (London, 1612).

——, *A Commentarie vpon the Fourth Booke of Moses, called Numbers* (London, 1618).

——, *A Continuation of the Exposition of the Booke of Numbers, or, The Historie of Balak the King and Balaam the False Prophet, or, An exposition vppon the xxij, xxiij, xxiiij, and xxv chapters of the booke of Numbers* (London, 1610).

——, *The Neuu Couenant, or, A treatise of the sacraments* (London, 1614).

Attree, F. W. T., and Booker, J. H. L. 'Sussex Colepepers', pt. 2, *Sussex Archaeological Collections*, vol. 48 (1905).

Aubrey, John, *The Natural History and Antiquities of the County of Surrey, begun in the year 1673* (London, 1719).

Aughterson, Kate (ed.), *The English Renaissance* (London, 2002).

Aveling, J. H., *The Chamberlens and the Midwifery Forceps* (London, 1882).

B. J., *A Faire in Spittle Fields, where all the knick knacks of astrology are exposed to open sale, to all that will see for their love; and buy for their money. Where, first Mr. William Lilley presents you with his pack, wherein he hath to sell. 1. The introduction, 2. Nativities calculated, 3. The great ephimeredies, 4. Monarchy, or no monarchy 5. The caracture of K. Charles, 6. Annus Tenebrosus. Second, Nicholas Culpeper, brings under his veluet jacket. 1. His chalinges against the docttors* [sic] *of phuisick,* [sic] *2. A pocket medicine, 3. An almanack, & conjuring circle* (London, 1652).

Barnard, John, 'London Publishing 1640–1660: Crisis, Continuity, and Innovation', *Book History*, vol. 4 (2001).

Bolnest, Edward, *Medicina instaurata, or, A brief account of the true grounds and principles of the art of physick* (London, 1665).

Bourgeois, Louise, *The Compleat Midwifes Practice* (London, 1656).

——, *The Compleat Midvvife's Practice Enlarged* (London, 1680).

Boynton, L., *The Elizabethan Militia 1558–1638* (London, 1967).

Brett-James, N. G., *Growth of Stuart London* (London, 1935).

Burton, Robert, *The Anatomy of Melancholy* (Oxford, 1621).

Calder, Isabel MacBeath, *The New Haven Colony* (New Haven, 1934).

Camden, William, *Britain, or, A chorographicall description of the most flourishing kingdomes, England, Scotland, and Ireland, and the islands adjoyning, out of the depth of antiquitie* (London, 1637).

Charles I, *By the King. A proclamation for the better ordering of those who repayrr to the Court for their cure of the disease called the King's Evill* (London, 1626).

——, *By the King. A proclamation for preuenting of the abuses growing by the vnordered retailing of tobacco* (London, 1633).

——, *By the King. A proclamation for suppressing of false rumours touching Parliament* (London, 1629).

——, *By the King: a proclamation restraining the abusive venting of tobacco* (London, 1634).

Clarendon, Edward Hyde, Earl of, *The History of the Rebellion and*

Civil Wars in England begun in the year 1641: with the precedent passages and actions that contributed thereunto, and the happy end and conclusion thereof by the King's blessed restoration and return, upon the 29th of May in the year 1660 (Oxford, 1702–4).

Clarke, Sir George, *History of the Royal College of Physicians* (London, 1964).

Clowes, William, *A Prooued Practise for all Young Chirurgians, concerning burnings with gunpowder, and woundes made with gunshot, sword, halbard, pyke, launce, or such other* ([London], 1588).

Cole, F. J., 'Harvey's Animals', *Journal of the History of Medicine*, vol. 12 (1957).

Coles, William, *The Art of Simpling* (London, 1656).

Cook, Harold J., *Decline of the Old Medical Regime in Stuart London*,

Coward, Barry, *The Stuart Age: England, 1603–1714* (London, 1994).

Crawfurd, Raymond, *The King's Evil* (Oxford, 1911).

——, *The Last Days of Charles II* (Oxford, 1909).

Cressy, David, *Literacy and the Social Order* (Cambridge, 1980).

Culpeper, Nicholas, *Catastrophe magnatum, or, The fall of monarchie a caveat to magistrates, deduced from the eclipse of the sunne, March 29, 1652, with a probable conjecture of the determination of the effects* (London, 1652).

——, *Culpeper's Astrologicall Judgment of Diseases from the Decumbiture of the Sick* (London, 1655).

——, *Culpeper's Last Legacy Left and bequeathed to his dearest Wife, for the publicke good* (London, 1655).

——, *Culpeper's School of Physick, or, The experimental practice of the whole art* (London, 1659).

——, *A Directory for Midwives, or, A guide for women, in their conception, bearing and suckling their children* (London, 1651).

——, *The English Physitian, or An astrologo-physical discourse of the vulgar herbs of this nation* (London, 1652).

——, *An Ephemeris for the Year 1652. Being leap year, and a year of wonders. Prognosticating the ruine of monarchy throughout Europe; and a change of the law* (London, 1652).

——, *An Ephemeris for the Yeer 1651. Amplified with rational predictions from the book of the creatures. 1. Of the state of the yeer.*

2. *What may probably be the effects of the conjunction of Saturn and Mars, July 9. 1650* (London, 1651).

——, *Galen's Art of Physic* (London, 1652).

——, 'The Life of the Admired Physician and Astrologer of our Times, Mr *Nicholas Culpeper*', *Culpeper's School of Physick* (London, 1659).

——, *Mr Culpepper's Treatise of aurum potabile* (London, 1656).

——, *Pharmacopoeia Londinensis or the London Dispensatory Further adorned* (London, 1653).

——, *A Physical Directory, or, A translation of the London dispensatory made by the Colledge of Physicians in London. Being that book by which all apothicaries are strictly commanded to make all their physick with many hundred additions which the reader may find in every page marked with this letter A. Also there is added the use of all the simples beginning at the first page and ending at the 78 page* (London, 1649).

——, *A Physical Directory, or, A translation of the dispensatory made by the Colledge of Physitians of London, and by them imposed upon all the apothecaries of England to make up their medicines by whereunto is added, the vertues of the simples, and compounds* (London, 1650).

——, *Semeiotica Uranica, or, An astrological judgment of diseases from the decumbiture of the sick (1) from Aven Ezra by the way of introduction, (2) from Noel Duret by way of direction . . . : to which is added, The signs of life or death by the body of the sick party according to the judgment of Hippocrates* (London, 1651).

Dekker, Thomas, *The Blacke Rod, and the VVhite Rod* (London, 1630).

——, *London Looke Backe at that Yeare of Yeares 1625* (London, 1630).

——, *A Rod for Run-aways* (London, 1625).

——, *The Wonderfull Yeare. 1603* (London, 1603).

Denne, Henry, *Grace, Mercy, and Peace* (London, 1645).

Devon, F., *Issues of the Exchequer* (London, 1836).

Digby, George, *A True and Impartiall Relation of the Battaile betwixt, His Majesties Army, and that of the Rebells neare Newbery in Berk-shire, Sept. 20. 1643* (Oxford, 1643).

Dobson, Mary J., *Contours of Death and Disease in Early Modern England* (Cambridge, 1997).

Edwards, Thomas, *Gangraena, or, A catalogue and discovery of many of the errours, heresies, blasphemies and pernicious practices of the sectaries of this time, vented and acted in England in these four last years* (London, 1646).

Eglisham, George, *A Forerunner of Revenge* (London, 1642).

England, Church of, *Articles, whereupon it was agreed by the archbishoppes and bishoppes of both prouinces, and the whole cleargie, in the Conuocation holden at London in the yere of our Lorde God 1562. according to the computation of the Churche of Englande* (London, 1571).

Evelyn, John, *Diary: Now first printed in full from the manuscripts belonging to Mr. John Evelyn*, ed. E. S. de Beer (Oxford, 1955).

Evenden, Doreen, *The Midwives of Seventeenth-Century London* (Cambridge, 2000).

'Evidence-Based Medicine, In its Place', *Lancet*, vol. 346: 8978 (23 September 1995).

D'Ewes, Sir Simonds, *The Journal of Sir Simonds D'Ewes, from the first recess of the Long Parliament to the withdrawal of King Charles from London*, ed. Willson Havelock Coates.

Felter, Harvey Wickes, *The Eclectic Materia Medica, Pharmacology and Therapeutics* (Cincinnati, 1922).

Fioravanti, Leonardo, *Three Exact Pieces of Leonard Phioravant Knight, and Doctor in Physick, viz. his Rationall secrets, and Chirurgery, reviewed and revived* (London, 1652).

Foster, Henry, *A True and Exact Relation of the Marchings of the Two Regiments of the Trained-Bands of the City of London . . . who marched forth for the reliefe of the City of Glocester from August 23 to Sept. 28* (London, 1643).

Friedlander, Walter J., *The Golden Wand of Medicine: A history of the caduceus symbol in medicine* (New York, 1992).

Fuller, Thomas, *The History of the Worthies of England* (London, 1662).

Gadbury, John, *Collectio geniturarum, or, A collection of nativities, in CL genitures, viz. princely, prelatical, causidical, physical, mercatorial, mathematical, of short life, of twins, &c* (London, 1662).

Galen, *On the Usefulness of the Parts of the Body*, tr. Margaret Tellmadge May (Ithaca, 1968).

Gardiner, S. R. (ed.), *The Constitutional Documents of the Puritan Revolution 1625–1660* (Oxford, 1951).

——, *History of the Great Civil War, 1642–1649* (London, 1987).

Garrison, Fielding H., *An Introduction to the History of Medicine with Medical Chronology, Suggestions for Study and Bibliographic Data* (London, 1929).

Gaskill, M., 'The Devil in the Shape of a Man: Witchcraft, Conflict and Belief in Jacobean England', *Historical Research*, vol. 71: 175 (June 1998).

Gauden, John, *Eikon Basilike* ([London], 1649).

Gee, John, *The Foot out of the Snare* (London, 1624).

Gell, Robert, *Stella Nova or A new starre leading wisemen unto Christ* (London, 1649).

Geneva, Ann, *Astrology and the Seventeenth-Century Mind: William Lilly and the language of the stars* (Manchester, 1995).

Gerard, Thomas, *Gerard's Herball: The Essence thereof distilled*, ed. Marcus Woodward (London, 1971).

Gillispie, Charles C., 'Physick and Philosophy: A Study of the Influence of the College of Physicians of London upon the Foundation of the Royal Society', *The Journal of Modern History*, vol. 19: 3 (September 1947).

Goodall, Charles, *The Colledge of Physicians Vindicated, and the true state of physick in his nation faithfully represented* (London, 1676).

——, *The Royal College of Physicians of London, founded and established by law* (London, 1684).

Goodwin, John, *Imputatio Fidei* (London, 1642).

——, *Anti-cavalierisme, or, Truth pleading as well the necessity as the lawfulnesse of this present warre for the suppressing of that butcherly brood of cavaliering incendiaries who are now hammering England to make an Ireland of it* (London, 1642).

Greaves, Richard L., 'Puritanism and Science: The Anatomy of a

Controversy', *Journal of the History of Ideas*, vol. 30: 3 (July–September 1969).

Grieve, Maud, *The Modern Herbal* (London, 1931).

Guybert, Philbert, *The Charitable Physitian*, tr. 'I. W.' (London, 1639).

Hacket, John, *Scrinia reserata* ([London], 1693).

Harvey, William, *Anatomical Exercitations, concerning the generation of living creatures* (London, 1653).

——, *The Anatomical Exercises of Dr William Harvey professor of physick, and physician to the Kings Majesty, concerning the motion of the heart and blood* (London, 1653).

——, *Lectures on the Whole of Anatomy*, tr. C. D. O'Malley, F. N. L. Poynter, and K. F. Russell (Berkeley, 1961).

Herring, Francis, *Certaine Rules, Directions, or Advertisements for this time of pestilentiall contagion* (London, 1636).

Heydon, John, *The Holy Guide, leading the way to vnite art and nature* (London, 1662).

——, *The Wise-Mans Crown* (London, 1664).

Hildanus, Wilhelm Fabricius, *Gulielm. Fabricius Hildanus, his experiments in chyrurgerie*, tr. John Street (London, 1643).

Hill, Christopher (ed.), *The Intellectual Revolution of the Seventeenth Century* (London, 1974).

——, *Puritanism and Revolution: Studies in interpretation of the English Revolution of the 17th century* (London, 1958).

——, 'William Harvey and the Idea of Monarchy', *Past and Present*, vol. 27 (April 1964).

——, *The World Turned Upside Down* (London, 1991).

Hirst, Derek, *England in Conflict 1603–1660: Kingdom, Community, Commonwealth* (London, 1999).

Historical Manuscripts Commission, *Calendar of the Manuscripts of the Most Honourable the Marquess of Salisbury* (London, 1906–40), vol. 14.

——, *Supplementary Report on the Manuscripts of the Earl of Mar & Kellie* (London, 1930).

Holinshed, Raphael, *The Third Volume of Chronicles, beginning at duke William the Norma, commonlie called the Conqueror* (London, 1587).

Houston, R. A., *Literacy in Early Modern Europe* (London, 1988).

Howell, James, *Londinopolis, an historicall discourse or perlustration of the city of London, the imperial chamber, and chief emporium of Great Britain* (London, 1657).

Hunnisett, R. F., *Sussex Coroners' Inquests, 1603–1688* (Lewes, 1998).

Huxley, Thomas, 'Address of Thomas Henry Huxley, President [to the British Association]', *Nature*, vol. 2 (1870).

Jacobs, J. (ed.), *Epistolae Ho-Elianiae: The familiar letters of James Howell* (London, 1890).

James I, *A Counterblaste to Tobacco* (London, 1604).

——, *By the King, a proclamation to restraine the planting of tobacco in England and VVales* (London, 1619).

——, *A Speech to the Lords and Commons of Parliament at White-Hall, on Wednesday the XXI. of March. Anno 1609* (London, 1609).

Johnson, Thomas, *The Herball or Generall Historie of Plantes . . . Very much enlarged and amended by Thomas Johnson* (London, 1633).

——, *Iter plantarum investigationis ergo susceptum a decem socijs* ([London], 1629).

Johnson, William, 'Agurto-Mastix' (London, 1665).

Jones, Rex F., *Genealogy of a Classic: 'The English Physitian' of Nicholas Culpeper*, Ph.D. thesis, University of California, San Francisco (1984).

Josten, C. H. (ed.), *Elias Ashmole (1617–1692): His autobiographical and historical notes, his correspondence and other contemporary sources relating to his life and work* (Oxford, 1966).

Kearney, H. F., 'Puritanism, Capitalism, and the Scientific Revolution', *Past and Present*, vol. 28 (July 1964).

Kenyon, John, and Ohlmeyer, Jane (eds.), *The Civil Wars : A military history of England, Scotland, and Ireland 1638–1660* (Oxford, 1998).

Keynes, Geoffrey, *The Life of William Harvey* (Oxford, 1966).

King, John, *King's American Dispensatory*, ed. and enlarged by Harvey Wickes Felter and John Uri Lloyd (Cincinnati, 1898–1900).

Kirby, David A., 'The Radicals of St Stephen's, Coleman Street, London, 1624–1642', *Guildhall Miscellany*, 3 (1970).

Laud, William, *A Sermon Preached on Munday, the seauenteenth of March, at Westminster* (London, 1628).

Lilly, William, *Anglicus, Peace, or no Peace. 1645. A probable conjecture of the state of England, and the present differences betwixt His Majestie and the Parliament of England now sitting at Westminster, for this present year, 1645* (London, 1645).

——, *England's Propheticall Merline, foretelling to all nations of Europe until 1663, the actions depending upon the influence of the conjunction of Saturn and Jupiter. 1642/3* (London, 1644).

——, *Merlinus Anglicus Junior; The English Merlin revived: or, his prediction upon the affaires of the English Commonwealth* (London, 1644).

——, *A Prophecy of the White King and Dreadfull Dead-man Explaned* (London, 1644).

——, *The Starry Messenger; or, an interpretation of that strange apparition of three suns seene in London, 19 Novemb. 1644, being the birthday of King Charles* (London, 1645).

——, *William Lilly's History of his Life and Times from the year 1602 to 1681* (London, 1822).

Lindley, Keith, *The English Civil War and Revolution* (London, 1998).

Lithgow, William, 'The Present Surveigh of London and England State', *Somers's Tracts*, second edition, ed. Walter Scott, vol. 4.

Liu, Tai, *Puritan London: A study of religion and society in the City parishes* (London, 1986).

Livy, Titus, *The Romane Historie vvritten by T. Livius of Padua. Also, the Breviaries of L. Florus: with a chronologie to the whole historie: and the Topographie of Rome in old time*, tr. Philemon Holland (London, 1600).

Lloyd Prichard, M. F., 'The Significant Background of the Stuart Culpepers', *Notes and Queries*, vol. 205 (November 1960).

Lockyer, Roger, *Buckingham: The life and political career of George Villiers, first Duke of Buckingham, 1592–1628* (London, 1981).

Lovelace, Richard, *The Poems of Richard Lovelace* (London, 1904).

Mabey, Richard, *Flora Britannica* (London, 1996).

Mackaile, Matthew, *Moffett-Well, Or a topographico-spagyricall description of the mineral wells at Moffet in Annandale of Scotland ... To these subjoined A character of Mr Culpeper and his Writings* (Edinburgh, 1664).

Maier, Pauline, 'Reason and Revolution: The Radicalism of Dr Thomas Young', *American Quarterly*, vol. 28: 2 (Summer 1976).

May, Edward, *A Most Certaine and True Relation of a strange monster or serpent found in the left ventricle of the heart of Iohn Pennant* (London, 1639).

Maynwaring, Roger, *Religion and Alegiance* (London, 1627).

McCarl, Mary Rhinelander, 'Publishing the Works of Nicholas Culpeper, Astrological Herbalist and Translator of Latin Medical Works in Seventeenth-Century London', *Canadian Bulletin of Medical History*, vol. 13 (1996).

McClure, Norman Egbert, *Letters of John Chamberlain* (London, 1939).

McKenzie, D. F. (ed.), *Stationers' Company Apprentices 1605–1640* (Charlottesville, 1961).

McKeown, T., Brown, R. G., and Record, R. G., 'An Interpretation of the Modern Rise of Population in Europe', *Population Studies*, vol. 26: 3 (November 1972).

Mercer, A. J., 'Smallpox and Epidemiological-Demographic Change in Europe: The Role of Vaccination', *Population Studies*, vol. 39: 2 (July 1985).

Milton, John, *Areopagitica: A speech of Mr. John Milton for the liberty of vnlicens'd printing, to the Parlament of England* (London, 1644).

Monardes, Nicolas, *Ioyfull Nevves out of the Newe Founde Worlde* (London, 1577).

Money, Walter, *The First and Second Battles of Newbury and the Siege of Donnington Castle during the Civil War A.D. 1643–6* (London, 1884).

Montagu, Richard, *Appello Caesarem* (London, 1625).

Munk, William, *The Roll of the Royal College of Physicians of London; compiled from the Annals of the College*, vol. 1 (London, 1861).

Needham, Marchamont, *Medela Medicinae* (London, 1665).

Orr, D. A., 'Sovereignty, Supremacy and the Origins of the English Civil War', *History*, vol. 87: 288 (October 2002).
Outwaite, R. B., *Inflation in Tudor and Early Stuart England* (London, 1982).

Parkinson, John, *Theatrum botanicum: The theater of plants. Or, An herball of a large extent* (London, 1640).
Pearl, Valerie, 'Change and Stability in Seventeenth-century London', *London Journal*, vol. 5 (1979).
——, *London and the Outbreak of the Puritan Revolution* (London, 1961).
Pease, Theodore Calvin, *The Leveller Movement: A study in the history and political theory of the English Great Civil War* (Washington DC, 1916).
Pelling, Margaret, *Medical Conflicts in Early Modern London: Patronage, physicians, and irregular practitioners, 1550–1640* (Oxford, 2003).
Pharmaceutical Society, *The British Pharmaceutical Codex* (London, 1911).
'Philaretes', *Culpeper Revived from the Grave, to discover the cheats of that grand impostor, call'd Aurum Potabile* (London, 1655).
——, *Work for Chimny-sweepers* (London, 1602).
'Philastrogous', *Lillies Ape Whipt* (London, 1652).
Plomer, Henry R., *A Dictionary of the Booksellers and Printers who were at work in England, Scotland and Ireland from 1641 to 1667* (London, 1907).
——, 'Secret Printing During the Civil War', *The Library*, 2nd ser., vol. 5 (1904).
Porta, John Baptista, *Natural Magick* (London, 1658).
Porter, Roy, *The Greatest Benefit to Mankind* (London, 1997).
——, *London and the Civil War* (London, 1996).
Poynter, F. N. L., 'Nicholas Culpeper and the Paracelsians', *Science, Medicine and Society in the Renaissance: Essays to honour Walter Pagel* (London, 1972), vol. 1.

Purkiss, Diane, 'Desire and its Deformities: Fantasies of Witchcraft in the English Civil War', *Journal of Medieval and Early Modern Studies*, vol. 27: 1 (1997).

Rachum, Ilan, 'The Meaning of "Revolution" in the English Revolution (1648–1660)', *Journal of the History of Ideas*, vol. 56: 2 (April 1995).
Rappaport, S., *Worlds within Worlds: Structures of life in sixteenth-century London* (Cambridge, 1981).
Razzell, Edward and Peter (eds), *The English Civil War: A contemporary account* (London, 1996).
Razzell, P. E., '"An Interpretation of the Modern Rise of Population in Europe" – A Critique', *Population Studies*, vol. 28: 1 (March 1974).
Read, Alexander, *An Alphabetical Book of Physicall Secrets* (London, 1639).
——, *The Chirurgicall Lectures of Tumors and Vlcers* (London, 1635).
——, *Manual of Anatomy of Man* (London, 1653).
——, *The Workes of that Famous physitian Dr Alexander Read, Doctor of Physick, and one of the fellows of Physitians-Colledge, London* (London, 1650).
Rive, Alfred, 'A Brief History of the Regulation and Taxation of Tobacco in England', *William and Mary College Quarterly Historical Magazine*, 2nd ser., vol. 9: 1 (January 1929).
Ross, Alexander, *Arcana microcosmi: or, The hid secrets of mans body disclosed* (London, 1651).
Rous, Francis, *A Brief Narrative of the Late Treacherous and Horrid Designe, which by the great blessing and especiall providence of God hath been lately discovered* (London, 1643).
Rushworth, John, *Historical Collections of Private Passages of State, weighty matters in law, remarkable proceedings in five Parliaments* (London, 1659).

Sackett, David L., et al., 'Evidence Based Medicine: What it is and what it isn't', *British Medical Journal*, vol. 312: 7023 (13 January 1996).
Saltmarsh, John, *A Peace but no Pacification. Or, An answer to that*

new designe of the oath of pacification and accomodation (London, 1643).

Sanderson, Jonathan, *Nicholas Culpeper and the Book Trade: Print and the promotion of vernacular medical knowledge, 1649–65*, Ph.D. thesis, University of Leeds (1999).

Schofield, John (ed.), *The London Surveys of Ralph Treswell* (London, 1987).

Schuler, Robert M., 'Some Spiritual Alchemies of Seventeenth-Century England', *Journal of the History of Ideas*, vol. 41: 2 (April–June 1980).

Scott, Susan, and Duncan, Christopher J., *Biology of Plagues: Evidence from historical populations* (Cambridge, 2001).

Seaver, Paul S., *Wallington's World: A Puritan artisan in seventeenth-century London* (London, 1985).

Sibbes, Richard, *'Philippians': An exposition of the third chapter of the Epistle of St. Paul to the Philippians* (London, 1639).

Smith, Steven R., 'The London Apprentices as Seventeenth-Century Adolescents', *Past and Present*, vol. 61 (1973).

Solt, Leo F., 'Puritanism, Capitalism, Democracy, and the New Science', *The American Historical Review*, vol. 73: 1 (October 1967).

Spalding, Ruth, *The Improbable Puritan: A life of Bulstrode Whitelocke, 1605–1675* (London, 1974).

Steiner, Bernard, *History of Guildford and Madison* (Baltimore, 1897).

Stetson, Sarah Pattee, 'American Garden Books Transplanted and Native, Before 1807', *William and Mary Quarterly*, 3rd ser., vol. 3: 3 (July 1946).

Stowe, John, *A Survey of London written in the year 1598* (London, 1997).

Stubbe, Henry, *Campanella Revived, or, An enquiry into the history of the Royal Society* (London, 1670).

Suetonius, *De Vita Caesarum*, tr. J. C. Rolfe (Cambridge, MA, 1920).

Taylor, John, *A Fearful Summer: or London's calamity* (London, 1625).

Thomas, Christopher, Cloane, Barney, and Phillpotts, Christopher, *Excavations at the Priory and Hospital of St Mary Spital* (London, 1997).

Thomas, Keith, *Religion and the Decline of Magic* (London, 1991).

Thompson, Lana, *The Wandering Womb: A cultural history of outrageous beliefs about women* (New York, 1999).

Thomson, George, *Galeno-pale* (London, 1665).

Thulesius, Olav, *Nicholas Culpeper: English physician and astrologer* (London, 1992).

Tobyn, Graeme, *Culpeper's Medicine: A practice of Western holistic medicine* (Shaftesbury, 1997).

Traister, Barbara H., 'New Evidence about Burton's Melancholy?', *Renaissance Quarterly*, vol. 29: 1 (Spring 1976).

Underwood, E. Ashworth, 'The Early Teaching of Anatomy at Padua', *Annals of Science*, vol. 19 (1963).

Urdang, George (ed.), *Pharmacopoeia Londinensis of 1618 Reproduced in Facsimile* (Madison, 1944).

Vaughan, William, *Directions for Health, naturall and artificiall* (London, 1626).

Venn, John, *Alumni Cantabrigienses: A biographical list of all known students, graduates and holders of office at the University of Cambridge, from the earliest times to 1900* (Cambridge, 1922–54).

Walker, George, *A Defence of the True Sence and Meaning of the Words of the Holy Apostle* (London, 1641).

Wall, Cecil, and Cameron, H. Charles, *A History of the Worshipful Society of Apothecaries of London, 1617–1815*, ed. E. Ashworth Underwood (London, 1963).

Wallington, Nehemiah, *Historical Notices of Events Occurring Chiefly in the Reign of Charles I*, ed. R. Webb (London, 1869).

Ward, John, 'Diary', Wellcome MS WMS 6170–6176.

Ward, T. O., 'The Effect of Malaria upon the Diffusion of Disease', *London Medical Gazette*, vol. 9 (1849).

Wear, Andrew, *Knowledge and Practice in English Medicine, 1550–1680* (Cambridge, 2000).

Webster, Charles, *The Great Instauration: Science, medicine and reform, 1626–1660* (London, 1975).

Wharton, George, *An Astrologicall Judgement vpon His Majesties Present Martch begun from Oxford, May 7* (London, 1645).

Whitelocke, Bulstrode, *The Diary of Bulstrode Whitelocke 1605–1675*, ed. Ruth Spalding (Oxford, 1990).

Willughby, Percival, *Observations in Midwifery. As also The Countrey Midwife's Opusculum* (Warwick, 1863).

Wolfe, Don M., *Milton in the Puritan Revolution* (New York, 1941).

Woodall, Thomas, *The Surgeon's Mate* (London, 1617).

Woodward, Marcus (ed.), *Gerard's Herball* (London, 1971).

Woolrych, Austin, *Britain in Revolution* (Oxford, 2002).

INDEX

Page references in *italics* denotes illustration

German, Simon 147
Giffard, John 85
Gifford, Dr 124
Glisson, Francis 297
Glover, Richard 126, 131
Goddard, Jonathan 344
Goddard's drops 344
Godorous, William 210
Goodwin, John 150, 154, 215–16, 240, 241,
    271, 282, 285
Goring, Sir George 79
Grand Remonstrance 187
Grant, John 7
Grant, William 207
Great Plague (1665) 341, 344
Grey, Lord 273
Grieve, Maud 2, 72, 304
Grocers' Company 35, 37, 55
guilds 36, 55, 94
Gurney, Lord Mayor Sir Richard 189

hallucinogenics 24
Hamey, Dr Baldwin 218–19, 339
Hamilton, James (Earl of Abercorn) 77
Hampden, John 190
Hart, Alexander 171–2
Hartland (Devon) 8
Harvey, Elizabeth 50–1
Harvey, Joan 47
Harvey, Matthew 218–19
Harvey, Michael 218–19
Harvey, Thomas 47
Harvey, William 46–54, 192, 285–6,
    332–4, 349, 350
  and anatomy 59–63
  and apothecaries 125–6, 127
  appearance and character 49–50
  awarded doctorate by Oxford
    University (1642) 218
  background and medical education
    47–8
  becomes Warden of Merton College
    220
  as censor for College of Physicians
    53–4, 93
  and Charles I 86, 103–4, 183
  circulation of blood theory 65–7, 69,
    179–82, 198, 286, 343
  and civil war 199, 201–2

De Generatione Animalium 184, 309,
    311, 312–13, 314–15
De motu cordis 180–2, *181*, 286
  death 333
  and death of Charles I 286
  dislike of war 201, 218
  dissections 63–5, 183
  experimentation on himself 312–13
  hospital physician at St Bartholomew's
    Hospital 51–2, 104
  investigation into embryos and
    fertilisation 183–4
  Latin skills 361n
  links with London severed 219
  losing of papers as apartment
    ransacked during civil war 198
  Lumleian lectures on anatomy 59,
    60–7, 68, 314
  member of King James's medical
    retinue 59
  and *Pharmacopoeia Londinensis* 59
  and poisoning of King James case
    81–3, 85–6
  seeking licence to practice from
    College of Physicians and success 46,
    48–50
  view of magic 108
  and William Smith case 360n
Haselrig, Sir Arthur 190
heart
  Galen on 64–6
  Harvey on 64–7
  Read on 155
hemlock (*Conium maculatum*) 161, 235–7
henbane (*Hyoscyamus nigra*) 161
Henrietta Maria, Queen 76, 86–7, 107,
    109, 112
Henry VIII, King 35
Herring, Francis 88–9
Heydon, John 323, 326, 328, 329, 332
  The Wise Mans Crown 324–5
Hicks, Thomas 128, 131
Hide, David 364n
Higgins, Stephen 144
Hildanus, Gulielm Fabricus 229–30
Hippocrates 42, 46
Holles, Denzil 190, 191
honeysuckle 19, 161
Hopkins, William 268